OLDER ADULTS

Understanding & Facilitating Transitions

— Second Edition —

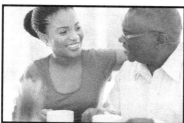

Annette M. Lane, RN, PhD
Athabasca University

Marlette B. Reed, BEd, MA
Community Chaplain and Pastor, Calgary, Alberta

Kendall Hunt
publishing company

Cover images © Shutterstock, Inc.

Kendall Hunt
publishing company

www.kendallhunt.com
Send all inquiries to:
4050 Westmark Drive
Dubuque, IA 52004-1840

To my husband, David R. Lane:
You are the absolute love of my life!

and to Jacquie Brezovski:
Thank you for over thirty years of cherished friendship.
(AML)

To my husband Brian and son Jonathan:
I love you guys more than I could express.
(MBR)

CONTENTS

PREFACE

It is truly a privilege to embark upon our second edition of this text. While the text remains largely the same, there are some distinct differences between the first and second editions that we believe will enhance the ease of use for students and educators.

As noted in the first edition, we structured this text in such a way that each chapter builds upon the previous one. In the first chapter, we lay the foundation by discussing transitions in general: What are transitions and how are they conceptualized? What are some examples of transitions across the life span? And what does the literature reveal about how children, adolescents, and adults progress through transitions? This allows the reader to consider how transitions have impacted her personally.[1] In Chapter 2, we address background information of why transitions are so difficult for older adults; in particular, we discuss demographic trends such as the aging of populations in developed countries, specific types of transitions faced by older adults, and we suggest why transitions can be so life changing for aging individuals. In Chapter 3, we discuss health transitions and how they impact the lives of older adults. We purposely focus on health transitions first, as they often precipitate other transitions, such as relocation to other living arrangements. Next, in Chapter 4, we concentrate on relocation transitions, including various options for older adults, as well as the impact of relocating upon aging adults. In Chapters 5 and 6, we discuss existential issues (those pertaining to meaning and purpose) and death and dying, respectively. If the reader is perusing various chapters out of order, we suggest that these chapters be read together, as existential issues related to transitions of life and dying/death often coincide. Chapter 7 covers challenging issues that health and human service professionals may encounter when working with older adults and their family members in transition. In Chapter 8, we offer future directions for research and professional practice that may benefit older adults (and their family members) as they experience the challenges of later life.

---

1. For ease of reading, we will avoid using the cumbersome juxtapositions *he/she* and *him/her*. Male and female pronouns will be used interchangeably throughout this text.

In terms of technicalities, a few points about how the chapters are configured may be helpful to the reader. Every chapter will have a case example in order to illustrate the challenges of transition, as well as how health and human service professionals can assess and intervene. When we offer examples throughout the text (including the case examples), we use pseudonyms to protect the identity of individuals. We also often change identifying information to further ensure anonymity of the situations described. At times, we use the acronyms AML (Annette Lane) and MBR (Marlette Reed) to refer to personal situations that one of us has encountered. These acronyms distinguish which author is referring to herself within the examples. We also use the term *health and human service professionals* to refer to a wide range of professionals such as registered nurses, social workers, chaplains, therapists, psychologists, and occupational and recreational therapists.

In this new edition, websites relevant to chapter material are listed at the end of each chapter. Also, ancillary materials—learning activities, PowerPoint slides, and multiple choice questions are available for each chapter for educators who are interested in using this text. This will facilitate the utilization of this text for instructors wishing to use it in coursework, as well as for aiding students in their learning of the material.

We want to stress that the purpose of this text is to illustrate the complexities of transitions faced by older adults and their family members and to offer some ideas for nurses, social workers, chaplains, and other health and human service professionals in working with vulnerable aging individuals. This is not a medical/surgical nursing text, a psychiatric/mental health text, a book on religion, or a volume addressing ethics. If readers want to delve more into the various health problems described, glean specifics on how to conduct a suicide risk assessment, or access greater detail on religion or ethical principles, we encourage you to seek out appropriate references.

So how did we come to be interested in how older adults process and progress through transitions? Our interest in and commitment to working with older adults spans many years and many different sites, including community agencies, hospitals, and hospice. AML has spent years teaching gerontological and mental health nursing to baccalaureate students, while MBR is a pastor and community chaplain, who for years has worked with dying individuals (in hospice and other settings) as well as with their families across the life span, including older adults. Within our work, we have observed that transitions, including those related to health, relocations (moves), and dying and death, evoke strong reactions in older adults and may trigger issues related to meaning and purpose. They also can result in great fear, frustration, anger, pain, and grief in family members. Personally, as identical twin sisters who have supported our aging parents through their final years, we have recognized how painful and even gut-wrenching transitions can be in older adulthood. Our writing reflects a mixture of personal and professional experience.

We would be remiss if we failed to mention the valuable expertise and contributions of our colleague and good friend, Dr. Sandra P. Hirst. Dr. Hirst was a co-author on the first edition of this text and graciously offered her chapters—1 and 4—for the second edition. Sandi, thank you!!

In closing, we wish to thank the team at Kendall Hunt for their support and guidance throughout the initial writing of this text and now, in the second edition. They have expressed belief in the importance of this topic, as well as in us as a writing team.

CHAPTER 1

INTRODUCTION

Nothing is secure but life, transition, the energizing spirit.
(Ralph Waldo Emerson, American essayist and poet)

Not in his goals, but in his transitions is man great.
(Ralph Waldo Emerson, American essayist and poet)

Reflective Questions

► What is the experience of human transition?

► How do stages of the life course influence and shape the experience of transition for health and human service professionals?

► What are my responsibilities in assisting older adults in their transitions?

By their very nature, transitions are enigmatic—mysterious, confounding, baffling! They are composed of multiple facets, may be expected or totally unexpected, may confuse or frighten some, but are critical in progressing successfully through life. While transitions are sometimes conceptualized as life's changes, they involve much more than that. They are those "in-between" stages that link the past to the future and determine that life will never be quite the same. The ability to navigate transitions depends upon more than the specifics of the various passages, but also is determined by the coping skills of the individuals negotiating them. And as noted in the first cited quote from the American essayist Ralph Waldo Emerson, transitions are inescapable. Even if individuals gamely try to avoid life's transitions, by the very process of attempting to escape them, these people will be changed. In the second cited quote of Emerson, he hinted at what transitions require of persons, but also how transitions may reveal individuals' characteristics. In other words, transitions may require much out of individuals and tax their coping abilities, and yet they also manifest the strength, the mettle of those experiencing them. Venture with us, please, through the dense forest of understanding transitions from a theoretical viewpoint, that is, frameworks within which to situate transitional experiences. Throughout this chapter, we will seek to narrow the focus of the dense forest, through specific examples of transition, in essence, flagging various trees of that timberland. It is our aim to assist readers with a framework as well as with illustrations to make the way clear. Slogging through the foundation of frameworks will enhance understanding in the upcoming chapters.

Our Changing Understanding of Human Transition

Etymologically, the word transition is derived from the Latin *transitio(n-)*, *transire* "go across." As a noun, the word *transition* refers to the process or a period of changing from one state or condition to another; as an example, *the students were **in transition** from one program to another* (Oxford dictionary). As a verb, it means "to undergo or cause to undergo a process or period of transition" (Oxford dictionary). Using the above example, but as a verb rather than a noun, the example would be, *the students **transitioned** from one program to another.* A perusal of a thesaurus reveals no adequate synonym for the depth of meaning found in the word, as the explanation below will reveal. Hence, we will use the term *transition* consistently in this text—avoiding synonyms such as "alteration" or "change" unless they appropriately convey our intent in representing that aspect of meaning in the word *transition*.

The term *transition* is used in diverse ways in the literature and is found in a number of disciplines, including molecular biology, sociology, anthropology, health care, and immigration planning. Within the literature, the word *transition* is used frequently to describe a process of change in life's developmental stages, or alterations in health and social circumstances, rather than individuals' responses to change. However, Bridges (2004; 2009) suggested that the term *transition* is not just another word for change, but also connotes the psychological processes involved in *adapting to* the change event or disruption. Similarly, transitions may be described as the ongoing processes characterized by changes *in* individuals during which a new situation or circumstance is incorporated into their lives (Kralik, Visentin, & van Loon, 2006). As such, transitions are not just changes per se, or even changes that occur over time, but are processes that require individuals to incorporate new knowledge and change behaviors, thus resulting in an alteration in how individuals define themselves within the new context. For example, a wife who has just lost her husband of 35 years needs to learn the tasks that her husband took care of for decades; she may need to learn, for the first time in her life, to pay the bills. And, she is now a widow: a very different identity than wife. Additionally, we posit that even when persons fail to confront the change event, such as commencing employment after post-secondary education, they are changed through the avoidance of the transition.

Transitions are often multiple and complex in nature; typically, they do not occur in isolation. Given the complexity and interrelatedness of transitions, individuals may experience different transitions simultaneously or experience transitions in rapid succession one after another, like a domino effect. This can greatly complicate how individuals process the transition; specifically, they may need to untangle what is the most pressing transition and how best to address it—hence the words mysterious and confounding were used in the introduction to this chapter. "Even attending to one transition can take time, as transitions can be lengthy when they involve a period of anticipation and movement over time through states of instability, confusion and distress, and finally end with a period of stability (Meleis, Sawyer, Im, Messias, & Schumacher, 2000)." The periods of instability and confusion are particularly unsettling. In his seminal work on transition, Bridges (1980) began his commentary with the following passage from *Alice in Wonderland:*

"Who are you?" asked the caterpillar . . . "I—I hardly know,
Sir, just at present." Alice replied rather shyly,
"at least I know who I was when I got up this morning,
but I think I must have changed several times since then."
(Carroll, 1967, p. 47)

Through Alice, this quotation reveals how transitions can leave individuals feeling like they are in a disorienting state of flux; the change in circumstances results in individuals not knowing who they are. As noted by Bridges (1980), transitions leave individuals in a "confusing nowhere of in-betweenness" (p. 47).

While some transitions can be anticipated, others cannot be foreseen. These can occur suddenly and concurrently and can be confusing and traumatic to individuals and their families. In catastrophic situations, such as major car accidents that occur suddenly, individuals' lives can change abruptly and permanently, with no time to foresee or prepare for a new and different future. Health and functional abilities can be greatly compromised, affecting the ability of those injured to work and perform regular activities of daily living. These kinds of transitions can be especially challenging for persons to face, as life is forever changed in a brief moment, and individuals have not had time to prepare for an altered body image or to develop mechanisms by which they can cope with their new life circumstances. As is sometimes said, "My life changed forever when this happened . . ."

How Transitions Are Conceptualized

Our understanding of transitions can be broadly categorized or organized in different frameworks. These frameworks include understanding transitions as specific types of changes (Meleis et al., 2000), transitions as involving not just events, but also individuals' responses to these events (Blair, 2000), as well as conceptualizing transitions through the lens of the life course perspective. Each of these frameworks can shed light on how transitions impact individuals, and why similar transitions can impact individuals very differently. As such, we briefly discuss each framework below.

Transitions as Types of Changes

Meleis and colleagues (2000) utilized an understanding of transitions that focuses on specific kinds of changes. Within this conceptualization, they identified four specific types of transitions. These transitions include health/illness transitions, developmental transitions, situational transitions, and organizational transitions. Health/illness transitions refer to changes in the health status of individuals; examples of this kind of transition include adapting to a chronic illness, returning home from hospitalization, or recovering from surgery. Developmental transitions occur due to standard or usual changes in developmental stages of life, such as adolescence, parenthood, or aging. Situational transitions pertain to environmental, contextual, and social changes; examples include adjustments such as changing educational or professional roles, and undergoing alterations in family situations, such as a divorce. Organizational transitions reflect changes in leadership, policies, or organizational structures, affecting both personnel and clients of an organization (Meleis et al., 2000). An example may be a change in administrative personnel or the introduction of a new policy regarding sick leave. Conceptualizing transitions according to the aforementioned types has been used by numerous authors and researchers.

Transitions as Events and Individuals' Responses to the Events

Another framework for categorizing transitions focuses upon events, including their predictability, as well as individuals' sense of control of the events (Blair, 2000). Within this framework, four primary types of events/responses are outlined. First, there are transitions that are *predictable-voluntary*. In these situations, the event is predictable and under the control of individuals; for example, moving to another house. Second, the *predictable-involuntary* type refers to transitions that are predictable, but over which individuals have no control. Mandatory retirement is an example of this type of event; while retirement is predictable, the choice and control over when to end employment is removed. Third, individuals may experience a type of transition that is *unpredictable-voluntary*. In these situations, the event may not have been predicted, but individuals may choose how they respond; for example, whether to apply for or accept a new job opportunity. The fourth category is labeled *unpredictable-involuntary*. These events are not predictable and individuals do not have control or choice in the event. Accidents are examples of this kind of event. This framework describes transitions as more than events, but also as how individuals conceptualize these events and respond to them; it has a focus upon coping strategies that may be available, including advance planning, to gain a sense of control over the situation that the individual is undergoing (Blair, 2000).

Transitions Within the Life Course Perspective

Another framework within which to conceptualize transitions is the life course perspective.[1] This perspective extends the element of time in considering transitions, and includes the interaction of individuals' lives, historical events, and the interdependence of people's lives (Hutchison, 2008). Traditionally, transitions were conceptualized as occurring with the onset of certain discrete events, such as the birth of a child, the first day of school, marriage, or retirement. As such, there were limitations in how long transitions lasted. Within the life course perspective, however, *current* transitions are located within the *larger historical context* of individuals' lives. Thus, transitional experiences in childhood and adolescence may impact how individuals face into transitions in the future. As an example, an aging woman—Mary—experienced childhood transitions in two orphanages as frightening and traumatic; she now feels a similar sense of dread and fear in an upcoming move to an assisted living facility. This feeling of foreboding is present, even though this woman has chosen to move to the new accommodations and finds the residents friendly and the surroundings aesthetically pleasing. She expresses pure befuddlement as to why she should feel so terrified by the move. The answer, in part, may be found within the life course perspective. When Mary was born (in the United Kingdom prior to 1950), she was considered "illegitimate," because her mother was not married. As Mary was not adopted into a family, she spent her first five years in an orphanage near her birth location. However, it was decided that that orphanage would be closed, and so at 7 years of age, Mary was relocated to another facility. At 14 years of age, she left the orphanage and spent several years working for various families in a nearby community. Although the first facility was not pleasant, she realized in hindsight that it was better than the subsequent orphanage. She never felt safe in her childhood, did not know who she could trust, and had little chance to make decisions or exercise some degree of choice.

Understanding Mary's previous transitional history sheds light on why the current transition is so difficult for her. Not only did her previous experiences of transition impact her current sense of dread, but her past transitions were shaped by trends and practices of that historical era, such as placing children of unwed mothers into orphanages. The life course perspective also emphasizes the interdependence of individuals (Hutchison, 2008). Although Mary never knew her parents, her entire life history is

---

1. Glen Elder, a sociologist, was one of the first authors to write about a life course perspective (Hutchison, 2008). For an example of his writing on this subject, see Elder (1998).

inextricably tied to the parents she never knew, as the *lack of familial support* impacted how she formed relationships with others. As well as the emphasis on historical events and interdependence of human lives upon individuals' behaviors, the life course perspective also emphasizes human agency (Hutchison, 2008). Thus, within reason, Mary was able to make some choices when she left the orphanage, such as working hard all of her adult life and being responsible to others around her. Despite her childhood trauma, Mary has constructed her life as best as she could, and even now, is trying to exercise some good decision-making in the current transition.

Domains of Transition

In addition to the aforementioned frameworks within which to understand transitions, literature in this area covers specific domains within which transitions occur, irrespective of the framework used. The primary domains identified in the literature include age-specific stages, education, employment, marriage and parenthood, retirement, the health care system, family caregiving, and death and dying. Within this chapter, we will not specifically address death and dying as a domain, because this will be explored in depth within Chapter 6 of this book.

Age-Specific Stages

Within the literature on age-specific stages, research is conducted on *normal* (expected) transitions as well as *traumatic* (unexpected) experiences within particular age groupings. The literature on expected transitions that involve age-specific stages addresses changes within the individual, such as the onset of menstruation, or changes in living circumstances, such as a move out of the parental home.

Expected transitions

Literature on expected changes within age-specific stages commonly focuses on transitions particular to adolescence. This is understandable, because adolescence is a period in life marked by multiple transitions. Not only is this the stage in which biological changes transform a child into an adult, it is also a period of transition in terms of emotional development, growth in cognitive skills, and further development of social roles and personal identity (Kaufman, 2006). And, to which many parents can attest, it can be a stage in which adolescents express their need for personal growth and identity in ways that may be contrary to their parents' wishes.

Another age-specific expected transition involves the transition from adolescence into adulthood. Arnett (2004) described the transition to adulthood in Western society as involving processes of both exploration and identity consolidation. It is also a period marked by relative freedom from clearly defined roles and responsibilities. Beyond the physical, psychological, and spiritual growth that adolescents experience, they also gain some sense of who they are in relation to others within the world. These multiple transitions are inherently stressful, challenging the adolescent's ability to solve problems and cope (Rasmussen, Ward, Jenkins, King, & Dunning, 2011). An age-specific transition that is expected in early adulthood involves the move out of the parents' home. With an assumption that adolescent transitions impact relationships between parents and children, a Dutch longitudinal study followed 1064 adolescents and young adults over a six-year period (Bucx & van Wel, 2008). The researchers found that adolescents reported a close bond with their parents; however, after leaving their parents' home, this bond weakened. The authors noted that their findings are consistent with theories about individualization, whereby the need for autonomy in young adult children causes some distancing in the parent–child relationship (Bucx & van Wel, 2008). An extreme example of this transitional adolescent/young adult distancing in the parent-child relationship can be found in the research of Tyler and Schmitz (2013). They explored the early family history of homeless young adults, the type and number of transitions they experienced, and their journey to the streets. Findings revealed that young adults' family histories placed them on trajectories to early independence, evidenced by multiple transitions and numerous living situations, resulting in lack of a permanent place to call home.

Similarly, the transition into the larger adult world is very complex for adolescents transitioning out of foster care situations. They are at risk for homelessness, economic challenges, physical and mental health problems, and they may only achieve minimal post-secondary education (Osterling & Hines, 2006). In these situations, the childhood transition into foster care influences how these adolescents transition into adulthood. With recognition of the perilous situations some of these young adults face, research is now examining how to support the transition through mentoring programs (Greeson, Usher, & Grinstein-Weiss, 2010; Osterling & Hines, 2006) or supporting resilience, knowledge, and skill building (Keller, Cusick, & Courtney, 2007; Scannapieco, Connell-Carrick, & Painter, 2007).

An example of this concept—although differing in particulars—is an acquaintance of ours. She grew up attending international boarding schools. When she got married, she stated that she had little understanding of how to set up a home and create a nurturing environment; hence the transitions into being a wife and a mother were difficult. Consistent with the life course perspective, she was resilient and did learn. For many years she and her husband provided an especially nurturing environment in their home for foster kids (as she knew what it was like to be "homeless"); now, as a mother with adult children, she develops curriculum for Canada's aboriginal population (some of whom were raised in residential schools).

Other age-specific expected transitions for women in midlife involve menopause and the "empty nest" syndrome. Historically, both transitions were considered to be difficult and even traumatic for some middle-aged women. However, Dare (2011) interviewed forty Australian women between the ages of 45 and 55 years. She found that most of the women interviewed managed menopause and the launching of children quite well; in contrast, these women noted that transitions related to divorce, as well as the aging and death of older parents, were much tougher to handle. These women reported that divorce resulted in a poorer financial state and had a negative impact on their social network. Caregiving for one or more aging parents resulted in feelings of great responsibility and guilt over not being able to help enough, and when parents died, painful grief (Dare, 2011).

Similarly, Lim and Mackey (2012) interviewed 14 menopausal and postmenopausal Chinese Singaporean women to understand the meaning they attach to menopause. The women interviewed spoke of the symptoms they experienced, such as abnormal bleeding, hot flushes, and emotional changes. Like Dare's study (2011), most participants described their transition to be uneventful and a normal process of aging: ordinary. The women utilized both Western and Chinese strategies to manage their symptoms and sought support from family and friends. Even though the findings of this study are similar to some other studies, the significance of this research is that the meaning of the transition of menopause is examined in women who are from a different ethnicity than those in Western cultures. It is important that research examining transitions includes individuals from varied ethnic backgrounds. Health and human service professionals need to be aware that findings from research conducted with participants from Western countries do not necessarily apply to individuals from other regions of the world. As well, the meaning that one attaches to transition impacts how one copes with it.

Traumatic transitions

Researchers examining age-specific stages often explore the impact of unexpected, traumatic experiences within childhood and how these transitions influence the life course. One example is childhood trauma related to the death of a parent. In a classic study, Brown and Harris (1979) traced the impact of parental loss during childhood on adult outcomes. Using data from a sample of working-class women in London, England, they found that parental loss during childhood was associated with increased risk of clinical depression, lower socioeconomic achievements, and poorer quality of marriage during adulthood. Additional analysis suggested that the effects of parental loss were mediated by the quality of care the child received after parental loss. Fewer negative outcomes were observed among women who as children received high-quality care from parental substitutes.

Not only can traumatic childhood transitions result in difficulties navigating future transitions, but such experiences may trigger psychological challenges for children in the present. Recent research into the effects of the terrorist attacks in New York City on 9/11 has confirmed this, including the detrimental effects of New York mothers' post traumatic stress disorder (PTSD) and depression upon their preschoolers after September 11 (Chemtob, Nomura, Rajendran, Yehuda, Schwartz, & Abramovitz, 2010). These children were more likely to have severe behavioral issues, because their mothers' sensitivity meters were altered through the trauma (PTSD), leading their children to feel unsafe; and these moms were not able to attend to their children as they would have normally, because of their depression.

These findings dovetail into an interesting study by van Wesel, Boeije, Alisic, and Drost (2012), where the researchers found that children who had experienced trauma, such as death of a sibling, witnessing war, being a victim of abuse or of an accident, all had the need to process the event; some engaged in the psychological work of understanding the meaning of the transition (also termed *existential work*) and how this impacted their sense of identity. van Wesel and colleagues found that if parents were able to help their children work through a traumatic transition, the effects of it could be mitigated.

With the lens of the life course perspective, we suggest that how children process traumatic transitions in childhood impacts how they manage transitions in the future, whether the transitions are expected and desired (such as marriage), or whether they are unexpected and traumatic (such as a serious accident).

Education

The education domain includes the diversity of transitional experiences across the academic years. Transitions within the educational system are influenced by the structure of the available academic facilities and how the school system is organized; for example, when students transition from grade school to junior high school. The transition from high school into further educational experiences may be positive and even exciting, but is often stressful (Suldo, Shaunessy, Thalji, Michalowski, & Shaffer, 2009). Stresses include leaving home and friends, the need to develop new friends, discovering how to learn and study in a different way (university expectations as opposed to those in high school), as well as the increased responsibility and autonomy—all combined with decreased parental supervision. These linked stresses can lead to mental health problems, or exacerbate pre-existing ones (Cleary, Walter, & Jackson, 2011). Writers now address the importance of starting transition planning and services for students early within their high school experience, because the services provided are free and accessible, and youth have time to participate in these opportunities (Izzo & Lamb, 2003).

Employment

Within the employment domain, most of the literature is focused upon the transition from academic institutions to formal work. School-to-work transition generally refers to the period between approximately 18 to 24 years of age. O'Regan (2010), in her work on the employment transition, commented that there were two key questions often asked by those in transitions: "Who am I?" and "What do I want to do?" Twenty-two undergraduate students were interviewed just prior to graduation. O'Regan (2010) categorized the participants into four categories. One year later, she re-interviewed the participants. The participants that found employment commensurate with their education were those who fit within her instrumental category. These former students were goal-oriented, strategic, and motivated to learn for the specific purpose of their upcoming career. Students who were placed in other categories, such as those who were oriented to learning for the sake of learning, or who were hesitant or introspective (e.g., anxious) about their university experience, were less likely to have found work associated with their university degree. Along a similar vein, Brown and Hesketh (2004) argued that with the rising numbers of university students, the number of employment opportunities that match the level of education are limited, thus resulting in student struggle and angst to secure the best of colleges and employment. And so the questions "Who am I?" and "What am I going to do?" may continue for these young adults.

It is understandable that the transition from school to work is challenging because many young people begin employment while in school, migrate out of their communities, work in low-paying and minimal hour situations, and may perhaps be discouraged by unsuccessful job searching. Some of the most immediate considerations of this period in a young person's life include issues related to adequacy of existing education and skills development, job search, labor market entry, occupational matches, stable employment, and adequate income.

Marriage and Parenthood

Although marriage is usually a desired transition, it is inherently stressful. On the classic Holmes and Rahe (1967) stress scale, which rates life stressors with a point system so that individuals can add up their points to see if they are at risk for illness, experiencing the death of a spouse scores 100 points, serving jail time scores 63 points, and getting married scores 50 points! The transition to marriage is stressful because during the first several years of marriage, the spouses are getting to know each other's habits, the rhythms of how they do things around the house, their moods, patterns in handling finances, and other such parameters. However, studies generally show that married men and women are happier than their single counterparts. Stack and Eshleman (1998) examined national surveys from seventeen countries. They found that within sixteen of seventeen countries, being married was associated with greater happiness. They concluded that men and women may be happier in marriage because this bond facilitates two processes: financial stability and health. Similarly, in an analysis of 27 countries, Lee and Ono (2012) compared ratings of happiness among married individuals, those who cohabitate, and individuals who are single. They found that married individuals are happier than couples who cohabitate, and couples who cohabitate are happier than single individuals.

Better health experienced by married individuals may be in part related to the state of marriage itself, which often results in a reduction in risky health behaviors, including problem drinking, drug use, and smoking (Bachman et al., 2002). Studies reveal that, in general, the married engage in less risky health behaviors compared with the unmarried. This generalization does not hold true for weight gain, however. Studies show

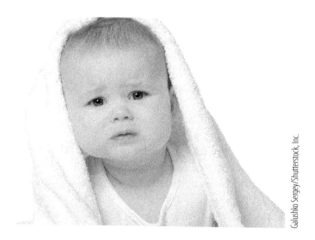

Galushko Sergey/Shutterstock, Inc.

that married individuals weigh more and exercise less than their unmarried counterparts. Interestingly, in one study it was found that having an obese spouse increased's one's own obesity risk by 37 percent (Smith & Christakis, 2008).

Transition into parenthood, the process that consists in discovering that a baby is expected and assuming the parenting role after the birth of that child, can be a very stressful time. Mothers and fathers have to review their lifestyles and redefine their relationships to work and daily life. In general, this transition is characterized by a decrease in relationship satisfaction, a lack of couple time, fewer leisure activities, reduced sexual relations, and a reorganization of the tasks of every member of the new family (Lawrence, Rothman, Cobb, Rothman, & Bradbury, 2008; Mortensen, Torsheim, Melkevik, & Thuen, 2012). The parenthood transition involves the acquisition of new knowledge. As suggested by Goodman (2005), in order for fathers to have a sense of parenting efficacy, they need to attain new knowledge and skills. They also need to be involved in the parenting role in order to perceive themselves as competent with their children (de Montigny, Lacharité, & Devault, 2012).

Couples who adopt children undergo unique transitions to parenthood. Each adoption is different, and each comes with a full spectrum of emotions, from elation to grief (Baldo & Baldo, 2003). While adoption can build strong family ties, numerous challenges can develop both during and after the adoption process. Parents and adopted children face a variety of challenges within the newly formed family unit. Parents struggle with the adoption process, while adoptees from various backgrounds often wrestle with identity development. For adopted children, the process of wrestling with and working through identity development can become particularly problematic during adolescence. The challenge of developing an identity in adolescence is magnified by being raised by non-biological parents, and parents may be bewildered as to how to help their adopted child.

Retirement

Retirement is another transitional experience. This transition brings the loss of a work role and often a substantial drop in income. Retirement is especially hard in Western societies, where great value is placed upon one's productivity. When work is a person's primary interest, activity, and source of social support, its loss can leave a significant void in life. In the past, retirement, with its benefits and challenges, was the domain of men; today, more and more women are working throughout their adult years, and this transition is now impacting them. "I've always looked forward to retirement," stated one such woman. "But I could not have imagined how this would impact my life, how to fill my days, and how I feel about myself!"

Although retirement has been extensively studied, we know relatively little about what predicts different retirement transitions and adjustment patterns. Some researchers have found that retirees, in comparison with workers, often report poorer physical health, greater depression and loneliness, lower life satisfaction, a less positive view about retirement, and lower activity levels (Kim & Moen, 2002). In contrast, others have found retirement to have a positive impact on life satisfaction, health, and stress level (Calasanti, 1996). Wang (2007) found that retirees do not follow a uniform adjustment pattern during the retirement process.

Similar findings were found in the work of Potocnik, Tordera, and Peiro (2013). They examined retirement satisfaction using the dynamic model of job satisfaction (Bussing, Bissels, Fuchs, & Perrar, 1999). Instead of examining job satisfaction with three criteria—degree, changes in level of aspiration, and problem-solving behavior—they applied these criteria to examine satisfaction with retirement. In the job satisfaction model, degree refers to the degree of satisfaction or dissatisfaction with a job; this satisfaction is contingent upon how a person's expectations and needs correspond to the actual work situation. The changes in level of aspiration pertain to three types of job satisfaction: progressive satisfaction, stabilized satisfaction, and resigned satisfaction. Last, an individual's problem-solving behavior is categorized as constructive dissatisfaction or fixated dissatisfaction (Bussing et al., 1999).

Using the dynamic job satisfaction model, Potocnik and colleagues (2013) applied the concept of satisfaction to retirement. They postulated that an individual develops a degree of retirement satisfaction or dissatisfaction contingent upon her expectations of retirement and the actual retirement situation. Additionally, an individual's level of aspiration regarding retirement, as well as her problem-solving abilities, can influence the level of satisfaction she actually experiences in this transition. As such, they proposed five types of retirement satisfaction, including progressive satisfaction (an individual is satisfied with retirement and endeavors to increase levels of aspiration and satisfaction), stabilized retirement (individual is satisfied with retirement and is determined to sustain satisfaction), resigned retirement satisfaction (individual is ambiguous about retirement and lowers her level of aspiration to adapt to the unpleasant facets of retirement), constructive retirement dissatisfaction (individual is dissatisfied with retirement but tries to maintain her level of aspiration and problem-solve), and fixated retirement dissatisfaction (the individual is dissatisfied with retirement and sustains her level of aspiration, but does not try to problem-solve to improve her experience) (Potocnik et al., 2013).

The researchers administered questionnaires to 270 Spanish retirees. They found that 41% of their sample could be categorized as stabilized-progressive retirement satisfaction, 27% as resigned-stabilized retirement satisfaction, 14% as resigned retirement satisfaction, and almost 18% as constructive-fixated retirement dissatisfaction. A good number of their sample was satisfied with retirement and maintained their level of aspiration and even reached for personal growth. They found, however, that involuntary retirement negatively impacted retirement satisfaction, as did gender. While men may be more likely to fall in the resigned retirement satisfaction, women were more likely to be dissatisfied with retirement (constructive-fixated retirement satisfaction) (Potocnik et al., 2013).

We would like to suggest several more points regarding the retirement transition. First, the process of retirement is often not linear. Thus, it is often not an abrupt transition, whereby an individual moves from a full-time work position or career one day to no employment the next day. Increasingly today, perhaps due to lengthening life spans, as well as economic downturns in developed countries, many individuals return to some form of employment after retirement. Second, retirement is broader than the cessation of work. Individuals can also "retire" from other activities that were key to their identity in adulthood. For instance, some individuals need to give up driving; this form of retirement is very difficult for older adults and has been found to result in feelings of loss of control and independence (Choi, Adams, & Mezuk, 2012; Fonda, Wallace, & Herzog, 2001). Further, retiring from volunteer positions or church attendance, due to poor health or the need to provide care, is another form of retirement that can cause much grief in some aging adults (Herrera, Lee, Nanyonjo, Laufman, & Torres-Vigil, 2009).

Health Care Systems

Literature on health care/medical service transitions (transfer of care) abounds in a number of countries (Bell, 2007; Binks, Barden, Burke, & Young, 2007; Freed & Hudson, 2006; Kaufman & Pinzon, 2007; Kingsnorth, Healy, & Macarthur, 2007; Radovick & DiVall, 2007; Tanner, Glasby, & McIver, 2014). Health care transitions are particularly precarious due to the *number of* and *variance in* kinds of transitions within the health care system itself (for example, an individual may transition from the emergency department to a hospital unit, and then to another unit within the same hospital and perhaps again to a rehabilitation facility), the critical nature of some transitions (such as moving from hospital to live permanently in a long-term care facility), as well as the significant vulnerability of some patients (for example, older adults may have numerous health problems, be taking multiple medications, and have cognitive or sensory deficits).

Furthermore, transitions are complicated by how health care services are structured. Health care systems are often configured according to discrete loci of care that function in isolation from each other (Coleman & Williams, 2007). This *silo effect* contributes to poor communication between professionals working in different specialties, yet for the benefit of the same individual. The lack of communication can have a serious impact upon the health of vulnerable individuals. In the following section, we will address transitions between medical services (e.g., adult to geriatric services), between home and facilities (e.g., home to hospital and hospital to home; home to long-term care), between facilities (e.g., hospital to long-term care facility and long-term care to hospital), as well as the role of transition professionals who aid clients and families with health care transitions.

Transitions between medical services

Transitioning between medical services can be difficult for some individuals, particularly if they have received health care for years from one primary service. Often, the transition across services is due to changing age groupings, rather than significant changes in needs: for instance, the transition of young adults with special health care needs from pediatric-oriented to adult-oriented care. In a qualitative study, Reiss, Gibson, and Walker (2005) examined the process of health care transition for youths and young adults with disabilities and special health care needs, their family members, and health care providers. Using both interviews and focus groups, they discovered that important reciprocal relationships, based upon mutual trust between providers and families, are developed in the process of caring for these children. This finding was noteworthy, as pediatric- and adult-oriented services represent two different medical subcultures; therefore, how care is delivered to children with special health care needs may differ from how care is delivered to these same individuals within the adult system (e.g., professionals working in adult services often expect greater autonomy out of youth than those who provide care in pediatric services). Additionally, Garvey and colleagues (2013) found that a lack of preparation for entry into the adult system contributed to transition problems in young adults with Type 1 diabetes. For people with mental illness, transitioning from adult to geriatric mental health services, just because they have turned 65 years of age, may not be a welcomed transition. Some of these individuals may have been seen by the same psychiatrist or community mental health nurse for years and feel comfortable and safe within those relationships. The transition to a new care provider is perceived as a loss, and it may take some time for a client to adjust and to forge new relationships.

Similarly, one study examined the transition of adolescents who were infected (in utero) with HIV—from pediatrics to adult services (internal medicine) (Vijayan, Benin, Wagner, Romano, & Andiman, 2009). The researchers interviewed 18 adolescents with HIV, 15 of their parents, and 9 pediatric health care professionals about their concerns regarding the transition. In addition to concerns about adolescent sexuality and compliance with medication regimes, adolescents, parents, and health care providers expressed concern about letting go of their relationships. Those interviewed described a familial quality to their health-focused relationships and experienced anxiety in anticipating termination (Vijayan et al., 2009).

Transitions between facilities

There is much literature that examines transitions between various kinds of health care facilities. Individuals can transition between hospital units (Beach et al., 2012), between hospitals and long-term care facilities (Callahan et al., 2012) or off-site rehabilitation units, and between acute care hospitals and hospices. Depending upon the vulnerability of the population, such as older adults with dementia, as well as the number of moves, transitions between facilities can be enormously stressful for older adults and family members and have detrimental effects upon the well-being and health of older adults (Naylor & Keating, 2008).

Transitions between health care facilities, such as transitioning from hospital to a long-term care facility, can be precarious. Not only do older adults experience psychological difficulty adjusting to the transition between facilities, the period of transition also represents a time where medication errors may be made (Desai, Williams, Greene, Pierson, & Hansen, 2011), which can result in serious health consequences. Or important health care information, which should have been passed from the staff in one facility on to the staff in the next facility, may be unwittingly omitted.

Another transition event is discharge from hospital to home. Even though the transition from hospital to home is usually eagerly anticipated by patients and family members, like other transitions between facilities, the nature of the transition experience is disruptive and can have negative consequences. Despite the abundance of research studies related to hospital discharge planning, transition care from hospital to home remains problematic. Problems include lapses in quality of health care and patient safety, gaps in communication between hospital and professional home care providers, ill-prepared family members, and confusion regarding coordination of care (Coleman & Williams, 2007). It is understandable then, that family caregivers often feel a tremendous burden of responsibility for the care of their relative (Plank, Mazzoni, & Cavada, 2012).

Transition facilitator

With an understanding that navigating through the health care system can be difficult, particularly for individuals with cognitive impairment, developmental disabilities, or extreme frailty, the value of the role of a transition facilitator is increasingly being discussed. The transition facilitator usually helps patients moving from hospital to home (Newbold, Schneidermann, & Horton, 2012), but may also help individuals navigate the health care system in the community (Boult et al., 2008). Although the transition facilitator is usually a registered nurse, the facilitator may also be a social worker (Manderson, McMurray, Piraino, & Stolee, 2012). The transition facilitator can help individuals and their families to connect with needed health care services within the community, as sometimes, despite the best intents of health care professionals across services, linkages on behalf of individuals fail.

How effective is a transition facilitator? Although the role of the transition facilitator is relatively new, early research results generally prove the value of this role to assist vulnerable individuals transitioning from hospital to home (Manderson et al., 2012). Results show that the use of a facilitator results in an increased adherence with taking medications at home (Newbold et al., 2012), greater patient and physician satisfaction (Boult et al., 2008), and in some cases, decreased length of hospital stay and fewer visits to the emergency department and hospital readmission (Cameron, Birnie, Dharma-Wardene, Raivio, & Marriott, 2007). It can be argued that the use of a transition facilitator encourages and empowers patients and family members to take responsibility for their care, thereby achieving better health outcomes.

Family Caregiving

It is only recently that the concept of transition has emerged in the caregiving literature (Seltzer & Li, 1996). The term *caregiver* is often used to describe the unpaid relatives or friends of a disabled individual who help that individual with his activities of daily living. For some, the transition into the caregiver role becomes all-consuming and other aspects of their lives, such as social events and leisure activities, are sacrificed for the benefit of the family member. Becoming a caregiver is a transition *in and of itself*; however, another aspect of caregiving involves helping a family member through various health and health care transitions.

Family caregivers encounter numerous difficulties supporting older adults during and through care transitions, such as moves from acute care to home and from home or hospital into long-term care. They report not feeling prepared for the transition and describe frustration over a lack of communication with health care providers, as well as difficulty obtaining needed information and access to resources (Davies & Nolan, 2004; Grimmer & Moss, 2004). These difficulties contribute to family caregivers' negative experiences of care transitions. The experiences of caregivers during a transition from home or hospital to a long-term care facility may, unfortunately, spill over into the early months of placement in the institution. The helplessness, anger, guilt, and frustration that may have been experienced during the transfer to long-term care may now be expressed by caregivers to staff in the facility. Caregivers may communicate these emotions through their hypervigilance about the care of their older adult, and through their verbal expressions of displeasure over the care their older member receives.

Current approaches to transitional care focus primarily on patients' and families' experiences of moving between the span of health care settings. However, Shyu, Chen, Chen, Wang, and Shao (2008) examined the outcomes of a caregiver-oriented care transition intervention for family caregivers of individuals who had suffered a stroke. They found that their intervention resulted in higher self-evaluations of preparation and better satisfaction of discharge needs in the caregivers, in comparison to a control group who received only routine care. Care for the caregiver in transition makes a significant difference!

As stated earlier in this chapter, we will not explore the transitional domain of death and dying until Chapter 6. However, before we examine how individuals cope with transitions, we would like to mention an important caveat. That is, although reasonable predictions can be formulated about the impact of expected events, the reality of the effect of change is *different for each individual*. What one individual considers impactful, whether in a positive or negative sense, another may experience as relatively inconsequential. To illustrate, in one study, individuals were asked to reflect upon their lives and name the major occurrences that changed the course of their lives. Some of the events frequently recognized in the transition literature as important were not identified by participants (Ronka, Oravala, & Pulkkinen, 2003), thus indicating that some individuals find commonly noteworthy transition experiences to be relatively unremarkable. As mentioned earlier, it is not simply the transition experienced, but the *meaning attached to it* that determines the effect upon those going through it.

Coping With Transitions

Because life course transitions can vary greatly, broad frameworks have been developed to describe the ways in which individuals cope with changes. Bridges (1980) developed a framework to explain the emotions that accompany transitions; each transition is composed of three stages: (1) "endings," which produce sadness, anger, and remorse; (2) "neutral zone," which brings fear and confusion accompanied by a potential for creativity; and (3) "new beginning," a mixture of confidence over what has been gained and anxiety about slipping backward.

The first stage begins with the acknowledgment that the change is real; "the way things were" is no longer possible. There is a sense of loss that is accompanied by mourning. An ending in the present may bring back memories from past losses and the resulting surge in feelings can overwhelm a person and trigger behavior that is hard for others, or the individual in transition, to understand and accept. Eventually, ending means letting go and saying goodbye to both the old identity and the old way of doing things.

In the second stage, an individual is confused, anxious, and perhaps defensive. People around the individual in this stage of transition may become impatient; they might express such comments as "you need to move on" or "get over it." While the neutral zone creates space for creativity and growth, the loss of familiar boundaries and supports creates the temptation to return to that which feels familiar. An individual needs to get through this uncomfortable in-between zone, when the old way is gone but the new way does not as yet feel truly comfortable. Even when the change seemed good initially, an individual may feel lost and confused at times. Yet, by experiencing fear and confusion, an individual may do her best problem solving. She may be able to explore a variety of paths to new beginnings (Bridges, 1980).

The third stage of Bridges' model (1980) of coping with transitions is "new beginning." In this stage, an individual is emotionally ready to do things in an entirely new way. The new beginning is reached after an individual has parted with the old and crossed the neutral zone. The past is not forgotten or discarded, but is understood as part of the individual, *in a new way*. Interestingly, an individual may believe that a new beginning can happen when he wants it to, but in actuality, the new beginning will happen when the person is inwardly ready.

Factors That Influence the Transition Experience

The literature offers a great deal of evidence about the different factors that influence the transition process. Any one factor can be perceived as either a barrier or support, depending on the situation. However, further study is required to determine the extent of the influence of these factors upon the transition process and outcomes, and how they interact with each other.

Individual Factors

There are a number of factors specific to individuals, which may influence successful navigation through the transition experience. Hopwood and colleagues (2011) noted that genetic factors are important for understanding personality stability and changes during the transition to adulthood. As such, a person's genetic makeup influences how she responds to the transition from adolescence into adulthood. Additionally, O'Regan (2010) stated that how an individual copes with a new identity is influenced by how secure he is in the epicenter of his identity. Presumably, the security of identity is not just related to genetic factors, but also to the individual's past history of learning to cope with difficulties and transitions.

Jim was a kind hearted man in his early 30s who was very attached to his mother. She had, over the course of Jim's childhood, struggled with severe multiple sclerosis; Jim's father left the family when Jim was in his late teens, and Jim had functioned as his mother's caregiver ever since. Jim lived within the family home and did not work outside of it. He had few friends and no goals other than caring for his mother to the best of his ability. When the disease took her life, he was devastated. Applying Hopwood and colleagues' (2011) concept of genetic factors influencing how one deals with transition, Jim's naturally sensitive personality played into his difficulty with his mother's passing. And utilizing O'Regan's (2010) understanding of security within the epicenter of one's identity, one could say that part of Jim's struggle with his mother's death is that Jim did not have a deeply rooted sense of identity. Other than being his mother's son and caregiver, he did not know who he was. These factors, combined with social isolation, lack of family support, and a history of depression, over-whelmed him. Sadly, Jim took his own life six months after she passed— not nearly enough time in which to discover who he was.

Physical or mental disabilities

As an individual factor, physical, mental, behavioral, sensory, intellectual, and learning disabilities are strongly correlated with school non-comple-tion and other negative outcomes of transition (Binks et al., 2007; Learning Disabilities Association of Canada, 2007; Vander Stoep et al., 2000). The influence of the type of disability has been reported in several published studies, and statistical evidence indicates that type of disability can affect the process and outcomes of adult transitions (Caton & Kagan, 2007; Van Naarden Braun, Yeargin-Allsopp, & Lollar, 2006). Some literature reports increased risk of negative outcomes with a high level of severity of differ-ent types of disability (Bowe, 2003; Caton & Kagan, 2007; Wong, 2004). However, it should be recognized that some believe that disability is only one factor in a complex process. Disabilities can greatly impact how indi-viduals move through transitions, but the evidence to date seems inconclu-sive about the influences of specific types of disabilities.

That being said, disabilities can be compounded with other factors that increase the challenges in successfully moving through transitions. Literature about Aboriginal, Hispanic, and African American youth with disabilities speaks to the "double jeopardy": risk factors of disability *and* ethnicity (Blacher, 2001; Hussain, 2003) put individuals at greater disadvantage. As an example, we know of an Aboriginal family that moved from one district to another in a large city. One of the teenage children had a debilitating disease and went to a special school. The arrangement for permanent transportation had not yet been established, and so the family arranged for a taxi to pick this boy up from home, take him to school, and then pick him up from school again and bring him home. In this transition, the taxi driver took advantage of this young man, both verbally abusing him and taking the long route home (running up the costs). With his vulnerabilities, this young man's transition from one home to another, and from one mode of transportation to another (no matter how short the duration), was difficult.

In understanding the impact of disabilities upon transitioning, some researchers have found that disabilities, in conjunction with gender, may influence *how* individuals cope with transitions, as well as *how well* they cope (Berge, Patterson, Goetz, & Milla, 2007; Powers, Hogansen, Geenen, Powers, & Gil-Kashiwabara, 2008). For instance, in an interesting study by Berge and colleagues (2007), adolescents with cystic fibrosis (CF) who were transitioning into adulthood were interviewed. The researchers identified that females coped with the transition differently than males. As an example, the female participants wanted others to hold them accountable for following their CF treatment regimes, while the males felt they needed to be responsible. Further, while both females and males reported the importance of a positive outlook, the males spoke of how the illness had developed their character, while the females took a more passive role and noted that they just had to accept the illness. Berge and colleagues (2007) concluded that a passive coping style may have influenced the mental health of the participants, because the female participants experienced greater mental health difficulties.

Environmental Factors

There is some discussion in the literature that specifically addresses environmental factors and their influence upon the transition experience. For illustration, recent studies have found that some youth with disabilities may become involved in criminal behavior and substance abuse (Baltodano, Mathur, & Rutherford, 2005). The influence of others (as an environmental factor) upon these youth in encouraging substance abuse and criminal behavior increases the complexity of their situations, and may result in negative outcomes of school failure and unemployment.

Maddalena, Kearney, and Adams' (2012) qualitative study examined factors influencing the quality of work life of Canadian novice nurses (less than two years' experience). In transitioning to their new role, they encountered numerous sources of environmental stress, including "difficult personalities," inadequate orientation and mentoring, and horizontal violence from nursing and medical colleagues. These stressors were compounded by staffing shortages and heavy workloads. Addressing the environmental factors by offering supportive mentoring and adequate orientation helped these beginning nurses' transition into their new role.

Nalder and colleagues (2012) investigated perceived success of the transition from hospital to home after traumatic brain injury. Among participants, sentinel events such as returning to work and independent community access, as well as changing life situations, were associated with greater perceived success; financial strain and difficulty accessing therapy services were associated with less perceived success. These findings were consistent with the earlier work of Cornwell and colleagues (2009) who reported that restricted access to community services, as well as organizational issues such as poor communication, limited funding, and inadequate availability of staff, influenced the transition experience for a similar client group.

Case Example

In order to illustrate some of the concepts previously discussed within this chapter, as well as to link into the following topic of interventions during transitions, we now present a case example.

Dwayne is a 20-year-old young man. He recently left his home in a large urban center in Eastern Canada to go to university in the United States. His adjustment thus far into university life has been difficult. Although his marks are very good, he is hardly eating, has returned to a previous behavior of cutting himself, and is isolating himself from others. Dwayne did not want to go to university, despite his great interest in the biological sciences, because he worried that he would find this transition difficult. His parents, worried about how Dwayne would "make it in life," strongly encouraged him and even pushed him to apply; hence his transition to a university student has been enigmatic!

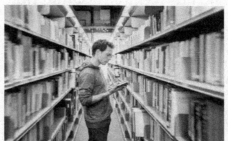

Ditty_about_summer/Shutterstock, Inc.

For his initial weeks on campus, Dwayne sat alone in his dorm room on campus, ruminating on how he ended up in this situation. In his mind he repeatedly has thought back on his junior and senior high school days. School was always a bitter experience for him, despite, and maybe in part because, of his stellar marks. His fellow students never liked him and repeatedly taunted him, first for being too heavy, then for being too skinny (his weight fluctuated greatly). He felt like he never fit in with his peers, or even his family, because he could not come to grips with his biological mother's giving him up for adoption. Off and on throughout his school career he cut himself in order to deal with the stresses of being disliked and lonely.

About halfway through the term, Dwayne decided that he needed to do something. In speaking with a kind professor, he was directed to go to Student Counseling. The student counselor talked with Dwayne about his transition to university life, as well as other concurrent transitions. She questioned Dwayne about the self-harming behavior and purposefully inquired if the self-harming was related to suicidal ideation, was done to relieve stress, or was caused by self-loathing. She examined Dwayne's coping methods, as well as who he has for support, both at home and on campus. Together they constructed a plan to help him, including ongoing appointments for counseling, as well as arranging an appointment with a doctor in the university health clinic to get a thorough checkup and be assessed regarding whether he should receive medication. Although still feeling worried about his ability to get through the semester, Dwayne feels less alone and a little more hopeful that he can continue.

Assessment and Interventions During Transitions

Transitions are difficult, in part, because of unknowns in *how they unfold*, as well as because of the uncertainties of how *individuals will react* throughout the transitional experiences. This may produce wariness and even fear in individuals as they approach transitions; the concern may even be extended to family members as they watch a member face into a transition and wonder how best to support the individual. Health and human service professionals need to recognize the importance of addressing the underlying individual and environmental factors, as well as the quality of supportive relationships (e.g., family and friends), in understanding and supporting individuals during transitions. We now address interventions to assist individuals through transitions, and where possible, will apply the situation of Dwayne in the discussion.

Awareness of the Impact of Transitional Experiences

It is important that health and human service professionals recognize the impact of transitions upon individuals. Even if transitions are expected, some individuals will struggle with facing into and getting through the changes. Particularly if past transitional experiences were difficult, present or future experiences may also be challenging. As part of understanding transitions, self-awareness among professionals cannot be overstated. Professionals who understand their own responses to transitions will be better able to be empathetic; they will understand the connection between transitions and personal identity, and that transitions can lead to uncertainty and even fear as individuals wonder *who they are* during these times. They will be able to understand the powerful emotions that emerge, and even the sometimes inappropriate expressions of anger, such as swearing at a health care professional or failing to show up for an appointment. These types of behaviors can be understood as expected and, indeed, *human* responses to the disorienting effects of transition.

Assessment of Past Transitional Experiences

In order to understand how individuals experience transitions, health and human service professionals may assess how individuals have processed and progressed through previous transitions. If individuals have perceived past transitions to be frightening, current or future transitions may be viewed as fear-provoking. Hence, Dwayne's counselor may ask about previous transitions that he experienced, including how he progressed through his school years. She may ask Dwayne about what worked for him when he faced difficulties and what strategies were not effective. The counselor should be mindful of how emotional reactions to past transitions faced by Dwayne may impact how he is making sense of this transition to university life.

Understanding That Transitional Experiences May Influence a Sense of Identity

Some transitional experiences can impact identity. At times, the impact can be positive; for instance, the change from single status to married can be positive and affirming for individuals. However, some transitions can rattle how persons perceive or define themselves. This may be the case when individuals move from one profession to another. The change may be unsettling, as how they have defined themselves has now changed (e.g., lawyer to homemaker). This can also occur in retirement, when adults leave specific careers that have given them status and a feeling of importance, as well as have largely defined who they have been as individuals. The impact of transition upon persons' sense of identity can be even greater if they struggle with who they are as human beings. As in the situation with Dwayne (case example), his wrestling with the transition of becoming a university student is exacerbated by his questions around who he is as an individual; his questions about who he is as an individual have been negatively impacted by his questions and emotional pain regarding being adopted (Kerr-Edwards, 2011).

The astute professional working with someone like Dwayne will ask him how he defines himself, what he is particularly proud of as an individual, and what are his strengths as well as areas for growth. The professional can then sensitively inquire about whether the current transition is affecting how he sees himself as a person and ascertain if there are past and current issues of personal identity that are being aggravated by the situation. If warranted, the health and human service professional can refer an individual like Dwayne to a support group, such as a group for those struggling with having been adopted (Kerr-Edwards, 2011).

Assessment of Mental State

Transitional experiences, if very difficult, may influence individuals' mental health. Irrespective of age, children, adolescents, adults, and older adults may respond with depressed mood and increased anxiety. Thus, health and human service professionals should routinely assess the mental health impact of transitions upon their clients. When presented with evidence of self-harm, health and human service professionals should assess individuals, such as Dwayne, for suicidal ideation. The knowledgeable professional will understand that sometimes acts like cutting are intended for suicide, but in other cases, such acts may be the means to relieve stress, to purge oneself of bad feelings, or to physically punish the self for perceived badness (Hill & Dallos, 2011; Rissanen, Kylma, & Laukkanen, 2011). When mental health is a concern, individuals should be referred to a physician or psychiatrist for assessment.

Assessment of Coping Strategies and Support Systems

In order to intervene with individuals experiencing transitions, health and human service professionals will assess coping strategies. Coping strategies include how individuals mentally process or appraise situations. For instance, individuals who look upon transitions as frightening and insurmountable may unwittingly, through rumination on negative thoughts, paralyze themselves with fear. The work of the professional involves helping individuals examine how they face transitions, to alter their thinking into more productive and positive patterns.

Other coping strategies involve finding social support through family or friends, clubs or groups; for some individuals, religious involvement is an important resource during periods of transition. Depending upon the type of transition, individuals may seek new support systems, such as support groups. Health and human service professionals should assess the support systems (Wright & Leahey, 2013) of those experiencing difficulties in managing transitions—both informal (family and friends) and formal (professional)—and encourage them not to separate themselves from that support. In particular, some age groups may have fewer social supports, such as older adults (Gillath, Johnson, Selcuk, & Teel, 2011), and some individuals, under stress, may have the tendency to isolate themselves.

Dwayne's counselor is aware that he has used cutting as a coping strategy to relieve stress (Hill & Dallos, 2011). Understanding, however, that while cutting may relieve stress for Dwayne, it can also create new stress when others question why he is covered in scars; the counselor will work with him to uncover old coping methods that have worked in the past (but are not being utilized in the present) and to discover new strategies to cope. His counselor will also consider who he has for support and will encourage him to connect with his parents and other support systems regularly during this time.

Knowledge of and Participation in Development of Community Services and Programs

It is helpful for professionals to be aware of services and programs that have developed to assist individuals experiencing transitions. For example, a number of promising practice models in education feature programs to include students in school meetings, as well as school-supervised work experiences, and functionally oriented curricula (Carnaby, Lewis, Martin, Naylor, & Stewart, 2003). Further, in the United Kingdom, transition guidelines have been developed to assist students going to university (Cook, Rushton, McCormick, & Southall, 2005). Additionally, models have been developed to facilitate the age-appropriate participation of youth with developmental disabilities in post-secondary classes (Dolyniuk et al., 2002). In these programs, students in transition receive guided experience in their new settings, support, and information.

For adults, there are a number of strategies/services to assist through transitions. For instance, many churches offer premarital counseling for couples who are getting married. Within these counseling sessions, couples are encouraged to talk about issues such as finances (and debt), expectations, and conflict resolution. These are topics that they might not address on their own, but in a session they are provided the opportunity to discuss these important and potentially "hot" topics. Further, for adults in their fifties and sixties, there are pre-retirement courses aimed at assisting them in examining financial implications of retirement, as well as considering the need to plan ahead (Hewitt, Howie, & Feldman, 2010).

There are now online support systems that help individuals, such as older adults. Some agencies provide means for online support for older adults who are housebound. Older adults can either access help for their health transitions (resulting in being homebound) through phone support, or can offer support to others through phone or "virtual" support (Cattan, Kime, & Bagnall, 2011; Mukherjee, 2010). Professionals who recognize the importance of programs that help individuals during transitions can refer their clients to relevant programs, or if unavailable, can be involved in the creation of such programs within their region.

SUMMARY

Human transition entails change and adaptation: developmentally (for example teenager to young adult), personally, within relationships, and situations. The literature provides a clear picture of the experiences, challenges, and desired outcomes for individuals of all ages and their families. Some literature also identifies experiences and perspectives of service providers and community members who are part of the transition process. To date, many of the studies and review articles focus on experiences of transitioning or transferring from one service system to another, for example, from pediatric to adult services. A shift in focus is evident in recent literature that focuses more on a holistic, life course perspective. Understanding the personal and environmental conditions that facilitate or hinder movement through a transition is critical to describing the experience of transition.

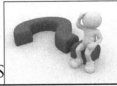

CRITICAL THINKING EXERCISES

▶ What does the word *transition* mean to you? How does your view of transition compare with what you have learned in this chapter?

▶ Transition is a central concept to understanding human behavior. Based upon your reading to date, assess your own understanding of transitions. Write down your experiences and feelings as you identify a specific experience of transition.

▶ Interview a professional colleague (e.g., faculty member, university classmate) and ask about a specific experience of transition. Compare his experience with your own.

INTERESTING WEBSITES

▶ Center for Parent Information and Services: http://www. parentcenterhub.org/repository/transitionadult/

▶ Easter Seals Ontario: http://www.easterseals.org/services/parent-resources/transitions

▶   The Network on Transitions to Adulthood: http://www.
transitions2adulthood.com/

▶   YoungMinds: http://www.youngminds.org.uk/training_services/
young_minds_in_schools/wellbeing/transitions

REFERENCES

Arnett, J. J. (2004). *Emerging adulthood: The winding road from the late teens through the twenties.* New York: Oxford University Press.

Bachman, J. G., Schulenberg, J., Johnston, L. D., Bryant, A. L., Merline, A. C., & O'Malley, P. M. (2002). *The decline of substance use in young adulthood: Changes in social activities, roles, and beliefs.* Mahwah, NJ: Lawrence Erlbaum Assoc.

Baldo, A. J., & Baldo, T. D. (2003). A dual-career couple's experience with adoption: The dramatic impact of moving from couple to instant parenthood. *The Family Journal, 11*(4), 400–403. doi:10.1177/1066480703255388

Baltodano, H. M., Mathur, S. R., & Rutherford, R. B. (2005). Transition of incarcerated youth with disabilities across systems and into adulthood. *Exceptionality, 13*(2), 103–124. doi:10.1207/s15327035ex1302_4

Beach, C., Cheung, D. S., Apker, J., Horwitz, L. I., Howell, E. E., O'Leary, K. J., Patterson, E. S., et al. (2012). Improving interunit transitions of care between emergency physicians and hospital medicine physicians: A conceptual approach. *Academic Emergency Medicine, 19*(10), 1188–1195. doi:10.111/j.1553-2712.2012.01448.x

Bell, L. (2007). Adolescents with renal disease in an adult world: Meeting the challenge of transition of care. *Nephrology Dialysis Transplantation, 22*(4), 988–991. doi:10.1093/ndt/gfl770

Berge, J. M., Patterson, J. M., Goetz, D., & Milla, C. (2007). Gender differences in young adults' perceptions of living with cystic fibrosis during the transition to adulthood: A qualitative investigation. *Families, Systems, and Health, 25*(2), 190–203. doi:10.1037/1091-7527.25.2.190

Binks, J. A., Barden, W. S., Burke, T. A., & Young, N. L. (2007). What do we really know about the transition to adult-centered health care? A focus on cerebral palsy and spina bifida. *Archives of Physical Medicine and Rehabilitation, 88*(8), 1064–1073. doi:10.1016/j.apmr.2007.04.018

Blacher, J. (2001). Transition to adulthood: Mental retardation, families, and culture. *American Journal of Mental Retardation, 106*(2), 173–188. doi:10.1352/0895-8017

Blair, S. E. (2000). The centrality of occupational life transitions. *British Journal of Occupational Therapy, 63*(5), 231–237.

Boult, C., Reider, L., Frey, K., Leff, B., Boyd, C. M., Wolff, J. L., Wegener, S., et al. (2008). Early effects of "guided care" on the quality of health care for multimorbid older persons: A cluster-randomized control trial. *Journal of Gerontology: Series A, Biological and Medical Sciences, 63*(3), 321–327.

Bowe, F. G. (2003). Transition for deaf and hard-of-hearing students: A blueprint for change. *Journal of Deaf Studies and Deaf Education, 8*(4), 485–493. doi:10.1093/deafed/eng024

Bridges, W. (1980). *Transitions: Making sense of life's changes.* Reading, MA: Addison-Wesley.

Bridges, W. (2004). *Transitions: Making sense of life's changes (Rev. ed.).* Cambridge, MA: Da Capo Press.

Bridges, W. (2009). *Managing transitions: Making the most of the change (3rd ed.)* Cambridge, MA: Da Capo Press.

Brown, G. W., & Harris, T. O. (1979). *Social origins of depression: A study of psychiatric disorders in women.* London: Tavistock.

Brown, P., & Hesketh, A. (2004). *The mismanagement of talent: Employability and jobs in the knowledge economy.* Oxford: Oxford University Press.

Bucx, F., & van Wel, F. (2008). Parental bond and life course transitions from adolescence to young adulthood. *Adolescence, 43*(169), 71–88.

Bussing, A., Bissels, T., Fuchs, V., & Perrar, K. M. (1999). A dynamic model of work satisfaction: Qualitative approaches. *Human Relations, 52*(8), 999–1028.

Calasanti, T. M. (1996). Gender and life satisfaction in retirement: An assessment of the male model. *Journal of Gerontology: Social Sciences, 51B*(1), S18–S29. doi:10.1093/geronb/51B.1.S18

Callahan, C. M., Arling, G., Tu, W., Rosenman, M. B., Counsell, S. R., Stump, T. E., & Hendrie, H. C. (2012). Transitions in care for older adults with and without dementia. *Journal of the American Geriatrics Society, 60*(5), 813–820. doi: 10.1111/j.1532-5415.2012.03905.x

Cameron, C. L., Birnie, K., Dharma-Wardene, M. W., Raivio, E., & Marriott, B. (2007). Hospital-to-community transitions: A bridge program for adolescent mental health patients. *Journal of Psychosocial Nursing & Mental Health, 45*(10), 24–30.

Carnaby, S., Lewis, P., Martin, D., Naylor, J., & Stewart, D. (2003). Participation in transition review meetings: A case study of young people with learning disabilities leaving a special school. *British Journal of Special Education, 30*(4), 187–193. doi:10.1111/j.0952-3383.2003.00309.x

Carroll, L. (1967). *Alice in Wonderland.* London, UK: Dobson.

Cattan, M., Kime, N., & Bagnall, A. M. (2011). The use of telephone befriending in low level support for socially isolated older people—An evaluation. *Health and Social Care in the Community, 19*(2), 198–206. doi:10.1111/j.1365-2524.2010.00967.x

Caton, S., & Kagan, C. (2007). Comparing transition expectations of young people with moderate learning disabilities with other vulnerable youth and with their non-disabled counterparts. *Disability and Society, 22*(5), 473–488. doi: 10.1080/09687590701427586

Chemtob, C. M., Nomura, Y., Rajendran, K., Yehuda, R., Schwartz, D., & Abramovitz, R. (2010). Impact of maternal Posttraumatic Stress Disorder and depression following exposure to the September 11 attacks on preschool children's behavior. *Child Development,* (July–Aug), *81*(4):1129-1141. doi: 10.1111/j.1467-8624.2010.01458.x

Choi, M., Adams, K. B., & Mezuk, B. (2012). Examining the aging process through the stress-coping framework: Application to driving cessation in later life. *Aging & Mental Health, 16*(1), 75–83. doi:10.1080/13607863.2011.583633

Cleary, M., Walter, G., & Jackson, D. (2011). "Not always smooth sailing": Mental health issues associated with the transition from high school to college. *Issues in Mental Health Nursing, 32*(4), 250–254. doi:10.3109/01612840.2010.548906

Coleman, E. A., & Williams, M. V. (2007). Executing high quality care transitions: A call to do the right thing. *Journal of Hospital Medicine, 2,* 287–290. doi: 10.1002/jhm.276

Cook, A., Rushton, B. S., McCormick, S. M., & Southall, D. W. (2005). *Guidelines for the management of study transition. The STAR (Student Transition and Retention) Project.* [Internet] Retrieved February 6, 2015, from: www.ulster.ac.uk/star/resources/star_guidelines.pdf

Cornwell, P., Fleming, J., Fisher, A., Kendall, M., Ownsworth, T., & Turner, B. (2009). Supporting the needs of young adults with acquired brain injury during transition from hospital to home: The Queensland service provider perspective. *Brain Impairment, 10*(3), 325–340.

Dare, J. S. (2011). Transitions in midlife women's lives: Contemporary experiences. *Health Care for Women International, 32*(2), 111–133. doi: 10.1080/07399332.2010.500753

Davies, S., & Nolan, M. (2004). Making the move: Relatives' experiences of transition to a care home. *Health and Social Care in the Community, 12*(6), 517–526. doi:10.111/j.1365-2524.2004.00535

de Montigny, F., Lacharité, C., & Devault, A. (2012). Transition to fatherhood: Modeling the experience of fathers of breastfed infants. *Advances in Nursing Science, 35*(3), E11–E22. doi:10.1097/ANS.0b013e3182626167

Desai, R., Williams, C. E., Greene, S. B., Pierson, S., & Hansen, R. A. (2011). Medication errors during patient transitions into nursing homes: Characteristics and association with patient harm. *The American Journal of Geriatric Pharmacotherapy, 9*(6), 413–422.

Dolyniuk, C. A., Kamens, M. W., Corman, H., DiNardo, P. O., Totaro, R. M., & Rockoff, J. C. (2002). Students with developmental disabilities go to college: Description of a collaborative transition project on a regular college campus. *Focus on Autism and Other Developmental Disabilities, 17*(4), 236–241.

Elder, G. H., Jr. (1998). The life course as developmental theory. *Child Development, 69*, 1–12.

Fonda, S. J., Wallace, R. B., & Herzog, A. R. (2001). Changes in driving patterns and worsening depressive symptoms among older adults. *Journal of Gerontology: Social Sciences, 56*(6), 343–351. doi:10.1093/geronb/56.6.S343

Freed, G. L., & Hudson, H. J. (2006). Transitioning children with chronic diseases to adult care: Current knowledge, practices, and directions. *Journal of Pediatrics, 148*(6), 824–827. doi:10.1016/j.jpeds.2006.02.010

Garvey, K. C., Finkelstein, J. A., Laffel, L. M., Ochoa, V., Wolfsdorf, J. I, & Rhodes, E. T. (2013). Transition experiences and health care utilization among young adults with type 1 diabetes. *Patient Preferences and Adherence, 7*, 761–769. doi:10.2147/PPA.S45823

Gillath, O., Johnson, D. K., Selcuk, E., & Teel, C. (2011). Comparing old and young adults as they cope with life transitions: The links between social network management skills and attachment styles to depression. *Clinical Gerontologist, 34* (3), 251–265. doi:10.1080/07317115.2011.554345

Goodman, J. H. (2005). Becoming an involved father of an infant. *Journal of Obstetric, Gynecologic, & Neonatal Nursing, 34*(2), 190–200. doi:10.1177/0884217505274581

Greeson, J. K., Usher, L., & Grinstein-Weiss, M. (2010). One adult is crazy about you: Can natural mentoring relationships increase assets among young adults with and without foster care experience? *Children and Youth Services Review, 32*(4), 565–577. doi:10.1016/j.childyouth.2009.12.003

Grimmer, K., & Moss, J. (2004). The development, validity and application of a new instrument to assess the quality of discharge planning activities from the community perspective. *International Journal of Allied Health Sciences & Practice, 2*(4). Retrieved February 6, 2015, from: http://ijahsp.nova.edu/articles/Vol2number3/pdf/grimmer_printversion.pdf

Herrera, A. P., Lee, J. W., Nanyonjo, R. D., Laufman, L. E., & Torres-Vigil, I. (2009). Religious coping and caregiver well-being in Mexican-American families. *Aging and Mental Health, 13*(1), 84–91.

Hewitt, A., Howie, L., & Feldman, S. (2010). Retirement: What will you do? A narrative inquiry of occupation-based planning for retirement: Implications for practice. *Australian Occupational Therapy Journal, 57*(1), 8–16. doi:10.1111/j.1440-1630.2009.00820.x

Hill, K., & Dallos, R. (2011). Young people's stories of self-harm. A narrative study. *Clinical Child Psychology and Psychiatry, 17*(3), 459–475. doi:10.1177/1359104511423364

Holmes, T. H., & Rahe, R. H. (1967). The social readjustment rating scale. *Journal of Psychosomatic Research, 11*(2), 213–218.

Hopwood, C. J., Donnellan, M. B., Blonigen, D. M., Krueger, R. F., McGue, M., Iacono, W. G., & Burt, S. A. (2011). Genetic and environmental influences on personality trait stability and growth during adulthood: A three way longitudinal study. *Journal of Personality and Social Psychology, 100*(3), 545–556. doi:10.1037/a0022409

Hussain, Y. (2003). Transitions into adulthood: Disability, ethnicity and gender among British South Asians. *Disability Studies Quarterly, 23*(2), 100–112.

Hutchison, E. (2008). *Dimensions of human behavior: The changing life course.* Thousand Oaks, CA: Sage.

Izzo, M. V., & Lamb, P. (2003). Developing self-determination through career development activities: Implications for vocational rehabilitation counselors. *Journal of Vocational Rehabilitation 19*(2), 71–78.

Kaufman, M. (2006). Role of adolescent development in the transition process. *Progress in Transplantation, 16*(4), 286–290.

Kaufman, M., & Pinzon, J. (2007). Transition to adult care for youth with special health care needs. *Paediatrics & Child Health, 12*(9), 785–788.

Keller, T. E., Cusick, G. R., & Courtney, M. E. (2007). Approaching the transition to adulthood: Distinctive profiles of adolescents aging out of the child welfare system. *Social Service Review, 81*(3), 453–484.

Kerr-Edwards, S. (2011). Group work with adopted adolescents. *Adoption & Fostering, 35*(3), 50–60.

Kim, J., & Moen, P. (2002). Retirement trends, gender, & psychological well-being: A life-course, ecological model. *Journal of Gerontology: Psychological Sciences, 57B* (3), P212–P222.

Kingsnorth, S., Healy, H., & Macarthur, C. (2007). Preparing for adulthood: A systematic review of life skill programs for youth with physical disabilities. *Journal of Adolescent Health, 41*(4), 323–332. doi:10.1016/j.jadohealth.2007.06.007

Kralik, D., Visentin, K., & van Loon, A. (2006). Transitions: A literature review. *Journal of Advanced Nursing, 55*(3), 320–329. doi:10.1111/j.1365-2648.2006.03899.x

Lawrence, E., Rothman, A. D., Cobb, R. J., Rothman, M. T., & Bradbury, T. N. (2008). Marital satisfaction across the transition to parenthood. *Journal of Family Psychology, 22*(1), 41–50. doi:10.1037/0893-3200.22.1.41

Learning Disabilities Association of Canada. (2007). *Putting a Canadian face on learning disabilities.* Retrieved February 6, 2015, from: www.pacfold.ca/what_is/index.shtml

Lee, K. S., & Ono, H. (2012). Marriage, cohabitation, and happiness: A cross-national analysis of 27 countries. *Journal of Marriage and Family, 74*(5), 953–972. doi:10.1111/j.1741-3737.2012.01001.x

Lim, H., & Mackey, S. (2012). The menopause transition experiences of Chinese Singaporean women: An exploratory qualitative study. *Journal of Nursing Research, 20*(2), 81–89. doi:10.1097/jnr.0b013e318254eb25

Maddalena, V., Kearney, A. J., & Adams, L. (2012). Quality of work life of novice nurses: A qualitative exploration. *Journal for Nurses in Staff Development, 28*(4),74–79. doi:10.1097/NND.0b013e31824b41a1

Manderson, B., McMurray, J., Piraino, E., & Stolee, P. (2012). Navigation roles support chronically ill older adults through healthcare transitions: A systematic review of the literature. *Health and Social Care, 20*(2), 113–127. doi:10.1111/j.1365-2524.2011.01032.x

Meleis, A. I., Sawyer, L. M., Im, E. O., Messias, D. K., & Schumacher, K. (2000). Experiencing transitions: An emerging middle-range theory. *Advances in Nursing Science, 23*(1), 12–28.

Mortensen, O., Torsheim, T., Melkevik, O., & Thuen, F. (2012). Adding a baby to the equation: Married and cohabiting women's relationship satisfaction in the transition to parenthood. *Family Process, 51*(1), 122–139. doi: 10.1111/j.1545-5300.2012.01384.x

Mukherjee, D. (2010). An exploratory study of older adults' engagement with virtual volunteerism. *Journal of Technology in Human Services, 28*(3), 188–196. doi:10.1080/15228835.2010.508368

Nalder, E., Fleming, J., Foster, M., Cornwell, P., Shields, C., & Khan, A. (2012). Identifying factors associated with perceived success in the transition from hospital to home after brain injury. *Journal Head Trauma Rehabilitation, 27*(2), 143–153. doi:10.1097/HTR.0b013e3182168fb1

Naylor, M., & Keating, S. A. (2008). Transitional care: Moving patients from one care setting to another. *American Journal of Nursing, 108*(9 Suppl), 58–63. doi:10.1097/01.NAJ.0000336420.34946.3a

Newbold, E., Schneidermann, M., & Horton, C. (2012). The Bridge Clinic. *American Journal of Nursing, 112*(7), 56–59. doi: 10.1097/01.NAJ.0000415966.23169.7e

O'Regan, M. (2010). Graduate transition to employment: Career motivation, identity, and employability. University of Reading. Retrieved February 1, 2015, from: http://www.reading.ac.uk/web/FILES/ccms/Graduate_transitions_to_employment.pdf

Osterling, K. L., & Hines, A. M. (2006). Mentoring adolescent foster youth: Promoting resilience during developmental transitions. *Clinical and Family Social Work, 11* (3), 242–253.

Oxford dictionary. (-). Retrieved November 12, 2014, from: http://oxford dictionaries.com/definition/english/transition

Plank, A., Mazzoni, V., & Cavada, L. (2012). Becoming a caregiver: New family carers' experience from hospital to home. *Journal of Clinical Nursing, 21*(13–14), 2072–2982. doi:10.1111/j.1365-2702.2011.04025.x

Potocnik, K., Tordera, N., & Peiro, J. M. (2013). Truly satisfied with your retirement or just resigned? Pathways toward different patterns of retirement satisfaction. *Journal of Applied Gerontology, 32*(2), 164–187. doi:10.1177/0733464811405988

Powers, K., Hogansen, J., Geenen, S., Powers, L. E., & Gil-Kashiwabara, E. (2008). Gender matters in transition to adulthood: A survey study of adolescents with disabilities and their families. *Psychology in the Schools, 45*(4), 349–364. doi:10.1002/pits.20297

Radovick, S., & DiVall, S. (2007). Approach to the growth hormone-deficient child during transition to adulthood. *Journal of Clinical Endocrinology and Metabolism, 92*(4), 1195–1200. doi:10.1210/jc.2007-0167

Rasmussen, B., Ward, G., Jenkins, A., King, S. J., & Dunning, T. (2011).Young adults' management of Type 1 diabetes during life transitions. *Journal of Clinical Nursing, 20*(13–14), 1981–1992. doi:10.1111/j.1365-2702.2010.03657.x

Reiss, J. G., Gibson, R. W., & Walker, L. R. (2005). Health care transition: Youth, family, and provider perspectives. *Pediatrics, 115*(1), 112–121. doi:10.1542/peds.2004-1321

Rissanen, M. L., Kylma, J., & Laukkanen, E. (2011). A systematic literature review: Self-mutilation among adolescents as a phenomenon and help for it—What kind of knowledge is lacking? *Issues in Mental Health Nursing, 32*(9), 575–583. doi:10.3109/01612840.2011.578785

Ronka, A., Oravala, S., & Pulkkinen, L. (2003). Turning points in adult lives: The effects of gender and the amount of choice. *Journal of Adult Development, 10*(3), 203–215.

Scannapieco, M., Connell-Carrick, K., & Painter, K. (2007). In their own words: Challenges facing youth aging out of foster care. *Child & Adolescent Social Work Journal, 24*(9), 423–435. doi:10.1007/s10560-007-0093-x

Seltzer, M. M., & Li, L. W. (1996).The transitions of caregiving: Subjective and objective definitions. *The Gerontologist, 36*(5), 614–626. doi:10.1093/geront/36.5.614

Shyu, Y. L., Chen, M., Chen, S., Wang, H., & Shao, J. (2008). A family caregiver-oriented discharge planning program for older stroke patients and their family caregivers. *Journal of Clinical Nursing, 17*(18), 2497–2508. doi:10.1111/j.1365-2702.2008.02450.x

Smith, K. P., & Christakis, N. A. (2008). Social networks and health. *Annual Review of Sociology, 34*, 405–429. doi:10.1146/annurev.soc.34.040507.134601

Stack, S., & Eshleman, J. R. (1998). Marital status and happiness: A 17 nation study. *Journal of Marriage and the Family, 60*(2), 527–536.

Suldo, S. M. Shaunessy, E., Thalji, A., Michalowski, J., & Shaffer, E. (2009). Sources of stress for students in high school college preparatory and general education programs: Group differences and associations with adjustment. *Adolescence, 44* (176), 925–948.

Tanner, D., Glasby, J., & McIver, S. (2014). Understanding and improving older people's experiences of service transition: Implications for social work. *British Journal of Social Work*, (-), 1–6. doi:10.1093/bjsw/bcu095

Tyler, K. A., & Schmitz, R. M. (2013). Family histories and multiple transitions among young adults: Pathway to homelessness. *Children and Youth Services Review, 35*, 1719–1726.

Vander Stoep, A., Beresford, S. A. A., Weiss, N. S., McKnight, B., Cauce, A. M., & Cohen, P. (2000). Community based study of the transition to adulthood for adolescents with psychiatric disorder. *American Journal of Epidemiology, 152*(4), 352–362. doi:10.1093/aje/152.4.352

Van Naarden Braun, K., Yeargin-Allsopp, M., & Lollar, D. (2006). A multi-dimensional approach to the transition of children with developmental disabilitiesintoyoungadulthood:Theacquisitionofadultsocialroles.*Disability and Rehabilitation, 28*(15), 915–928. doi:10.1080/09638280500304919

van Wesel, F., Boeije, H., Alisic, E., & Drost, S. (2012). I'll be working my way back: A qualitative synthesis on the trauma experience of children. *Psychological Trauma: Theory, Research, Practice and Policy, 4*(5), 516–526. doi:10.1037/a0025766

Vijayan, T., Benin, A. L., Wagner, K., Romano, S., & Andiman, W. A. (2009). We never thought this would happen: Transitioning care of adolescents with perinatally acquired HIV infection from pediatrics to internal medicine. AIDS Care, 21(10), 1222–1229. doi:10.1080/09540120902730054

Wang, M. (2007). Profiling retirees in the retirement transition and adjustment process: Examining the longitudinal change patterns of retirees' psychological well-being. *Journal of Applied Psychology, 92*(2), 455–474. doi:10.1037/0021-9010.92.2.455

Wong, M. E. (2004). Higher education or vocational training? Some contributing factors to post-school choices of visually impaired students in Britain. Part 1, Great Britain. *British Journal of Visual Impairments, 22*(1), 37–42. doi:10.1177/026461960402200107

Wright, L. M., & Leahey, M. (2013). *Nurses and families: A guide to family assessment and intervention* (6th ed.). Philadelphia: F.A. Davis.

CHAPTER 2

TRANSITIONS AND OLDER ADULTS: AN OVERVIEW

*Old age. We dread becoming old almost as much
as we dread not living long enough to reach old age.*
(Walsh, 1989, American family therapist and writer)

Reflective Questions

- ► What aspects of aging make transitions more complex and difficult to manage than in younger adulthood?

- ► What demographic trends in North America, as well as developed countries throughout the world, complicate how older adults manage transitions?

- ► What are some challenges that health and human service professionals face in assisting older adults through transitions?

The pervasive dread of old age within developed countries was poignantly expressed by Walsh (1989). With raw honesty, she articulated the sentiments of numerous individuals in the United States, Canada, and other countries. Many individuals within developed countries do not eagerly anticipate getting old. In fact, through means such as plastic surgery and permanent makeup, some try gamely to resist reflecting their advancing years. Why is old age so feared? What is it about the changes and challenges experienced in older age that frightens many adults? We suggest that some of these changes and challenges involve transitions. While some of these transitions may be readily embraced, for example retirement, a number of them present obstacles to enjoyable and independent living.

Within the first chapter, we addressed the concept of transitions and how transitions may be experienced across the life span. Within this second chapter, we consider the types of transitions that older adults face and why these transitions are so daunting. We examine demographic changes in North America and other developed areas of the world that may impact how older adults experience passages. We also highlight the challenges that health and human service professionals may face when working with older adults and their family members who are experiencing these life transitions. While we cover illnesses that older adults face, our focus is purposefully on how older adults and their family members face these illnesses **as transitions,** and how these illnesses may precipitate other transitions; our focus is not to offer an in-depth examination of pathophysiology, pharmacology, or medical treatment.

Intentionally, this chapter is an overview for the subsequent chapters, wherein specific transitions, such as the transition to hospital and then a long-term care facility, will be explored in greater depth. In ensuing chapters we will address the complexities of how experiences of transition in the past color and impact how older adults face current transitions (life course perspective), the circular nature of the influence of transition upon older adults and older adults' responses to the transitions, and the existential impact of later life transitions upon older adults. Within this chapter we lay a foundation by simplistically pulling out and explicating contextual factors and transitions one by one.

Why This Is an Important Topic

Understanding the transitions faced by older adults and the reasons why these transitions can be so difficult is important, in part, due to contextual factors. These contextual factors shape how older adults experience transitions related to age and age-related conditions and include demographic changes such as the explosive growth of our older adult population, the low birth rate, and the substantial geographical mobility in American and Canadian societies and other developed nations, as well as the heterogeneity of the older adult age grouping. In particular, these demographic changes converge to greatly change how older adults experience aging, compared to older adults of earlier generations.

Numbers of Older Adults

The population of North America, and indeed, worldwide, continues to age. As such, the percentage of the population experiencing older age is expected to grow significantly. For instance, in 2014, older adults represented approximately 15.7% of the entire population of Canada. This proportion was 10.0% in 1984 (Statistics Canada, 2014). The proportion of older adults within Canadian society will continue to increase dramatically; it is projected that by 2063, older adults will comprise somewhere between 24% and 28% of the entire population of Canada (Statistics Canada, 2014). Similarly, within the United States, older adults comprised 13% of the population in 2009. However, the percentage of older Americans is projected to jump to 20% by 2050 (Jacobsen, Kent, Lee, & Mather, 2011). Perhaps even more significant is that the number of the *oldest-old*—those 85 years of age and older—is expected to increase dramatically in North America and the developed world (NIH, 2011; Statistics Canada, 2008). As the very old generally experience far more physical and cognitive health problems and often require greater amounts of health care, this stark increase in the very old demographic will place added importance in supporting the transitions necessary at that stage of life.

Birth rates

Within the past half century, Canada and the United States, as well as other developed countries, have experienced a drastic plunge in birth rates. In 1960, Canadian women gave birth to an average of four children. By 1997, the birth rate dropped to approximately 1.5 children (George, Loh, Verma, & Shin, 2001). Currently, the birth rate in Canada is estimated to be 1.59 children per woman, and in the United States of America, 2.06 children per woman (CIA–The World Factbook, n.d.). This means that in Canada, the birth rate is not sufficient to simply replace the existing population.[1] As adult children, particularly adult women, provide the bulk of informal support to their aging parents, this drop in available adult children to help aging parents as they experience transitions is significant. Additionally, the

---

1. A related concept to birth rate is termed *replacement rate*. This construct factors in the mortality rates of children within a country, as well as accounts for women who choose not to, or are unable to, have children. In developed nations, the generally accepted replacement rate is 2.1 children per woman, so that a society will replace itself, resulting in "zero population growth." In developing nations, where mortality rates of infants/children are higher, the replacement rates are also greater (Rosenberg, 2009).

geographical mobility of adults in developed countries further complicates the ability of family members to support older adults through transitions.

Geographical Mobility

Generations ago, it was not unusual for adult children to live in close proximity to their parents. This meant that adult children could attend, even daily, to the concerns and health needs of aging parents. Their close proximity meant that they could be physically present to provide care and to monitor changes in their parents' well-being. However, as many adult children now move away from their parents for education and employment, the ability to provide hands-on care or attention is hampered (Jutras, 1988). This is not to deny that many adult children valiantly attempt to provide some measure of watchfulness and assistance from a distance, but the opportunities to recognize subtle or not so subtle changes in parents is compromised by geographical distance. And, to further compound the issue of monitoring, older adults may hesitate to share their worries regarding health or other transitions, for fear of worrying adult children who are unable to physically address their concerns in the immediate.

Employment Rate of Women

As mentioned previously, adult women typically provide the vast amount of care to aging parents. Their availability to provide care is now often impacted by employment. Prior to the 1970s, many women were homemakers. For example, in 1970, roughly 40% of North American women with children were employed outside the home (Cohn, Livingston, & Wang, 2014; Statistics Canada, 2010a). This meant that a large number of women could care for their children, but also have some flexibility in providing care to aging parents, especially when their children were in school. However, the availability of women to attend to aging parents has changed considerably, as in the past 5 years, just over 70% of Canadian and American women with children under the ages of 16–18 were employed (Cohn et al., 2014; Statistics Canada, 2010a). The considerable increase in women's employment status has reduced the discretionary time available in women's schedules to provide care for their parents. Despite the reduction in flexible time, however, adult women still provide the majority of caregiving for older parents; this is reflected in terms such as the *sandwich generation* (coined by Dorothy Miller in 1981) and *women in the middle* (Dautzenberg, Diederiks, Philipsen, & Stevens, 1998). The toll this takes upon women in this category is being increasingly recognized; their health and well-being is affected by the demands of being in the sandwich generation. Reciprocally, this impacts the care they can provide to one or more aging family members (Kind, 2010).

The Heterogeneity of This Age Grouping

The term *heterogeneity* refers to "the quality of being diverse and not comparable in kind" (Free Online Dictionary, 2015). Older adults, as an age grouping, are the most heterogeneous grouping of all age populations. This means that the degree of differences in older adults is greater than any other age grouping; for example, children or adults. How can this be? First, the classification of old age is somewhat arbitrary and, within developed countries, is often tied to when individuals can access government pensions (Hirst, 1990). Currently, then, older age commences around age 65 in some developed countries. With individuals living so much longer, and the oldest-old (those 85 years of age and older) being the fastest growing group of older adults within Canada (Statistics Canada, 2008), adults may be considered "old" for 20 years or longer. The sheer length of time older adults are considered "old" allows for great diversity in how individuals function and where they live.

Second, there are sub-populations of older adults who are older much earlier than the 65 years of age demarcation, such as those with intellectual disabilities (Hirst, Lane, & Seneviratne, 2013), those with HIV/AIDS (Lane, Hirst, & Reed, 2013), older incarcerated individuals (Beckett, Peternelj-Taylor, & Johnson, 2003), and aboriginals within Canada (Grose & Pravikoff, 2012)[2] or Australia (Caple & Schub, 2012). For these older adults, either disease processes or, in the case of HIV/AIDS, disease processes coupled with the long-term effects of HIV medications, have resulted in these individuals being much older physically, at a much younger age (Lane et al., 2013). These individuals are often considered older adults in their 50s and may require assistance with stable housing, such as group homes, housing support, or eventually, long-term care facilities. The difficulty in transitioning to other accommodations for this sub-population is that they often do not "fit" with the other residents within these settings. For instance, older adults with HIV/AIDS may find themselves homeless, but accessing a home-

2. Aboriginal people in Canada have a higher frequency of cardiovascular diseases, diabetes, and HIV/AIDS than the general Canadian population. Their life span is significantly shorter than the national average; on average they die 5 to 17 years earlier than non-Aboriginals (Grose & Pravikoff, 2012).

less shelter is not a suitable option due to potential exposure to infection (Furlotte, Schwartz, Koornstra, & Naster, 2012). Similarly, accessing long-term care facilities is not ideal for individuals with HIV/AIDS or for those with intellectual disabilities, as these older adults are significantly younger than most of the residents within these settings.

Third, there is often a sharp discrepancy in the level of health between those who are in their late 60s and those who are in their mid 80s or older. As an example, the incidence of Alzheimer's disease or related dementias is approximately 11% for individuals 65 years of age and older. However, by 85 years of age and older, the incidence jumps to almost one third (32%) (Alzheimer's Association, 2014). A 68-year-old man, in good physical shape and with intact cognitive abilities, is in a much different stage in his life than an 85-year-old woman with moderate stage Alzheimer's disease who is transitioning to a long-term care facility. The 68-year-old man will most likely be living in his home, will require little to no support with activities of daily living, may still be working part-time or volunteering, and will manage his life independently. However, the 85-year-old woman with moderate-stage dementia will need assistance with activities of daily living, such as bathing, dressing, and eating, will not be able to manage her finances and may not recognize family members (Alzheimer Society of Ontario, 2015). The difference between these two individuals is enormous, and by extension, there is a stark difference in the demands placed upon the family members of these older adults.

What Are the Transitions Faced by Older Adults?

There are multiple transitions that occur in older age. Some of these transitions are related to societal expectations, such as retirement, and others relate to physiological changes in older adults or their spouses, such as illness or death. Transitioning to an assisted living facility or long-term care may be precipitated by illness in the older adult, the death of a spouse, or significant cognitive impairment (Buhr, Kuchibhatla, & Clipp, 2006). Transitioning to other living situations may trigger existential issues and cause older adults to consider the meaning of their lives and what it means to die.

Retirement

Retirement—the cessation of part-time or full-time paid employment—marks a major life transition for many aging adults. Although viewed as "normal," or even "desirable," this transition is far more complex than may appear. There are a number of factors that impact how older adults experience retirement. For instance, is retirement voluntary or forced? Some evidence suggests that older adults cope better with retirement if it is voluntary and anticipated (Hardy & Quadagno, 1995; Reitzes & Mutran, 2006); in these situations, adults specifically *choose* to leave work. The ability to choose preserves, to some degree, the sense of identity and control in life. Second, are there financial concerns about retirement? Some older adults experience significant concern about how they will cope with the reduced income that comes from retirement (Nuttman-Shwartz, 2004). While these older adults may have enough money to pay their bills, will they be able to afford the activities that they find meaningful? If newly retired individuals cannot afford to engage in the activities they once did, how will they manage the boredom of being at home all day and the stress of being in the constant company of their spouses (Nuttman-Shwartz, 2004)?[3]

Third, are there health issues that trigger the retirement, either of a working older adult, or his or her spouse (Hardy & Quadagno, 1995)? While an older man may feel some sense of relief to retire when struggling with a chronic illness, he may also feel that his choice to retire was taken away, not by a company, but rather by illness and life. In these situations, the perceived lack of control over an illness may result in him feeling demoralized upon retirement. A similar process may occur when leaving work to care for an ailing spouse. When an older woman leaves a job that she loves to care for her ill husband, she may resent being pulled away from the perks of her work: structure in her life, social contact, purpose, and a sense of pride and accomplishment in earning money. If her husband was hospitalized for a serious illness and now is being discharged home, she may feel unprepared and even frightened to be the person solely responsible for her husband's care (Plank, Mazzoni, & Cavada, 2012). Retirement may affect not only how she views herself, it may impact how she views her spouse.

Regardless of the reasons for this transition, retirement can have a profound effect upon individuals' sense of personhood and identity, upon social contacts, and upon daily structure and finances. Older adults may wonder what purpose their life has since they retired, and this question may cause them to reflect back and wonder if their life had meaning prior to this point in time (Gaede, 2010). Although some older adults welcome

---

3.   A variation on this theme is that a number of older adults in North America, for financial reasons, *cannot* retire at the time they would like to (Sterns & Dawson, 2012). The other transitions of old age, such as illness, make this situation particularly difficult.

retirement and truly flourish during this time, others struggle. Decades ago, some adults held the belief that once retirement came, death followed shortly thereafter. Also, as practitioners working with older adults, we know of situations where retirement has precipitated a suicide attempt in an older adult. The loss of identity and daily structure was too much to bear. Within the upcoming chapters, we will continue to address some concerns related to retirement, including the need for financial planning, as well as for aging adults to give some consideration to issues of purpose and meaning in life.

Illness

Older adults often experience life-changing illnesses. These illnesses can cause profound transitions. Health crises, such as heart attacks, may be life-threatening or can cause significant changes in the physical functioning of older adults. Older adults who suffer ischemic strokes, without receiving timely thrombolytic therapy, experience significant changes in functional abilities (Smeltzer & Bare, 2004). For example, the older man may become hemiplegic (paralyzed on one side) and have great difficulty in dressing himself and bathing; he may no longer be able to manage independently within his home. Arthritis, as the most common disability reported by older adults in North America (Centers for Disease Control and Prevention, 2014; Turcotte & Schellenberg, 2007), may hinder an older woman from maintaining her home and yard; climbing stairs may no longer be possible. If her spouse is having difficulty providing care for her due to the extent of her disabilities and structural issues within their home—such as steep staircases—this couple may need to move to a seniors' complex or an assisted living facility. While some older adults look forward to moving to an assisted living facility where their meals are prepared, many grieve the loss of their home. Their home represents more than a physical locality; it incorporates the deeper and richer meanings of comfort, security, and community (Gillsjo & Schwartz-Barcott, 2011). The grief, as well as powerful and conflicting emotions experienced (e.g., ambivalence), may be even greater when the move is to long-term care, rather than an assisted living facility (Davies, 2005; Gill & Morgan, 2011; Kao, Travis, & Acton, 2004). The grief and emotional response associated with the loss of an independent dwelling will be addressed further in Chapter 4.

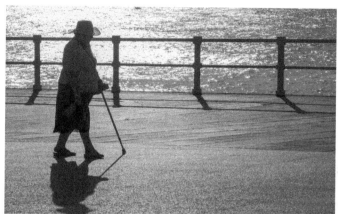

Marco Antonio/Shutterstock, Inc.

Widowhood: The Death of a Spouse

The death of a spouse is one of the most stressful and heart-wrenching transitions experienced by an adult (Holmes & Rahe, 1967). Sometimes it is assumed that the death of a younger spouse is more difficult than the death of an older spouse; the underlying premise in this assumption is that the older couple had many more years together and therefore the death of a younger spouse is more tragic. However, we suggest that advancing age does not necessarily make the death of a spouse easier. Often older couples have developed an *interdependence* whereby they assume different tasks and roles in their relationship; there is a wonderful sense of needing and being needed. The identity of each is intricately, and sometimes inextricably, entwined with the other; the "two have become one" (Genesis 2:24). Hence, the grief associated with the loss of a spouse can be profound. An older man who has lost his wife has not only lost his spouse of 55 years, but may also have lost his best friend, a confidante, and a cook and housecleaner (Gibson, 2012); he may feel like he has lost a part of himself, or himself completely. He may wonder why he should continue to exist when his spouse of many years has passed (Damianakis & Marziali, 2012). Social isolation may further complicate his transition to widowhood; he is no longer part of a "couple" and hence may lose social groups to which he and his spouse belonged.[4] Not only does loss have an

---

4. This complication to an older person's grief is particularly piercing for widowers, who may have solely relied upon their wives for meaningful relationship (Hart, 2001).

impact on the quality of life, it may also impact health. For instance, the social isolation and loneliness that come from the loss of a spouse can lead to poorer health outcomes (Working Together for Seniors, 2007).

Transitional Moves to Other Locations

Older adults may experience multiple moves within a very short time, and these moves may not be welcomed or planned. The relocations signify a leaving of home. As touched upon earlier in this chapter, and will be discussed in depth in Chapter 4, the "home" of an aging adult means much more than four walls; the concept of home is imbued with meaning and security (Gillsjo & Schwartz-Barcott, 2011). An older adult may move from her home to the hospital and reside on one or more hospital units during her hospital stay. It may be determined that due to confusion, she is not capable of living safely alone in her home, and she may be transferred to an assisted living facility or to long-term care (depending upon the assessment in hospital). Even when in a facility, she may still experience moves to another facility or back to the hospital. These relocations may cause significant emotional responses in older adults; they may experience grief in their moves, as well as anger, confusion, and a sense of being lost (Kao et al., 2004; Newson, 2008).

Death of the Older Adult: The Final Transition

Not only may an older adult face the death of a spouse, but by virtue of age, she faces her own impending death. For much of an adult's life, the aging process is either avoided through cosmetic procedures or poked fun at: "You're not 50; you're 41 with nine years' experience!" exclaims one "Happy Fiftieth Birthday" card. But over time, the reality of old age and its challenges, become unavoidable: "Old age is no place for sissies," Bette Davis poignantly stated (BrainyQuote, 2015).

The losses associated with the aging process can be preparatory in facing one's own passing. But the final transition, heretofore not experienced, can demand all the "tools in the toolbox" of the older adult whose resources may already be taxed. The mindset of North American culture, which is often described as "death denying" (Rando, 1984, pp. 5–8), may also hinder the older adult's preparation in dying; family members may avoid the topic of death, thinking they are being helpful. Unfortunately, it is a regular occurrence in palliative care to have family members ask staff not to tell the patient that she is dying: "We don't want Mom to give up hope," is often the rationale. Meanwhile, the older adult in the hospice bed will say confidentially to staff, "I know I'm dying, but my kids don't want to talk about it." How ironic and sad!

Old age and impending death can have profound impact upon a person existentially. *Who am I? What has this all been for? What comes next?* These questions are commonly asked. Belief systems at this point in life can be helpful or hindering in facing into death; in some cases, there is opportunity to do spiritual/existential work in preparation for the final transition. The internal resources the older adult has used in life for meaning and coping can play a large role in how he faces into mortality; the healthier the spiritual, psychological, and emotional resources, the smoother the process is likely to be. An exception to this may be in situations where the older adult is experiencing a dementia and the cognitive processes are hindered; but even then, some of the existential structures of the past can be accessed and utilized by family members and health care professionals to help bring comfort. Within Chapter 5 we will discuss the existential issues of dying in much greater depth. Also, an older adult's external resources—support systems—play a vital role in facing into death. Support systems within the family, as well as outside the family, such as friends and community contacts, can be significant. They can provide support, as well as infuse the dying person's journey with meaning.

We touched upon the changing older adult population in North America earlier in this chapter. As more adults live into very old age, the need for professional caregiving for the dying will become all the more vital. Hospitals, long-term care facilities, palliative home care, and hospices all play, and will continue to play, essential roles in providing care for older adults. Seniors living in larger urban centers are more likely to have access to specialized end-of-life care; unfortunately, those residing in rural areas may have less access to these services. Within Chapter 6 we will delve into the profound issues of death and dying for the older adult.

The Complexities of Transitions in Older Adulthood

Within this book, we aim not only to describe the transitions faced by older adults, but also to demonstrate how these transitions can be far more complex than those experienced in earlier years. These complexities impact not only older adults, but their family members too. Additionally, health and human service professionals may need to tailor assessments and interventions to acknowledge and address these intricacies. The following example illustrates in a brief manner why transitions can be so arduous for the older adult and her family members.

Case Example

Tina is a 75-year-old woman who is currently staying on a geriatric unit. She was brought to hospital against her will when police received a call from the manager of the apartment building where she had been residing. When the manager entered Tina's apartment, he noticed a foul smell. There were pots and pans scattered throughout the apartment that had been used as makeshift toilets. Papers were strewn all over the floor and the only food in the apartment was rotten. Tina looked disheveled with greasy hair; her clothing looked and smelled dirty. The manager informed police that while Tina's apartment was never clean, when her husband was alive he made sure that there was some semblance of sanitation and that Tina's hygiene was tended to. Sadly, however, Tina's husband passed away six months prior. As police determined that she was a hoarder and unable to safely care for herself, they brought her to hospital under the region's mental health act.

Initially, Tina spent several days in the emergency department of a hospital in a large urban center in Michigan. She was then transferred to a medical unit, but made life miserable for the staff. She swore at the nurses and threw her medications and food trays at them. The staff complained that they were not able to care for Tina, so she was then transferred to a geriatric unit.

Since being on the geriatric unit, Tina has been diagnosed with probable frontal lobe dementia and possibly some vascular dementia related to a previous small stroke. She continues to hoard papers, magazines, and food in her room. In fact, she hides food under her hospital mattress and in her clothing cupboard with soiled laundry. Her son and daughter, both in their early 50s, are extremely ambivalent about becoming involved in the care of their mother. While they care about the older woman who clearly needs help, the fear and even terror of the years spent being emotionally and physically abused have been re-evoked by being in her presence now. Although their father could act as an intermediary between the children and Tina, his death has meant that the "go-between" between them and their mother is gone.

The psychiatrist and staff are in a quandary. Tina clearly cannot care for herself and yet she seems too young and physically well for a long-term care facility. Her adult children, however, are adamant that they cannot take Tina home to live with them. The psychiatrist explains to Tina's children that although long-term care is not the best fit for Tina, this is where she will eventually be placed. However, the psychiatrist and staff know that it will take some time before they find a facility that will accept Tina.

Although Tina is a composite of older adults we have worked with, her situation illustrates some of the transitional issues faced by older adults and their family members. First, older adults often experience multiple transitions at once or within a relatively short period of time. In Tina's situation, the death of her husband may have exacerbated her hoarding tendency, and certainly, his death revealed her inability to care for herself. This then led to being taken to hospital against her will. Within the hospital, she experienced the transition of moving from the emergency room to a medical unit and then to a geriatric unit. The multiple moves within the hospital have, unfortunately, exacerbated her confusion (Detwiler, 2003) and anger.

Second, some of the physical and cognitive changes associated with illnesses in older age—such as heart attacks or dementia—represent transitions in and of themselves, but they also may trigger a new transition, such as retirement (Turcotte & Schellenberg, 2007) or placement into a long-term care facility (Alzheimer Society of Ontario, 2015). While the issue that triggered the call to police related to pungent odors wafting through the apartment hallways, Tina's inability to take care of hygiene needs and cook for herself resulted in the transition to hospital, and ultimately, to long-term care.

Third, older adults are more likely to experience widowhood than younger adults (Government of Canada, Newsletter of the National Advisory Council on Aging, 1998). In Tina's situation, her husband was a stable influence in her life. He made sure that she received proper nutrition and that she maintained some measure of hygiene. When he passed away, Tina not only lost her husband, but lost her partner who, through his efforts, allowed her to live in an independent dwelling. Six months after the transition of the death of her spouse, Tina is now residing in a hospital awaiting placement in long-term care. Hence, her move to a long-term care facility is being precipitated by the death of her husband. Like Tina, some seniors in North America are able to remain in their homes, as long as their spouses are able to compensate for their deficits by cooking, doing housework, assisting in hygiene, and providing continuous monitoring. When the spouses pass away, the functional weaknesses in individuals such as Tina are revealed and/or exacerbated, forcing transitions that are not necessarily welcomed by these older adults. The death of a spouse becomes much more than the death of a spouse; it often translates into a series of life-changing transitions.

Fourth, transitions faced by older adults may require the decision-making involvement of adult children, such as the move to long-term care or a hospice. The decision of adult children to place their parent can be extremely difficult and traumatic to make (Chang & Schneider, 2010; Noonan, Tennstedt, & Rebelsky, 1999; Silverberg, 2011). In some circumstances, such as with Tina, adult children may have great difficulty making decisions on behalf of their older parent, because that parent was abusive when the children were younger. Dealing with a parent's hospitalization and impending placement re-evokes painful childhood memories for the adult children. The current events are, in essence, retraumatizing them as they relive the memories of their childhood. Even if the relationship was not tainted by prior abuse or neglect, the decision on behalf of the children to place an older parent may negatively impact the child–parent relationship, at least temporarily (Gill & Morgan, 2011).

Fifth, when younger, some older adults may have developed and cultivated coping mechanisms, such as strenuous exercise, to decrease stress and enhance feelings of control and well-being. By the time some of these older adults reach their sixth and seventh decades, they may need to greatly curtail or adjust their level of exercise due to chronic pain and osteoarthritis (Statistics Canada, 2010b). For some older adults, the inability to utilize exercise as a coping mechanism can be a significant loss. While we do not know if Tina exercised or what coping methods she used, her husband provided some stability in her life, which may have enhanced her coping.

Finally, unhealthy coping methods in earlier years, such as the abuse of alcohol or other substances, may have more deleterious effects with advancing age. For instance, older adults may be less able to metabolize benzodiazepines (anti-anxiety medications) than in previous decades, and now may experience confusion or gait imbalances (Lilley, Harrington, Snyder, & Swart, 2011), which can lead to falls and fractured hips. Although we do not know whether Tina abused substances, or even whether she would admit to this if asked, this may not be a substantial problem for her, as she does not appear to have experienced withdrawal symptoms.

Underlying Assumptions in Working with Older Adults

As we begin to consider how health and human service professionals can work with older adults to assist them with life-changing transitions, we would like to address assumptions which underpin our discussion in the subsequent chapters. The underlying premises include:

- ▶ **Older adults are amazingly resilient, despite the multiple challenges they face.** To work effectively with older adults and their family members, health and human service professionals should adopt a strengths-oriented stance. This may involve a conscious choice on the part of professionals to view older adults as resilient, rather than as weak, full of deficits and problems (American Psychological Association, 2013). As noted by Hwang and Cowger (1998), many practitioners believe they operate out of a strengths-oriented approach, but in actuality may not.

- ▶ **Transitions in older adulthood may be more difficult to face than those in younger adulthood.** The multiplicity of health changes and illnesses that occur in advancing age, as well as the magnitude and permanence of changes (e.g., retirement, death of a spouse, death of friends), can converge to make transitions in older life extremely challenging. Not only may the older adult and family members feel befuddled as to how to make sense of the multitude of changes and which ones to address first, but health and human service professionals may also be at a loss on how to unravel the complexities of a situation.

- ▶ **Experiences with transitions in earlier life may influence how older adults manage current transitions.** This assumption is congruent with a life course perspective in which past situations and circumstances (both in terms of personal circumstances, as well as the historical context) impact how older adults face present situations. If aging adults experienced transitions in earlier life as negative or devastating, they may approach current changes with dread. Conversely, if transitions such as immigration, education, and marriage were experienced as challenging, but rewarding and even exciting, older adults may face present-day changes with greater optimism. Interestingly, older adults may not consciously tie their current dread of a transition to previous negative transitional experiences. They understand that they feel anxiety over the changes today, but they do not recognize that this fear is in part driven by traumatic transitional experiences in the past (as in the example of Mary in Chapter 1).

▶   **Illnesses, particularly those that impact physical or cognitive functioning, are transitions in and of themselves, and often lead to further transitions.** Although challenging, illnesses in adulthood often do not lead to significant changes in living locations or to changes in being able to care for self. In older adulthood, illnesses may lead to moves from home to hospital, to assisted living or long-term care facilities, or to hospices. In some cases, the move to long-term care or hospice represents a physical fracture in their primary relationship, as these older adults no longer share a bed or physical location with their partner. Even if a couple remains in the same physical locale, an illness may change the dynamic of the relationship, whereby the spousal relationship becomes a caregiver–care receiver relationship, rather than an interdependent marital partnership.

▶   **There can be a circular relationship between transitions and the responses of older adults** (Wright & Leahey, 2013). The influence of the transition(s) may lead an older adult to think, feel, and behave in certain ways, which can complicate or ameliorate the impact of the transition upon him. When the older adult perceives transitions to be devastating, he may become depressed and anxious and unable to exercise positive actions on behalf of himself. This may then exacerbate the impact of the transition. For instance, an 80-year-old man who is unable to cope with the death of his wife may become severely depressed and stop eating or caring for himself. This may cause his children to worry about his safety and question his ability to live alone. The children may then make plans for an assessment for long-term care placement, which further reinforces to the older man that life is not worth living. Thus, the circular relationship (Wright & Leahey, 2013) between this man's response to the initial transition of widowhood which precipitates further negative emotions, thinking, and actions (or inactions), and eventually leads to his children's initiation of an assessment for placement. This gentleman's response to one loss leads to other losses.

► **Transitions in older adults may influence their very sense of personhood and can lead to existential issues.** At any age, transitions can positively or negatively affect one's sense of personhood. However, the possibility of a negative impact upon personhood is greater for older adults, *due to the magnitude and sometimes permanence of transitions.* Transitions in older age often involve significant changes in functional abilities, and possibly, in areas that are quite personal and that, in the past, were associated with maturity and independence. For example, the mastery of bowel and bladder control in toddlers is typically seen as a sign of maturity. In advancing years, the loss of bowel and bladder control may be viewed as a return to a more infantile and dependent state, and hence viewed with humiliation and horror. Transitions related to changes in housing are not associated with moving to "bigger and better" like with younger adults, but rather for some aging adults, are associated with a downward progression toward dependence and death. "This is the last stop," said one older adult in response to the long-term care facility he was entering.

► **Transitions in older adults place enormous challenges upon family members.** As will be discussed throughout this book, the transitions faced by older adults result in major stressors for spouses and adult children. Not only do family members often step in to fill in the deficits in daily functioning—personal care, cooking, driving to doctors' appointments, and other such tasks—but present-day demands can re-evoke painful issues of the past. These painful issues may have occurred between parents and children, or they may have transpired between the siblings. Adult siblings, who for years communicated very little, now have to come together in some fashion for the care of aging adults. This can be positive and result in some measure of restoration of relationship, but it can also reinitiate feuds between siblings. We suggest one more point about the stressors experienced by adult children: that is, adult children may become frightened by the changes and challenges experienced by their parents. This is often the case when adult children are attending to a parent with dementia. The level of memory loss, behavioral changes, and total dependency may scare them. They understandably ask, "Will this be me in 20 years?"

Adult children may also wonder about the meaning and purpose of life, if all their years of hard work may amount to the fate of one or both of their parents: experiencing dementia, placement in long-term care, and death. They may question "the point" of their efforts now, if there may not be an experience of fulfillment, meaning, and joy at the end of their labors.

▶ **Health and human service professionals need to assess and intervene.** Professionals need to be especially astute about how the interactions of multiple transitions affect the abilities of older adults and their family members to cope. Sadly, health and human service professionals may view working with older adults as unappealing, requiring fewer clinical skills and not intellectually challenging (Happell & Brooker, 2001; Stewart, Giles, Paterson, & Butler, 2005; Swanlund & Kujath, 2012). Unwittingly, professionals have often assimilated the negative views on aging, even prior to entering work in the health care or human service sectors. We suggest that working with older adults experiencing transition requires highly sophisticated assessment and intervention skills, not just with the seniors, but also with their family members. It also requires a sensitivity toward, and willingness to discuss issues that are larger than life, and indeed, transcend the present understandings of reality. (This will be addressed further in Chapter 5.)

These underlying assumptions will be interwoven through the fabric of discussion in upcoming chapters.

Challenges for Health and Human Service Professionals

With these underlying assumptions made explicit, there are a number of challenges that health and human service professionals may encounter when assessing and intervening with older adults experiencing transitions. These challenges relate to the lack of educational preparation in Canada and the United States to work knowledgeably with older adults, the circumstances of the older adult, the inclusion of the family in working with the older adult, the personal/professional circumstances of professionals, as well as systems issues faced by those intervening on behalf of the older adult.

Lack of Undergraduate and Graduate Gerontological Content

Many nursing, social work, medicine, and psychology programs have a limited amount of gerontological content within their programs (American Psychological Association, 2013; Baumbusch & Andrusyszyn, 2002; Grocki & Fox, 2004; McCleary, McGilton, Boscart, & Oudshoorn, 2009; Roberts & Blieszner, 2007). Pathophysiology, mental health, and pharmacology are taught within the adult context, but not necessarily the *older adult context*. The underlying assumption is that disease processes and life stressors affect older adults the same way as they do younger adults. Unfortunately, this is not true. For instance, many health care professionals are not aware that older adults may have significant infections, but not register as febrile (feverish) (Smeltzer & Bare, 2004). Further, many professionals are not aware of how older adults with depression can present differently than their younger counterparts (American Psychological Association, 2013; Mood Disorders Society of Canada, n.d.).

To illustrate, approximately three decades ago, a call went forth in the nursing literature to educate nurses in gerontology in order to meet the changing demographics—the boom of the older adult population. What has been the response to this call? A study done by Hirst, Lane, and Stares (2012) regarding nurses and social workers investigated the reply, and arrived at the following two conclusions (we generally use the present tense in discussing these two conclusions, because we believe that the results still apply).

First, despite the recognition that knowledge about older adults is absolutely crucial to provide good care to our aging population, interest in and commitment to this specialty is relatively small in comparison to the need for knowledge; and there is no agreement upon how to increase student knowledge. There appears to be confusion surrounding how best to teach gerontological concepts within nursing and social work programs. There are differences in position as to whether it is best to teach gerontological content within an integrated approach (where content is assimilated into existing courses), or to offer stand-alone courses. While students may like an integrated approach, the challenge is to monitor *how much* gerontological content is being taught and *how it is* being taught. Some researchers call for a mixed approach where there are stand-alone courses and integrated content (Gebhardt, Sims, & Bates, 2009). However, the trend seems to be toward integrated curriculums. In their 2008 survey of undergraduate and graduate nursing and social work programs in Canada, Hirst and colleagues (2012) found that 79% of programs reported that gerontological content was assimilated into the curriculum.

Second, despite the attempts of nursing and social work programs to bolster gerontological content within their programs (Hirst et al., 2012), there are very few faculty members that report gerontology as their specialty and relatively few students that indicate a commitment toward working with older adults. In the above cited survey, only 2.4% of master's prepared faculty and 6% of doctorally prepared faculty had a gerontological focus. Correspondingly, only 6% of students chose a gerontological setting for their final practicum experience (Hirst et al., 2012).

How do these Canadian results compare with other countries? There are similar results from the United States. In 1996 only 3% of Master's of Social Work students identified older adults as their population of focus (Scharlach, Damron-Rodriguez, Robinson, & Feldman, 2000). In a pilot study of American nursing students, Swanlund and Kujath (2012) found that gerontology tied with psychiatry for seventh place out of a possible 10 placements to work. Placements such as pediatrics, obstetrics, intensive care, the operating room, and oncology took precedence over working with older adults. Similarly, in an Australian study, very few students

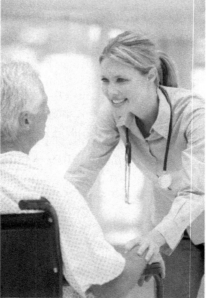

Monkey Business Images/Shutterstock, Inc.

entering nursing chose gerontology as a preferred area to work in the future. Rather, most students chose obstetrics, pediatrics, and critical care (Happell, 1999).

There are extrapolations that can be made from the lack of expertise among faculty and the lack of interest in gerontological work among students in developed countries. With few faculty members in all health and human services disciplines truly excited to work with older adults, how can programs ensure that content about older adults will be taught in an accurate and effective manner? Also, how will students become interested in this specialty? In our teaching experience, students often choose an area of specialty when they are taught and mentored by faculty who are knowledgeable and enthusiastic about an area of expertise. Once in the work environment, will these new graduates be able to find mentors that are committed to working with older adults? If these students return to graduate school, how will they find appropriate faculty supervisors if there are a limited number of professors specializing in the care of older adults?

Circumstances of Older Adults

Some aging adults experience life circumstances that complicate how they experience transitions, and thus add to the complexity of the work of health and human service professionals. Some of these life circumstances include the multiplicity of transitions that can occur concurrently or in rapid succession, the compromised mental status of some older adults, inexperience with new systems (for example, the professional trying to find placement for the older adult "stuck" on an over-crowded hospital ward until a long-term care bed becomes available; the older adult trying to cope with how to manage in that over-crowded hospital ward), the impact of transitions upon older adults' perceptions of personhood and the sense of hopelessness in some older adults.

Multiple transitions

For older adults, one transition often involves multiple transitions. As mentioned earlier, a serious illness may result in involuntary retirement or in a move to a facility, such as an assisted living facility, a lodge, or long-term care. In these situations, the first transition, that of experiencing a serious and life-changing illness, directly impacts other life circumstances, such as work or living location. Not only does the older adult need to contend with changes in his physical or cognitive status, but he also now has to cope with a change in his social contacts. If this older adult is no longer employed, not only does he lose the structure of going to work on a regular basis, he may lose collegial relationships; the context for his relationships—the work environment—is no longer available to him. Even if this man continues contact with these work colleagues, he can no longer share in the camaraderie of present-day work strategizing or gossip.

Additionally, depending upon how he defines himself as a person, he may wonder who he is in relation to others and how he can now define himself. In this situation, the professional working with this man needs to consider not just the physical illness, such as cardiac problems, but also how he is holistically impacted by retirement. Is this older adult depressed, not just because of the health problems, but because he does not know how to make use of his days in a meaningful and productive manner and is feeling isolated from others? If this is the case, the assessment of health and human service professionals will need to be more comprehensive, with interventions focused not solely on his illness. Professionals may also need to consider the impact of his health upon his marriage and social life.

The professional needs to consider if there are other transitions besides the most obvious change: are more transitions occurring—like a domino effect—because of the first one, or are unrelated transitions occurring concurrently? The professional then needs to untangle from this complex ball of yarn the transition(s) that is/are causing the greatest adjustment difficulties for the older adult, isolating the following threads: what are the adjustment challenges, how can they be addressed in the immediate, and what issues can be targeted in the long run? This may take some time as the professional may view the situation differently than the older adult.

Mental status

Another circumstance that may impact how older adults manage transitions involves mental status. If older adults experience cognitive decline related to a dementia, their ability to utilize coping strategies to process transitions will be diminished (Haase, 2010). Hence, an individual who could mentally strategize how to navigate through a difficult transition in years past, or who could restructure his thoughts (as part of cognitive restructuring) (Austin & Boyd, 2010) to reconceptualize strenuous circumstances, will no longer be able to tap into these mechanisms. In order to assist cognitively impaired older adults, health and human service professionals must expand their assessment and interventions to include family members of these individuals, as well as the environments in which they live. A key goal of professionals will be to ensure the safety of older adults who cannot singly negotiate the transition to, for example, a long-term care facility, and to support the older adult, as well as family members, in the transition; this will decrease the stress upon the older adult with dementia, as well as family members (Haase, 2010).

Inexperience with societal norms of relating

There is a small sub-population of older adults that have been incarcerated for many years. In their older years (50s and 60s), they may face a transition into the community to live in group homes or long-term care facilities (Snyder, van Wormer, Chadha, & Jaggers, 2009). These older adults may be very fearful and uncertain about the move into the community (Beckett et al., 2003). In part, they may have protected themselves within the prisons by withdrawing or becoming as inconspicuous as possible; now they may feel uncertain as to how to relate to others within mainstream society. There are other aspects that can complicate the transition for these older adults. Receiving facilities within long-term care may be very reluctant to accept someone who has been imprisoned for many years (Beckett et al., 2003). Also, family members who could offer support in the transition to a group home or long-term care facility may no longer be accessible; family members may have abandoned the relationship with the incarcerated member years before (Snyder et al., 2009). Finally, older adults who have been incarcerated for years often have significant health problems at a much earlier age than individuals in the general population. Thus, they may have mental health issues, such as depression, as well as substantial physical health issues, which may hinder their ability to form relationships with others and adjust in the new setting.

Responding to the impact of transitions upon sense of personhood

As has been mentioned, in older age, transitions can significantly impact how older adults view themselves—their sense of personhood. Personhood can be defined as "the state or condition of being a person" (Free Online Dictionary, 2015). This definition, however, does not reflect the intangible aspects of personhood, such as identity, self-expression, and decision-making (Hirst, Lane, & Reed, 2013). Older adults who can no longer bathe on their own or dress themselves may feel a deep sense of shame. ("This has got to be the worst day of my life!" exclaimed a woman who, due to her disease process, had lost control of her bowels for the first time.) They may feel that they have become burdens and have little to offer to their families or society. An important aspect of working with these individuals is to encourage them to do whatever they can do for themselves, rather than quickly taking over the acts of dressing or bathing. Also, health and human service professionals need to look for areas of strength in these older adults and verbally acknowledge these strengths to them.

As another example, moving to a long-term care facility can be traumatic for older adults, as who they were in the past may not be recognized by staff; instead, staff may view them as decrepit and dependent. Staff members need to make a conscious effort to understand who their residents were in the past, and who they are today (Greenfield, 1984); there is more to the older adult than their physiological challenges! This knowledge can help staff tailor activities to the interests and abilities of individual residents. Also, independent homes or apartments are often viewed by older adults as a reflection of their personhood—their walls, shelves, and cabinets display pictures and items that reflect who they are and what they enjoy. Staff may need to encourage older adults and family members to bring cherished items from home that reflect the personhood of the older adults and that help them feel more "at home" within their new residence (Cook, 2010).

Hopelessness: How do you instill hope?

In my work in geriatric mental health (AML), one of the most difficult aspects of the work involved the instillation of hope, or perhaps the *reinstallation* of hope (Bergin & Walsh, 2005). Hope is absolutely critical, not only to quality of life, but to life itself. Individuals who experience great degrees of hopelessness are at greater risk for suicide (Uncapher, Gallagher-Thompson, Osgood, & Bongar, 1998). Even if individuals do not commit suicide, a loss of hope can be associated with illness and death. For example, within concentration camps in World War II, individuals who lost hope were prone to suffer illness and die more quickly than those who held steadfastly to hope (Fink, 2000, p. 391).

When older adults have lost so much to declining functional abilities, illness, and the deaths of loved ones, how do health and human service professionals help them rediscover meaning, hope, and purpose in their lives? This is especially problematic when individuals' sources of hope are found in the "here and now," and are not partially rooted in an afterlife or in spiritual beliefs. It can also be difficult when the hopeless older adult is cognitively impaired and cannot participate in cognitive therapy to re-engage with life (Cutcliffe & Grant, 2001), or finds himself in difficult circumstances, such as the incarcerated older adult (Duggleby, 2005).

For health and human service professionals, the struggle with hopelessness of older adults can impact their own sense of personhood. Despair can result. These professionals may wrestle greatly with how to bring purpose to their patients' lives, or help them reconnect with purpose. They may try to avoid speaking of issues of meaning. In health care settings where there is an interprofessional staff, these duties can be delegated. Spiritual care and social work referrals are common. For the home care nurse, she often wears more than one hat in her role; how can she bring hope to elderly patients who are struggling? Beyond the despair of not being able to help her patients/clients, existential questions of the professional may be evoked and re-evoked. Some professionals leave the specialty within their field for this reason. More than one hospice nurse or chaplain has left that arena because the issues of their patients hit too close to home. The need for professionals to do their own spiritual work will be explored in Chapter 5.

Assessment Needs to Include Family Members, as Well as Older Adults

While a family approach to working with older adults in transition is imperative when there is cognitive impairment, as a basic tenet for professional practice, family members should be included, irrespective of the older adult's status. Family inclusion in assessment and intervention will allow the health or human service professional to understand the older adult within the context of her family (Wright & Leahey, 2013) and will also open up other possibilities for intervention—that is, with family members. While some professionals avoid family contact because of the amount of time it takes to interact with relatives, intervening with family members may consume more time in the immediate but *circumvent problems in the long run*; in the end this may save countless hours on the part of members of the health care team (Wright & Leahey, 2013).

Although including the family can bolster the support that relatives offer to older adults who are experiencing transitions, it can also unveil longstanding family issues (such as physical abuse or substance abuse) that impact how relatives are responding to and coping with the older adult's transition. This difficult circumstance was previously illustrated in the story about Tina. Issues from the past may also result in a stalemate between individuals within the family, whereby family members cannot come to an agreement on a plan of action for their elderly member and are vehemently opposed to working with each other. Professionals may become frustrated and even angry, as a family decision-making stalemate can result in a lengthier hospital stay for the older adult, and in effect, block a hospital bed from another older adult who needs to be admitted. These situations will be explored at greater length in Chapter 7.

The Challenges of Working on an Interprofessional Team

In a number of settings where professionals work with older adults, they function as part of an interprofessional team. This team may consist of a physician or psychiatrist, nurses, one or more social workers, an occupational and recreational therapist, a psychologist, and a chaplain. The benefit of such a team is that professionals assess different aspects of functioning in their older clients (Dyer et al., 2003). For instance, a physician or psychiatrist, as well as nurses, may assess the mental and physical functioning of an older adult. Social workers may assess the family situation, as well as explore discharge options; a chaplain may conduct a spiritual assessment. Further, there is often overlap in what the professionals assess. This provides for a rich texture of clinical opinions and options in terms of how the team can help their elderly client.

However, differing opinions on the interprofessional team may result in heated arguments about how the care of the client should be approached. In these situations, not only may professionals have differing life experiences that cause them to arrive at varied conclusions, but their professional discourses may influence their judgments. For instance, a prominent disciplinary discourse in nursing is that of safety; safety of the patient should be promoted at all costs (Lane, 2007). However, social work, as a profession, strongly promotes self-determination. In our experience, differences in disciplinary discourse can result in nurses and social workers, as well as other professionals, taking opposing sides in the decision to place an older adult in a long-term care facility. Nurses may argue for safety, while social workers may argue for self-determination, and therefore, a less restrictive environment for the client (Lane, 2007). Neither profession is wrong; they simply advocate for their older adults differently, depending upon the underlying tenets of their profession. Thus, members of interprofessional teams need to present their arguments to each other with maturity and respect, solid communication skills (Dyer et al., 2003; Junger, Pestinger, Elsner, Krumm, & Radbruch, 2007), and an understanding of each other's professional discourses (Lane, Waegemakers Schiff, Suter, & Marlett, 2010).

The Clashing of Professional and Personal Experiences

Health and human service professionals working with older adults bring into their work not just their professional experiences, but also their personal experiences. This can be very positive. Previous experiences with older adults, such as grandparents, may enhance the opinions of professionals toward older adults (Wesley, 2005). In our experience, some professionals working in gerontology specifically chose to work with older adults because of fondness toward and respect for older family members. However, there can also be a downside. When professionals have experienced personally traumatic experiences and a professional situation in some way mirrors those previous experiences, professionals can feel traumatized. For instance, caring for an older woman who is an alcoholic may trigger frightening memories of being raised by an alcoholic mother. In our experience, we have seen professionals weep over work situations that have triggered personal memories. Also, a current professional experience may trigger emotional responses from previous professional experiences; for example, working with an aggressive older adult in the present may re-evoke feelings of fear, even terror, because that situation resembles one in the past that caused the professional pain (Scott, Ryan, James, & Mitchell, 2011). Health and human service professionals working with older adults need to be mindful of how work experiences affect them professionally and personally.

Another issue related to the clash between personal and professional experiences involves compassion fatigue. Compassion fatigue refers to physical and psychological fatigue caused by extreme professional demands that sap the resources and reserves of professionals. It can result in professionals experiencing lowered levels of concern for patients or clients, exhaustion, lowered job satisfaction, and increased absenteeism (Leon, Altholz, & Dziegielewski, 1999). Within acute care settings, compassion fatigue is normally associated with professionals working in the emergency department (e.g., Hooper, Craig, Janvrin, Wetsel, & Reimels, 2010), critical care (e.g., Jenkins & Warren, 2012) or oncology (e.g., Aycock & Boyle, 2009); however, those working with older adults may also experience this.

There are a number of reasons why professionals may experience compassion fatigue in working with older adults. First, in working with older individuals, professionals may come face-to-face with their own fears about aging and death. These fears may especially be triggered if the professional is currently helping aging parents or family members. Second, depending upon the situation (hospital versus community, city versus rural), services for older adults may be relatively sparse, increasing the load upon the professionals that are working with these elderly folk. Third, as discussed earlier, older adults often have multiple illnesses and issues and dealing with the complexity of the situations may be physically and mentally exhausting for professionals (Leon et al., 1999).

Not only can helping aging parents trigger personal fears and issues regarding aging and death in health and human service professionals, the *actual physical work of caring for aging parents* can contribute to the physical and psychological exhaustion already experienced at work (Ward-Griffin, St-Amant, & Brown, 2011). Ward-Griffin and colleagues (2011) conducted a qualitative analysis of two previous studies of nurse–daughter caregivers.[5] In analyzing the data of 20 Canadian registered nurses who were also caring for aging relatives, they found that these women were at risk for compassion fatigue. Because of the context of being both daughters and nurses, there was a blurring of personal and professional boundaries. Further, the limited personal and professional resources of the nurses, combined with increasing expectations by health care providers on them to provide care to their aging family members, resulted in great burden upon these nurses (Ward-Griffin et al., 2011).

There is perhaps one more reason why health and human service professionals may experience compassion fatigue in working with older adults. Eric Gentry, an American psychotherapist suggested:

People who are attracted to caregiving often enter the field already compassion fatigued. They come from a tradition where they are taught to care for the needs of others before caring for themselves.
(ISNA Bulletin, 2012, p. 5, italics ours)

We agree wholeheartedly. Often individuals entering caring professions have already filled caring and caregiving roles within their families, churches, and communities. While their previous experiences can be beneficial, in that they bring insight and compassion, they can also be problematic. Some of these individuals may already be tired from years

---

5. In this specific study, all the nurses were female, hence the nurse–daughter categorization. It is noteworthy that just as the majority of nurses are female, so are the majority of caregivers!

of providing care to ailing family members. When they begin working as nurses, social workers, psychologists, and so on, they may find themselves intensely fatigued and not realize why (as some degree of compassion fatigue is their "norm"); they now have caregiving roles in their professions as well as within their families and communities. Occasionally, professions involving caregiving will attract individuals who experience great mental distress and who only feel acceptable when they give of themselves extensively and to their own detriment. When these individuals face compassion fatigue or great challenges in their work situations, they may undergo major existential and mental health crises.

Systems Issues

There are "systems issues" that can complicate the work of professionals on behalf of older adults. By using the term *systems issues*, we refer to the structure or processes within health care systems that make the work of professionals challenging. One such structural issue relates to the relatively few readily available options for older adults if they are not able to function independently within their homes. [6] Often, particularly if the older adult is currently in hospital and placement needs to occur quickly, the choices available boil down to long-term care or assisted living facilities. Assisted living facilities are often upscale and can be expensive, and some older adults do not have the financial resources to afford this option. Further, if older adults are experiencing mental illness that impacts how they dress and relate to others, staff in assisted living facilities may be reluctant to allow them entrance. And yet, these same individuals, if healthy physically, may not meet the necessary requirements for entrance into long-term care facilities (Lane, 2011; Lane, McCoy, & Ewashen, 2010). Thus, like in the case of Tina, professionals are in a quandary to find suitable placement options. Their older clients do not fit comfortably in any of the facilities that are available.

Another systems issue relates to the extreme acuity of patients in acute care environments and heavy workloads for health and human service professionals (Vander Zyl, 2002). High patient acuity coupled with weighty workloads results in professionals having less time than they

---

6. There are certainly more options available than assisted living and long-term care facilities. However, other options, such as low-cost seniors' complexes or lodges, may have long wait lists. Thus, for elderly individuals who are on a hospital unit awaiting placement, the major options include assisted living or long-term care facilities. This will be discussed in further detail in Chapter 4.

otherwise would for older individuals who may need extra time for bathing, dressing, eating, and talking. The older adult who might need more time to reflect, answer questions, and make connections between past life events and current situations may not be given the time that he needs, not because of indifference on the part of the professional, but due to the extreme demands on the professional's time. The professional who enters a caring profession to respond to the suffering of individuals may become disillusioned at not being able to provide the care that she feels is required. This may lead to compassion fatigue (as mentioned above) and can actually become a spiritual crisis for the professional. The professional is no longer able to find meaning and purpose in work (Vander Zyl, 2002) and may wonder what she should do next for employment, as well as for deriving meaning in her life.

SUMMARY

Within this chapter we presented an overview of the transitional challenges faced by older adults, as well as the demographic changes within North America that complicate how older adults experience these challenges. We offered the assumptions upon which we predicate our discussion about transitions in older adults. Finally, we briefly touched upon challenges that health and human service professionals may face in working with older adults experiencing transitions.

While "old age is not for sissies" (Bette Davis), neither is working with older adults! We suggest, however, that the impact upon these elderly patients, and the meaning for professionals working with them, can be profound. Within the next chapter, we address illnesses as transitions in older adults.

CRITICAL THINKING EXERCISES

► As you reflect on the various transitions experienced by older adults, what transition do you most fear? Why? How will you address this fear so that it does not impact the effectiveness of your work with older adults?

▶ As you consider how your work with older adults is shaped by your professional education, what disciplinary discourses guide your approach? How do you describe your professional decision-making with members of the interprofessional team who are influenced by other disciplinary discourses?

INTERESTING WEBSITES

▶ American Association of Retired Persons: http://www.aarp.org/

▶ Canadian Association of Retired Persons: http://www.carp.ca/

▶ Centers for Disease Control—Aging: http://www.cdc.gov/aging/

▶ National Institute for the Care of the Elderly (NICE)—Older adults and substance use: http://www.nicenet.ca/tools-introduction-to-older-adults-and-substance-use

REFERENCES

Alzheimer Society of Ontario. (2015). Caring for someone—long term care. Retrieved February 14, 2015, from: http://www.alzheimer.ca/en/Living-with-dementia/Caring-for-someone

Alzheimer's Association. (2014). Alzheimer's disease facts and figures. *Alzheimer's & Dementia, 10*(2). Retrieved February 10, 2015, from: https://www.google.ca/webhp?sourceid=chrome-instant&ion=1&espv=2&ie=UTF-8#q=2014%20alzheimer's%20disease%20facts%20and%20figures

American Psychological Association. (2013). Guidelines for psychological practice with older adults. Retrieved December 20, 2014, from: www.apa.org/practice/guidelines/older-adults.pdf

Austin, W., & Boyd, M. A. (2010). *Psychiatric & mental health nursing for Canadian practice* (2nd ed.). Philadelphia: Lippincott Williams & Wilkins.

Aycock, N., & Boyle, D. (2009). Interventions to manage compassion fatigue in oncology nursing. *Clinical Journal of Oncology Nursing, 13*(2), 183–191. doi:10.1188/09.CJON.183-191

Baumbusch, J. L., & Andrusyszyn, M. (2002). Gerontological content in Canadian baccalaureate nursing programs: Cause for concern? *Canadian Journal of Nursing Research, 34*(1), 119–129.

Beckett, J., Peternelj-Taylor, C., & Johnson, R. L. (2003). Growing old in the correctional system. *Journal of Psychosocial Nursing & Mental Health Services, 41*(9), 12–18.

Bergin, L., & Walsh, S. (2005). The role of hope in psychotherapy with older adults. *Aging & Mental Health, 9*(1), 7–15. doi:10.1080/13607860412331323809

BrainyQuote.com. Retrieved March 20, 2015, from: www.brainyquote.com/quotes/quotes/b/bettedavis126805.html

Buhr, G. T., Kuchibhatla, M., & Clipp, E. C. (2006). Caregivers' reasons for nursing home placement: Clues for improving discussions with families prior to the transition. *The Gerontologist, 46*(1), 52–61.

Caple, C., & Schub, T. (2012). Aborginal population, Australia: Providing culturally competent care. *CINAHL, January 06*, 1–4.

Centers for Disease Control and Prevention. (2014). Meeting the challenge of living well at a glance 2014—Arthritis. Retrieved February 9, 2015, from: http://www.cdc.gov/chronicdisease/resources/publications/aag/arthritis.htm

Chang, Y. P., & Schneider, J. K. (2010). Decision-making process of nursing home placement among Chinese family caregivers. *Perspectives in Psychiatric Care, 46*(2), 108–118. doi:10.1111/j.1744-6163.2010.00246.x

CIA—The World Factbook. (n.d.). Total fertility rate—country comparison. Retrieved October 10, 2014, from: https://www.cia.gov/library/publications/the-world-factbook/geos/xx.html

Cohn, D., Livingston, G., & Wang, W. (2014). After decades of decline, a rise in stay-at-home mothers. Washington, DC: Pew Research Center's Social & Demographics Project.

Cook, G. (2010). Ensuring older residents retain their unique identity. *Nursing & Residential Care, 12*(6), 290–293.

Cutcliffe, J. R., & Grant, G. (2001). What are the principles and processes of inspiring hope in cognitively impaired older adults within a continuing care environment? *Journal of Psychiatric and Mental Health Nursing, 8*(7), 427–436. doi:10.1046/j.1365-2850.2001.00399.x

Damianakis, T., & Marziali, E. (2012). Older adults' response to the loss of a spouse: The function of spirituality in understanding the grieving process. *Aging & Mental Health, 16*(1), 57–66. http://dx.doi.org/10.1080/13607863.2011.609531

Dautzenberg, M. G., Diederiks, J. P., Philipsen, H., & Stevens, F. C. (1998). Women of a middle generation and parent care. *International Journal of Aging and Human Development, 47*(4), 241–262.

Davies, S. (2005). Meleis' theory of nursing transitions and relatives' experiences of nursing home entry. *Journal of Advanced Nursing, 52*(6), 658–671. doi:10.1111/j.1365-2648.2005.03637.x

Detwiler, C. (2003). The client with a cognitive disorder. In W. K. Mohr (Ed.), *Johnson's psychiatric-mental health nursing* (5th ed.; pp. 607–640). Philadelphia: Lippinicott Williams & Wilkins.

Duggleby, W. (2005). Fostering hope in incarcerated older adult. *Journal of Psychosocial Nursing & Mental Health Services, 43*(9), 15–20.

Dyer, C. B., Hyer, K., Feldt, K. S., Lindemann, D. A., Busby-Whitehead, J., Greenberg, S., Kennedy, R. D., et al. (2003). Frail older patient care by interdisciplinary teams: A primer for generalists. *Gerontology & Geriatrics Education, 24*(2), 51–62. doi:10.1300/J021v24n02_05

Fink, G. (2000). *Encyclopedia of stress*. San Diego, CA: Academic Press.

Free Online Dictionary. (2015). Retrieved February 9, 2015, from: www.thefreedictionary.com

Furlotte, C., Schwartz, K., Koornstra, J. J. & Naster, R. (2012). "Got a room for me?" Housing experiences of older adults living with HIV/AIDS in Ottawa. *Canadian Journal on Aging, 31*(1), 37–48. doi:10.1353.cja.2012.0003

Gaede, B. A. (2010). What will I do next? Discerning God's callings for retirement. *Journal of Religion, Spirituality & Aging, 22*(1–2), 27–40. doi:10.1080/15528030903313847

Gebhardt, M. C., Sims, T. T., & Bates, T. A. (2009). Enhancing geriatric content in a baccalaureate nursing program. *Nursing Education Perspectives, 30*(4), 245–248.

George, M. V., Loh, S., Verma, R. B., & Shin, Y. E. (2001). *Population projections for Canada, provinces and territories, 2000–2026*. Ottawa: Statistics Canada.

Gibson, J. (2012). How cognitive behaviour therapy can alleviate older people's grief. *Mental Health Practice, 15*(6), 12–17.

Gill, E. A., & Morgan, M. (2011). Home sweet home: Conceptualizing and coping with the challenges of aging and moving to a care facility. *Health Communication, 26*(4), 332–342. doi:10.1080/10410236.2010.551579

Gillsjo, C., & Schwartz-Barcott, D. (2011). A concept analysis of home and its meaning in the lives of three older adults. *International Journal of Older People Nursing, 6*(1), 4–12. doi:10.1111/j.1748-3743.2010.00207.x

Government of Canada, Newsletter of the National Advisory Council on Aging. (1998). Bereavement: A life passage. *Expression, 12,* 1–8.

Greenfield, W. L. (1984). Disruption and reintegration: Dealing with familial response to nursing home placement. *Journal of Gerontological Social Work, 8*(1/2), 15–21.

Grocki, J. H., & Fox, G. E. (2004). Gerontology coursework in undergraduate nursing programs in the United States: A regional study. *Journal of Gerontological Nursing, 30*(3), 46–51.

Grose, S., & Pravikoff, D. (2012). Aboriginal people living in Canada: Providing culturally competent care. *CINAHL Nursing Guide, June 22,* 1–7.

Haase, M. (2010). Delirium, dementias, and other related disorders. In W. Austin and M. A. Boyd (Eds.), *Psychiatric & mental health nursing for Canadian practice* (2nd ed.; pp. 750–789). Philadelphia: Lippincott Williams & Wilkins.

Happell, B. (1999). When I grow up I want to be a . . .? Where undergraduate student nurses want to work after graduation. *Journal of Advanced Nursing, 29*(2), 499–505. doi:10.1046/j.1365-2648.1999.00913.x

Happell, B., & Brooker, J. (2001). Who will look after my grandmother? Attitudes of student nurses towards the care of older adults. *Journal of Gerontological Nursing, 27*(12), 12–17.

Hardy, M. A., & Quadagno, J. (1995). Satisfaction with early retirement: Making choices in the auto industry. *Journal of Gerontology: Social Sciences, 50B*(4), S217–228. doi:10.1093/geronb/50B.4.2217

Hart, A. D. (2001). *Unmasking male depression.* Nashville, TN: Thomas Nelson.

Hirst, S. P. (1990). Psychogeriatrics: What's in a name? *Perspectives, 14*(3), 10–12.

Hirst, S. P., Lane, A. M., & Reed, M. B. (2013). Personhood in nursing homes: Results of an ethnographic study. *Indian Journal of Gerontology, 27*(1), 38–54.

Hirst, S. P., Lane, A. M., & Seneviratne, C. C. (2013). Growing old with a developmental disability. *Indian Journal of Gerontology, 27*(1), 69–87.

Hirst, S. P., Lane, A. M., & Stares, B. (2012). Gerontological content in Canadian nursing and social work programs. *Canadian Geriatrics Journal, 15*, 8–15. doi:http://dx.doi.org/10. 5770/cgj.15.21

Holmes, T. H., & Rahe, R. H. (1967). The social readjustment rating scale. *Journal of Psychosomatic Research, 11*, 213–218.

Hooper, C., Craig, J., Janvrin, D. R., Wetsel, M. A., & Reimels, E. (2010). Compassion satisfaction, burnout, and compassion fatigue among emergency nurses compared with nurses in other selected inpatient specialties. *Journal of Emergency Nursing, 36*(5), 420–427. doi:10.1016/j.jen.2009.11.027

Hwang, S. C., & Cowger, C. D. (1998). Utilizing strengths in assessment. *Families in Society, 79* (1), 25–31. doi:10.1606/1044-3894.1797

Indiana State Nurses Association (ISNA). (2012). "I've fallen and I can't get up": Compassion fatigue in nurses and non-professional caregivers. *ISNA Bulletin, 38*(3), 5–12.

Jacobsen, L. A., Kent, M., Lee, M., & Mather, M. (2011). America's aging population. *Population Bulletin, 66*(1). Washington, DC: Population Reference Bureau.

Jenkins, B., & Warren, N. (2012). Concept analysis: Compassion fatigue and effects upon critical care nurses. *Critical Care Nursing Quarterly, 35*(4), 388–395. doi:10.1097/CNQ.0b13e318268fe09

Junger, S., Pestinger, M., Elsner, F., Krumm, N., & Radbruch, L. (2007). Criteria for successful multiprofessional cooperation in palliative care teams. *Palliative Medicine, 21*(4), 347–354. doi:10.1177/0269216307078505

Jutras, S. (1988). Formal and informal caregivers: Towards a partnership in prevention. *Health Promotion,* (Fall), 9–12.

Kao, H. F., Travis, S. S., & Acton, G. J. (2004). Relocation to a long-term care facility: Working with patients and families before, during and after. *Journal of Psychosocial Nursing & Mental Health, 42*(3), 10–16.

Kind, V. (2010). *The caregiver's path to compassionate decision making: Making choices for those who can't.* Austin, TX: Greenleaf.

Lane, A. M. (2007). *The social organization of geriatric mental health.* Unpublished doctoral thesis. University of Calgary.

Lane, A. M. (2011). Placement of older adults from hospital mental health units into nursing homes: Exploration of the process, systems issues and implications. *Journal of Gerontological Nursing, 37*(2), 49–55.

Lane, A. M., Hirst, S. P., & Reed, M. B. (2013). Housing options for North American older adults with HIV/AIDS. *Indian Journal of Gerontology, 27*(1), 55–68.

Lane, A. M., McCoy, L., & Ewashen, C. (2010). The textual organization of placement into long term care: Issues for older adults with mental illness. *Nursing Inquiry, 17* (1), 3–14. doi:10.1111/j.1440-1800.2009.00470.x

Lane, A. M., Waegemakers Schiff, J., Suter, E., & Marlett, N. (2010). A critical look at participation of persons with mental health problems in training mental health professionals within university education. *CURRENTS, 9*(2), 1–18.

Leon, A. M., Altholz, J. A., & Dziegielewski, S. F. (1999). Compassion fatigue: Considerations for work with the elderly. *Journal of Gerontological Social Work, 32*(1), 32–62.

Lilley, L., Harrington, S., Snyder, J. S., & Swart, B. (2011). *Pharmacology for Canadian health care practice* (2nd ed.). Toronto, ON: Elsevier Canada.

McCleary, L., McGilton, K., Boscart, V., & Oudshoorn, A. (2009). Improving gerontology content in baccalaureate nursing education through knowledge transfer to nurse educators. *Canadian Journal of Nursing Leadership, 22*(3), 33–46.

Miller, D. (1981). The 'sandwich' generation: Adult children of the aging. *Social Work, 26*, 419–423. Mood Disorders Society of Canada (n.d.). Depression in elderly: Getting old in our society is depressing, right? Retrieved February 9, 2015, from: http://www.mooddisorderscanada.ca/documents/Consumer%20and%20Family%20Support/Depression%20in%20Elderly%20edited%20Dec16%202010.pdf

National Institute on Health (NIH). (2011). Global health and aging. *NIH Publication no. 11-7737, October.* Retrieved February 10, 2015, from: http://www.nia.nih.gov/sites/default/files/global_health_and_aging.pdf

Newson, P. (2008). Relocation to a care home, part one: Exploring reactions. *Nursing & Residential Care, 10*(7), 321–324.

Noonan, A. E., Tennstedt, S. L., & Rebelsky, F. G. (1999). Getting to the point: Offspring caregivers and the nursing home decision. *Journal of Gerontological Social Work, 31*(3-4), 5–27. doi:10.1300/J083v31n03_02

Nuttman-Shwartz, O. (2004). Like a high wave: Adjustment to retirement. *The Gerontologist, 44*(2), 229–236. doi:10.1093/geront/44.2.229

Plank, A., Mazzoni, V., & Cavada, L. (2012). Becoming a caregiver: New family carers' experience during the transition from hospital to home. *Journal of Clinical Nursing, 21* (13/14), 2072–2082. doi:10.1111/j.1365-2702.2011.04025.x

Rando, T. (1984). *Grief, death and dying: Clinical interventions for caregivers.* Champaign, IL: Research Press Company.

Reitzes, D. C., & Mutran, E. J. (2006). Lingering identities in retirement. *The Sociological Quarterly, 47*(2), 333–359.

Roberts, J., & Blieszner, R. (2007). Infusion of gerontology content: An ethical imperative. *The Journal of Baccalaureate Social Work, 12*(2), 129–140.

Rosenberg, M. (2009). *Total fertility rate impacts a country's population. About. Com Guide, April 12*. Retrieved February 10, 2015, from: http://geography. about.com/od/populationgeography/a/fertilityrate.htm

Scharlach, A., Damron-Rodriguez, J., Robinson, B., & Feldman, R. (2000). Educating social workers for an aging society: A vision for the 21st century. *Journal of Social Work Education, 36*(3), 521–538.

Scott, A., Ryan, A., James, I. A., & Mitchell, E. A. (2011). Psychological trauma and fear for personal safety as a result of behaviors that challenge in dementia: The experiences of healthcare workers. *Dementia, 10*(2), 257–269. doi:10.1177/1471301211407807

Silverberg, E. (2011). Applying the 3-A grief intervention approach to nursing home placement. *Canadian Nursing Homes, 22*, 22–25.

Smeltzer, S. C., & Bare, B. G. (2004). *Textbook of medical-surgical nursing.* Philadelphia: Lippincott Williams & Wilkins.

Snyder, C., van Wormer, K., Chadha, J., & Jaggers, J. W. (2009). Older adult inmates: The challenge for social work. *Social Work, 54*(2), 117–124.

Statistics Canada. (2008). Census snapshot of Canada—Population (age and sex). Statistics Canada—Catalogue No. 11-008.

Statistics Canada. (2010a). Women in Canada: Paid work. Retrieved February 10, 2015, from: www.statcan.gc.ca/daily-quotidien/101209/dq101209a-eng.htm

Statistics Canada. (2010b). Pain or discomfort that prevents activities. Statistics Canada—82-229-X.

Statistics Canada (2014). Canada's population estimates: Age and sex. Retrieved February 10, 2015, from: http://www.statcan.gc.ca/daily-quotidien/140926/ dq140926b-eng.htm

Sterns, H. L., & Dawson, N. T. (2012). Emerging perspectives on resilience in adulthood and later life: Work, retirement, and resilience. *Annual Review of Gerontology and Geriatrics,32*(1), 211–230. http://dx.doi.org/10.1891/0198-8794.32.211

Stewart, J. J. Giles, L., Paterson, J. E., & Butler, S. J. (2005). Knowledge and attitudes towards older people: New Zealand students entering health professional degrees. *Physical & Occupational Therapy in Geriatrics, 23*(4), 25–36. doi:10.1300/J148v23n04_02

Swanlund, S., & Kujath, A. (2012). Attitudes of baccalaureate nursing students towards older adults: A pilot study. *Nursing Education Perspectives, 33*(3), 181–183.

Turcotte, M., & Schellenberg, G. (2007). *A portrait of seniors in Canada.* Statistics Canada. Catalogue no. 89-519.

Uncapher, H., Gallagher-Thompson, D., Osgood, N. J., & Bongar, B. (1998). Hopelessness and suicidal ideation in older adults. *The Gerontologist, 38*(1), 62–70. doi:10.1093/geront/38.1.62

Vander Zyl, S. (2002). Compassion fatigue and spirituality. *Nursing Matters, 13*(12), 4–14.

Walsh, F. (1989). The family in later life. In B. Carter and M. McGoldrick (Eds.), *The changing family life cycle: A framework for family therapy* (pp. 311–332). Toronto: Allyn & Bacon.

Ward-Griffin, C., St-Amant, O., & Brown, J. (2011). Compassion fatigue within double duty caregiving: Nurse-daughters caring for elderly parents. *Online Journal of Issues in Nursing, 16*(1), 1–21. doi:10.3912/OJIN.Vol16No01Man04

Wesley, S. C. (2005). Enticing students to careers in gerontology. *Gerontology & Geriatrics Education, 25*(3), 13–29. http://dx.doi.org/10.1300/J021v25n03_02

Working Together for Seniors. (November 2007). Working Together for Seniors—Federal/Provincial/Territorial Ministers Responsible for Seniors. Retrieved February 10, 2015, from: http://www.hss.gov.yk.ca/pdf/working_together.pdf

Wright, L. M., & Leahey, M. (2013). *Nurses and families: A guide to family assessment and intervention* (6th ed.). Philadelphia: F. A. Davis.

CHAPTER 3

HEALTH TRANSITIONS IN OLDER ADULTS

For age is opportunity no less
Than youth itself, though another dress
And as the evening twilight fades away
The sky is filled with stars, invisible by day.

(Henry Wadsworth Longfellow, American poet and professor)

Reflective Questions

► What are some of the physical, mental, and cognitive changes that older adults may experience?

► How do transitions in health affect the functional abilities, social abilities, and social contact with others?

► How should health and human service professionals assess and intervene with older adults experiencing health transitions?

The quote of American poet and professor Henry Wadsworth Longfellow expressed an important truth about advancing age. Although changes occur in later years, these changes can be meaningful and full of opportunity. That being said, older adults may face more transitional challenges in trying to keep life purposeful and rich. While many adults enter the older life stage in good health, significant numbers of older adults will experience some health problems as they enter their 70s and 80s. Depending upon the nature of the health issues, as well as the degree of disability that comes from these challenges, older adults may face other transitions related to the health concerns, such as moves from personal homes into assisted living or long-term care facilities. The compounding nature of the transitions can result in profound stress for older adults and demands significant resilience and adaptability on their part. If older adults do not possess this hardiness or adaptability due to extreme health conditions, such as dementia, then added responsibility is placed upon family members and professionals to support them in their health transitions.

Within this chapter we discuss some of the health challenges faced by older adults, such as physical illnesses, chronic illness and pain, addictions, mental illness, and dementias. We propose that life transitions, such as the loss of a spouse, can lead to illness in older adults, such as depression. However, we also suggest that illnesses, *in and of themselves*, are transitions for older adults; the ability of seniors to manage day-to-day functioning can decrease significantly and may even lead to other transitions, such as a move to a hospital, assisted living, or long-term care facility. While we document the prevalence of various illnesses, as well as symptoms, our purpose in doing so is to emphasize the *complexity of the emotional responses to the transition of illness* in older adults. Additionally, we address how health and human service professionals may assess and intervene with older adults experiencing significant issues in health.

Physical Illness: Chronic

Chronic illness or conditions refer to "long-term diseases that develop slowly over time, often progressing in severity, and can often be controlled, but rarely cured" (Ministry of Health and Long-Term Care, 2007). Common chronic illnesses in older adults include some forms of heart disease, cancer, diabetes, and arthritis. Other common illnesses such as strokes (cerebrovascular accidents) are acute in that they occur suddenly, but after the initial event, the changes incurred generally become constant or chronic. The impact of chronic illness in the United States and Canada, as well as worldwide, is astronomical. Chronic illnesses (also called noncommunicable diseases) are a significant cause of death and disability throughout the world, including North America; for instance, according to the World Health Organization (2014), 88% of deaths in North America are caused by chronic illness.

The presence of chronic illness can restrict the activities that older adults can take part in. Chronic illnesses may also lead to involuntary retirement in older adults; that is, some older adults need to retire because of health issues, rather than by choice. If the senior enjoyed work, cherished the camaraderie with colleagues, and appreciated the purpose and structure work gave, retirement can be a major loss (Smith, 2012). Not only can the cessation of work represent a loss for the older adult, finding an alternate purposeful and enjoyable replacement may be difficult due to the limitations caused by the illness. Lack of purpose in life results in an existential crisis (Frankl, 2006). The older adult may question, "What good is my life anymore?" He may live with chronic sorrow related to coping with the chasm between who he once was and who he is presently (Weingarten, 2012). And perhaps that chronic sorrow is also tied to the fear of who he will become. When chronic illness causes some sort of physical disability, for example, difficulties negotiating stairs due to cardiac problems or arthritis, then a move may be necessary. Older adults may move to a retirement community, a seniors' complex, or an assisted living facility. While some older adults find that they enjoy the newfound companionship that comes with living in an assisted living facility or a seniors' complex, others grieve the loss of their home (Pickersgill, 2001). They grieve because home represents much more than physical structure or a place to sleep. For some older adults, a lifetime of memories is ensconced within the walls of the home; the home is where they raised their families, cooked and entertained, cared for ailing parents, and dreamed of the future. Beyond a lifetime of memories, their homes have represented security and may also symbolize freedom and independence. Moving out of the home may be viewed as the first step down a slippery slope toward total dependence and mortality (Gill & Morgan, 2011). And, as will be discussed in Chapter 4, the concept of "home" represents more than simply a physical structure within which to sleep; it possesses a somewhat ethereal quality.

The previous section offered some common problems associated with chronic illness. In the following section, we will provide some statistics and specifically address what it is like for older adults to live with heart disease, strokes, diabetes, and arthritis.

Heart Disease and Strokes

Cardiovascular diseases are a significant problem amongst older adults in North America. For instance, more than one in three older Americans suffers from one or more types of cardiovascular disease. According to the American Heart Association (2013), the leading cause of death in older men and women (65 years of age and older) in 2009 was heart disease. Within Canada in 2008, cardiovascular diseases accounted for 29% of all deaths in Canada, of which 54% were attributed to ischemic heart disease (narrowing of the blood vessels of the heart), 20% to strokes (cerebrovascular accidents), and 23% to heart attacks (myocardial infarction) (Heart and Stroke Foundation of Canada, 2012).

Living with the impact of cardiovascular diseases in older adulthood can be difficult. Heart disease impacts all areas of life for older adults; they experience less energy, debilitating shortness of breath, and severe fatigue. Older adults, particularly those older than 75 years of age, often experience greater physical symptoms of heart failure than their younger counterparts. And emotionally they suffer as well, experiencing fear of becoming a burden, depression, and existential struggles (Falk, Ekman, Anderson, Fu, & Granger, 2013). Within their literature review examining older adults' experiences of heart failure, Falk et al. (2013) highlighted several studies revealing that symptom management by health care professionals is often inadequate, as is the self-monitoring of symptoms by these older adults. Interestingly, however, motivational interviewing has been found to be useful in improving older adults' abilities to manage their illness (Falk et al., 2013).[1]

Stroke

When older adults are left with functional deficits following a stroke, the sudden catastrophic event leads to life with significant changes. Older adults with deficits following a stroke often experience exhaustion, changes in physical abilities, such as difficulties in utilizing an affected hand for personal care or household duties, difficulties with mobility (walking and driving), changes in cognitive function, aphasia (problems with verbal communication), and changes in vision (Ekstam, Tham, & Borell, 2011; McKenna, Liddle, Brown, Lee, & Gustafsson, 2009; Northcott & Hilari, 2011). These changes can have a profound effect upon older adults' social lives, lead to a loss of friends, resulting in loneliness, which in turn, can precipitate depression. In their article entitled "Why do people lose their friends after a stroke?" Northcott and Hilari (2011) examined why strokes can damage friendships. The research participants spoke of their challenges following the stroke event, including the experiences listed above. However, they also reported that their friends offered unhelpful responses, such as ridicule, telling them how they should feel, or patronization. With

---

1. Motivational interviewing is often used in addiction counseling. It involves ascertaining individuals' willingness to change and making steps toward change.

all of these challenges following the acute stroke event, the research participants conveyed that they "closed in on themselves." The difficulties in communicating, exhaustion, and transportation challenges, as well as embarrassment of being seen as unwell, meant that getting together with friends was no longer enticing. Because of how they felt about themselves, as well as the responses of others, they simply withdrew (Northcott & Hilari, 2011).

Diabetes

Some older adults living with diabetes have managed their illness for years; for others, diabetes is a new experience. Living with diabetes includes dietary management, administration of insulin or oral hypoglycemics, blood glucose monitoring, and other tasks. Due to the changes of aging, successfully managing diabetes can pose problems that younger adults may not face. As well, co-morbidities (other concurrent illnesses) may impact how older adults deal with their illness. First, older adults may have visual problems that can influence medication administration, particularly the self-injection of insulin. Changes in daily exercise or physical activities can result in lower food intake, which can then result in hypoglycemia (low blood glucose). Developing cognitive impairment in some older adults can affect how they manage blood glucose monitoring, diet, and medication administration (George & Thomas, 2010).

Unstable or erratic blood glucose levels may result in older adults living with constant concern, or even fear, for their lives (Canadian Diabetes Association, 2015). For instance, if an older adult experiences very low blood sugars in the night, he might fear never waking up due to a severe hypoglycemic reaction. This can be especially frightening for the older adult who lives alone. An older woman who enjoys babysitting her grandchildren may have to cancel her cherished activity of looking after her young family members due to dizziness, trouble concentrating, and feelings of confusion caused by very low blood sugars. In both examples, there often are accompanying psychological reactions, such as fear, loss of control, and feelings of worthlessness. Loss of control and living with constant fear may lead to depression. And, unfortunately, depression in conjunction with diabetes may decrease the commitment of older adults to follow through with their daily self-care regimens (Jack, Airhihenbuwa, Namageyo-Funa, Owens, & Vinicor, 2004).

Further, living with diabetes may trigger existential issues in older adults. George and Thomas (2010) interviewed 10 older adults living in rural America about their experiences with insulin-dependent diabetes. The research participants had been diagnosed with diabetes 7–39 years previously. All had complications from the diabetes and each participant had one or more chronic illnesses in addition to the diabetes. The researchers concluded that the rural participants lived with fear of hypoglycemic reactions and subsequent death, a disconnect between what health care providers told them to do and how they actually managed their diabetes, a somber recognition that the only escape from diabetes involves death, as well as a stoicism to continue on. As the researchers noted, living with advanced diabetes caused older adults to ask existential questions (George & Thomas, 2010).

Arthritis

Although there are a number of forms of arthritis, the most common forms of arthritis are rheumatoid arthritis and osteoarthritis (The Arthritis Society, 2015). Arthritis is one of the most common causes of disability in older adults (Centers for Disease Control and Prevention—CDC, 2013); particularly rheumatoid arthritis results in physical disabilities (including problems with mobility and physical activities), decreased energy, and chronic pain (which can be severe in nature).

Understandably, living with chronic pain can result in despair and depression. In a recent study, older women who self-reported greater severity of pain and greater pain interference (the extent to which pain interfered

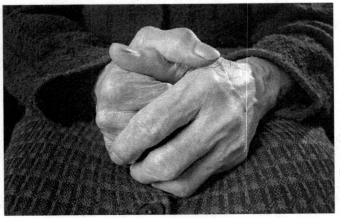

Sandra Matic/Shutterstock, Inc.

with activities of daily life) experienced more depression. Additionally, older men and women who had more co-morbidities (other concurrent illnesses in addition to the arthritis) experienced greater depression (Onubogu, 2014). Older adults who experience severe rheumatoid arthritis may live with the existential pain that comes from a lack of control and independence, as well as fear for the future due to the progressive nature of the disease. Depending upon the severity of the physical limitations, some older adults need to transition to seniors' complexes, assisted living, or long-term care facilities due to their inability to manage in their homes.

Chronic Pain

Chronic pain is pain that occurs for more than 12 weeks; it may, however, last for months or years (NIH Medline Plus, 2011a). It may be caused by chronic illnesses, such as arthritis (osteo or rheumatoid), neuropathic pain (related to nerve damage from diabetes), heart disease, and cancer; regardless of the cause, it can be debilitating. Estimates of the prevalence rates of chronic pain in older adults vary according to country. For instance, within Canada it is estimated that 27% of older adults living independently and 38% of those living within long-term care have chronic pain (Statistics Canada, 2010). Prevalence rates in the United States are even higher. The National Institute of Health (NIH) Medline Plus (2011b) reported that about 50% of older Americans living independently experience chronic pain, and the percentage climbs to 75–85% of those living in long-term care facilities.

Considerable consequences ensue from the presence of chronic pain in the lives of older adults. Living with persistent pain leads to problems sleeping, disabling fatigue, and a reduction in what older adults can accomplish in terms of household work and activities (Jakobsson, Hallberg, & Westergren, 2004). And the inability to accomplish household tasks often carries greater meaning for older adults than their younger counterparts; it is not simply the everyday business of getting the house cleaned, doing banking, and other chores, it is the structure these activities give to daily life. Because these activities need to be done, there is a reason to get out of bed in the morning, as well as a sense of a "job well done" when relaxing in the evening. Even more, it is the importance of these tasks to a sense of self—how older adults view themselves, their very personhood. If they cannot complete the most basic of duties—those they have completed since adolescence—what does that say about who they are as people? Older adults have described the experience of decreased mobility related to pain as not only frustrating, but tremendously *humiliating* and *demoralizing*. These feelings of incompetence and humiliation may cause some older adults to sequester themselves within their own homes, in a sense, to go into hiding (Smith, 2012). The loneliness that comes from living in isolation can then contribute to depression. However, when loneliness is coupled with persistent and longstanding pain, it is not uncommon for older adults to become very depressed. A complex entangled web of chronic pain, depression, loneliness, and social isolation may result. Some may medicate their physical and emotional pain with substances such as alcohol; sadly, for some, the end result of this web of despair is suicide (Conwell, Van Orden, & Caine, 2011).

In their review of studies examining barriers to the self-reporting of chronic pain by older adults, Gammons and Caswell (2014) found that there were internal barriers to self-reporting pain, one being older adults' desire to prevent pain from becoming the focus in their lives. The other barrier pertained to health care professionals and was site specific: whether the older adults lived in an institution or in the community. Seniors living in institutions experienced communication problems with health care professionals and stated that staff did not listen to them, nor understood their pain. Those living in the community also reported communication problems with health care professionals, in that they expected they would receive a prescription, but felt their stories were not heard (Gammons & Caswell, 2014). Additionally, some studies revealed the stoicism of older adults toward pain and that they believe that pain is a normal consequence of aging (Gammons & Caswell, 2014). When older adults do not feel that they can share their physical pain, or their stories about the pain, this can result in emotional pain, loneliness, and an uncomfortable predicament. To share physical pain and have it minimized will trigger emotional pain; however, to keep quiet and not share pain means that older adults are existentially alone with it: a double bind!

Chronic illness coupled with pain can result in suicide in older adults. In one Canadian study (Juurlink, Herrmann, Szalai, Kopp, & Redelmeier, 2004), researchers examined coroners' records of the suicides of older adults in Ontario, Canada from 1992–2000. They determined that of the 1354 older adults who committed suicide during this time period, a number of these individuals suffered from congestive heart failure, chronic obstructive pulmonary disease (COPD), anxiety disorders, depression (as well as other mental illnesses), and moderate or severe pain. The researchers noted that where individuals had multiple illnesses, the risk of suicide was higher. Sadly, almost 50% of these older adults had seen a physician in the week prior to committing suicide (Juurlink et al., 2004).

Mental Illness

Symptoms of mental illness are surprisingly common among older adults. And mental illness in older age can be heartbreaking for individuals and their family members. While older adults experience the same types of mental illnesses as younger adults do—including depression, adjustment disorders, anxiety, schizophrenia, and bipolar disorder—they may additionally develop Alzheimer's disease or other dementias.[2] Because the focus of this book is on transitions in older adults, and not specifically mental illness, we will focus on just depression, anxiety, dementias, and addictions.

Depression

Contrary to past societal beliefs, depression in older adults is not normal (NIH, n.d.). Depression may develop from the stress of dealing with a life-changing and gut-wrenching transition, such as the loss of a spouse; it can also occur in those who have had previous experience with depression in the past and in those who have illnesses that impact brain functioning (such as strokes or dementias); it can happen in response to chronic illness and pain; and it may occur as a result of medications (and/or medication misuse) or alcohol abuse. Much more than feeling "out of sorts" or "being moody," depression involves significant sadness, fatigue, anhedonia (a loss of pleasure in activities once considered enjoyable), concentration difficulties, guilt, and suicidal thoughts (American Psychiatric Association, 2013).

A significant number of older adults experience symptoms of depression (although they may not necessarily meet the criteria for Major Depressive Disorder within the *Diagnostic and Statistical Manual of Mental Disorders*). In Canada, it is estimated that up to 20% of older adults living in the community experience symptoms of depression. This percentage doubles to 40% for seniors living within long-term care facilities (Canadian Coalition for Seniors' Mental Health, 2009). For aging individuals, living with depression can make life miserable, and for some, even intolerable.

---

2.   We recognize that a small number of adults develop Alzheimer's disease or related dementias in their 40s or 50s; however, the vast number of individuals affected are considered older adults (Alzheimer's Association, 2014).

How painful and unbearable life can be for some depressed older adults is reflected in suicide rates of this age grouping. Older Caucasian men in both the United States and Canada have the highest rates of suicide in terms of population groups (CDC, 2012; Public Health Agency of Canada—PHAC, 2010). Further, the rates of suicide among older adults may actually be notably higher than reported. This is because judging the intentionality of the actions of individuals can be difficult. Particularly if the suicide is nonviolent, the death may be wrongly attributed to illness (Juurlink et al., 2004). Also, within Canada, when coroners perform autopsies, they may initially label the cause of death as "undetermined." However, after an autopsy is completed and the cause of death is confirmed as suicide, the change may not be registered in the mortality database (PHAC, 2014).

Suicide is not the only way in which older adults with depression may eventually die. The impact of depression upon older adults can shorten lives. One study (Reynolds, Haley, & Kozlenko, 2008) examined the effects of depression upon the active life expectancy of older Americans (70 years of age and older) who were living in the community. The researchers found that depressive symptoms decreased the life expectancy of young-old adults (70 years of age) by 6.5 years in men and 4.3 years in women, and by 3.2 years in the oldest-old men (85 years old and above) and 2.2 years in oldest-old women.

Anxiety

Like depression, anxiety is common in later life and can be extremely debilitating. Its prevalence is estimated to be double that of dementia and up to four to eight times more common than major depressive disorders (Cassidy & Rector, 2008). However, it is often not recognized by health and human service professionals and, as such, has been labeled the "silent geriatric giant" (Cassidy & Rector, 2008, p. 150).

What makes anxiety so "slippery" to recognize in older adults? First, anxiety may occur concurrently with other mental illnesses, such as depression. Or, anxiety can be a precursor to, or an initial symptom of, cognitive impairment (Potvin, Forget, Grenier, Preville, & Hudon, 2011). Second, older adults may express anxiety through a fixation on physical symptoms, or they may experience anxiety as a response to health conditions, such as cardiac disease (Grenier et al., 2012) or diabetes (Poulsen & Pachana, 2012). Further, older adults with anxiety often demonstrate anxiety differently than their younger counterparts, exhibiting far more physical symptoms of anxiety. As such, professionals may then focus on the physical concerns of their clients. Fourth, older adults suffering from anxiety are less likely to seek mental health services than older adults who are depressed (Scott, Mackenzie, Chipperfield, & Sareen, 2010).

The other challenging aspect of addressing this "geriatric giant" is treatment. As older adults absorb, metabolize, and excrete medications less effectively with age, pharmaceutical treatment becomes more challenging. Not only are there concerns about polypharmacy (see later in this chapter), but treatment with anti-anxiety agents, such as benzodiazepines, can lead to confusion and falls in older adults (Hirst, Lane, & Miller, 2015).

Alzheimer's Disease and Related Dementias

Alzheimer's disease and related dementias have a profound impact upon older adults, their spouses, and their family members. Alzheimer's disease refers to a progressive degenerative disease that results in memory loss (especially short-term memory loss), inability to make decisions, impaired ability to perform activities of daily living, changes in mood and behavioral problems, and communication problems that may lead to aphasia (loss of speech) (Alzheimer's Association, 2014). Alzheimer's disease is believed to be caused by neurofibrillary tangles and neuritic plaques. While Alzheimer's disease is the most common form of dementia, there are a number of other forms of dementia, including vascular dementia, frontal lobe dementia, Creutzfeldt-Jakob disease, and Lewy Body dementia (Alzheimer's Association, 2014).

The losses associated with dementias, such as Alzheimer's disease, are so profound and impact the very personhood of those affected; as such some have labeled the experience of Alzheimer's disease as "the loss of self" (Cohen & Eisdorfer, 2001). The person with Alzheimer's disease will eventually not be able to recognize family members or even him- or herself (in the mirror). By the middle stages of the illness, family members usually place the senior into a long-term care facility, as the care demands become too much. Death usually occurs somewhere between 7–10 years after the onset of the illness; however, some individuals live much longer (Alzheimer Society of Canada, 2012).

The stress upon family caregivers is enormous and cannot be overstated. In fact, it is not all that uncommon for a spousal caregiver of someone with Alzheimer's disease to die because of the stresses of caregiving. In one study (Schulz & Beach, 1999), 392 spousal caregivers were compared to 427 non-caregivers. All of the older adults were between the ages of

66–92 years of age. The results revealed that spousal caregivers had a 63% increased mortality rate over the non-caregivers. Schulz and Beach (1999) concluded that caregivers who experience emotional and mental stress related to caregiving have a greater likelihood of dying than non-caregivers. In situations such as illustrated by this study, Alzheimer's disease ends up taking two individuals: the older adult with the disease and the spousal caregiver. In our experience, caregiving may not only lead to increased mortality rates for spouses, but at times, spousal caregivers may actually pass away *before* the partner with Alzheimer's disease. And, in rare situations, an adult child may pass away before the parent with dementia.

I (AML) remember sitting at the unit desk (on a geriatric mental health unit) one morning reviewing a patient's chart when a caring psychiatrist entered the unit. She seemed upset. She told me that a particular person had died. I looked up, somewhat distracted, and said words to the effect of, "Well, she was very old." I was referring to the fact that our past patient was 95 years of age, if not by now, 96 years of age. The psychiatrist looked at me, paused, and said, "No, her *daughter* died." I was stunned. I asked what had happened. This psychiatrist then explained the circumstances of this adult daughter's death and her health challenges. I felt badly for the adult daughter, as well as for the psychiatrist, because the psychiatrist had worked hard to convince the daughter to scale back her efforts at caregiving and to consider placement in a facility, rather than solely providing help within her home. For various reasons, including cultural beliefs, the daughter could not accept help in caregiving and, ultimately, the stress involved in being the only person providing care may have shortened her life.

Grief is so intricately tied to seeing a family member (with dementia) not only progressively lose the ability to care for herself, but also in seeing the personality characteristics, that uniquely defined her as a person, disintegrate (Rolland, 1993). And that grief is complex and unresolved, in that the person with Alzheimer's disease has not passed away, but the person the caregiver knew is gone. Pauline Boss (1999) termed this situation "ambiguous loss." Initially, she coined this term to refer to American soldiers who were missing in action. Although they were presumed dead, family members could not see a dead body. Hence, they were physically absent (presumed dead), but psychologically present to family members. Boss (1999) then applied this expression to individuals experiencing dementias, but flipped the meaning. Because individuals with Alzheimer's disease or related dementias are not dead, they are physically present. However, as their personalities have changed and they forget who others are, they are psychologically dead (Boss, 1999). This results in complicated grieving

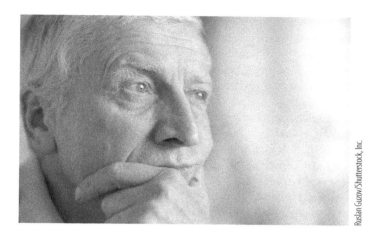

for family members, because they grieve the loss of the older adult with Alzheimer's disease, but the individual has not yet died. "I lost my mom a long time ago," is a common sentiment of an adult child coping with her parent's dementia and the demands of caregiving.

The notion of anticipatory grieving is somewhat different, but also related to the concept of ambiguous loss. Anticipating the death of a spouse with a progressive illness, such as Alzheimer's disease, can be as painful as the actual physical death of the individual (Rolland, 1993). While awaiting an eventual death, spouses and family members grieve each downward drop in functioning. They often feel as if they are losing their older adults "one piece at a time." Because the course of Alzheimer's disease is generally somewhere between 7–10 years, but can be longer, family members live in a state of grief for a long period of time. This is both emotionally and physically exhausting. In our experience, by the time older adults with Alzheimer's disease pass away, spouses and family members often admit that much of their grieving is done. This is not an indication that a spouse or family members did not love the older adult, but rather, that they carried their grief for a long period of time and now were ready to set this grief down. More will be discussed on the grief associated with ambiguous loss in Chapter 6.

Medication Usage and Addictions

Medication usage, in and of itself, is not a sign of addiction in older adults. However, prescribed and over-the-counter medications can cause significant problems for older adults, leading to hospitalization or place-ment in a long-term care facility. Older adults may suffer adverse drug reactions related to physiological changes that come with aging (and hence, a decreased ability to metabolize and excrete medications), and due to inappropriate dosages of medications or interactions between medica-tions (Berryman et al., 2012). The more medications taken by older adults the greater the chances for adverse drug reactions (Rochon, Schmader, & Sokol, 2014). Depending upon the survey, almost 40% to over 50% of older adults in North America take five or more prescribed medications yearly (Canada Safety Council, 2012; CDC, 2010).

Concurrently, older adults consume over-the-counter medications, often to a great extent. Commonly, they consume cold medications, decongestants, antihistamines, analgesics, and laxatives. Older adults may presume that these medications are harmless, as they are sold without a prescription; however, they are not benign for older adults.

For instance, older adults taking antihistamines may experience con-fusion (Berryman et al., 2012). Medications, particularly the adverse inter-actions between multiple medications, can lead to hospitalization because of a delirium. Delirium can be life threatening and includes symptoms such as confusion, disorientation, delusions and hallucinations, and agita-tion. Older adults hospitalized with delirium have a greater length of stay in hospital than their counterparts who are not experiencing delirium, and, tragically, have increased rates of death (Hirst, Lane, & Miller, 2015). While older adults living in the community may experience a delirium, those residing in long-term care are at particular risk. This risk is in part due to the fact that by the time older adults enter these facilities, they are often more frail, cognitively impaired, unable to effectively manage conti-nence, and thus, more prone to infections (another cause of delirium).

There is another significant adverse effect of some medications in older adults. Some medications affect balance and gait and can result in falls in seniors. Falls may cause fractured hips and may lead to disability or death (Huang et al., 2012). Even if older adults survive a fall and possible surgery, disabilities related to that fall may result in loss of independent living and possible transition to assisted living or long-term care.

The preceding discussion about medications, including the physio-logical changes in older adults that make them particularly susceptible to complications from medications and potential adverse effects, is presented with the underlying assumption that medications are taken as prescribed and that there are no intents to misuse or be psychologically reliant on substances. However, substance abuse can be a problem for some older adults and, combined with the number of over-the-counter and prescription medications ingested, can be dangerous or even deadly.

Substance abuse is included in the *Diagnostic and Statistical Manual of Mental Disorders* (DSM V) (American Psychiatric Association, 2013). And unraveling the reasons behind substance abuse is complicated. Substance abuse by older adults may be an attempt to self-medicate depression, anxiety, sleep problems, physical pain, and boredom; or, substance abuse may have caused depression and other health problems (Reardon, 2012). Like the proverbial cart and the horse, sometimes it is difficult to know which has come first.

There is another possible explanation, however. Aging individuals may abuse substances to deal with existential issues. In an interesting study, Wiklund (2008) explored the experiences of individuals living with addictions, with a focus upon existential issues. She interviewed nine individuals between the ages of 35–46. Although the research participants were not seniors, the findings may be considered relevant to the situations of some aging adults. Some of Wiklund's (2008) participants described experiencing life as meaningless and as a battle between life and death. However, when they took drugs, they felt alive, even if this type of existence was not really who they were as individuals. Could it be that some retired, chronically ill older adults are confused about their identity within a world where youth and productivity are revered, and find that alcohol or drugs not only quells loneliness and emotional pain, but on some level, makes them feel alive? However comprehensible the reasons for using/abusing substances in advancing years, the results can be deleterious and even dangerous.

The most commonly abused substance among older adults in North America is alcohol (Health Canada, 2005; Substance Abuse and Mental Health Services Administration—SAMHSA, 2009). The National Institute on Alcohol Abuse and Alcoholism (n.d.) reported that in 2008, 40% of older Americans drank alcohol. While older adults are generally considered less likely to be heavy drinkers (five drinks or more at one time at least once a month over a 12-month period), some older adults do consume amounts of alcohol considered to be problematic. For instance, in 2003, 12% of Canadian older men and 3% of Canadian older women were rated as heavy drinkers (Turcotte & Schellenberg, 2006). Risk factors for alcohol abuse among older adults includes those who experienced involuntary retirement and have had problems with alcohol abuse in the past (Kuerbis & Sacco, 2012), as well as those with mental health problems.

While the rates of alcohol abuse are not extreme, there is evidence that current rates of older adults abusing illicit substances is significantly higher than older adults in the early 1990s (SAMHSA, 2010). For example, between the years of 1992 and 2008, the rates of admission to hospital for heroin abuse among older Americans doubled (SAMHSA, 2010). This changing trend is attributed to the aging of the baby boomers (Reardon, 2012); this generation of individuals used illicit substances when younger and has continued to use these substances.

The use of substances such as alcohol or other illicit drugs, in conjunction with other prescription medications, can have dangerous effects. For instance, alcohol has a depressant effect upon the central nervous system (CNS). In combination with other medications, such as benzodiazepines (anti-anxiety medications), which also have a CNS depressant effect, can magnify or potentiate the depressant effect. This can lead to respiratory depression and death (Berryman et al., 2012). Older adults who may have combined prescribed medications, over-the-counter medicines, and alcohol younger in life may not be aware of the dangers of mixing substances in their advancing years. And, if they are bored or depressed due to the activity restrictions from chronic pain or chronic illness, or feeling empty due to forced retirement, they may be prone to use alcohol or other substances to numb their feelings (Reardon, 2012). While retirement or chronic illness does not cause a person to abuse substances, if the inclination to use substances is there and the senior is depressed, lonely, or bored, substances may be used to fill the void.

Framework Within Which to Understand Illness

Before presenting a case study and addressing assessment and intervention, we believe it is useful to offer some insights from Rolland's work on the psychosocial typology of illness (1987, 2005). These insights reveal the degree of challenges and suffering faced by older adults and their family members.

Psychosocial Typology of Illness

Rolland's psychosocial typology of illness (1987, 2005) assists professionals in understanding the unique challenges that come with managing varying illness trajectories associated with some of the diseases previously discussed in this chapter. This typology classifies illnesses according to onset, course, outcome, incapacitation, and uncertainty (1987). In this typology, Rolland differentiated between the demands and challenges experienced with an acute onset illness as compared to those with a chronic illness.

Depending upon the onset, course, and outcome, individuals and families will face specific challenges that will impact how they respond psychologically. For instance, Rolland (1987) included two categories under onset: acute and gradual. An acute onset can include such events as strokes or myocardial infarctions (heart attacks); gradual onset can include such illnesses as Parkinson's disease or multiple sclerosis. In illnesses that present with an acute onset, family members need to mobilize crisis management skills and support in a short period of time. Although dealing with a chronic illness demands just as many psychosocial resources in individuals and family members, the gradual onset of such illnesses offers time within which to adjust to the changes in health (Rolland, 1987).

Rolland (1987) conceptualized the illness course as generally taking three types: progressive, constant, and relapsing/episodic. Alzheimer's disease (and many related dementias) falls under the progressive course. When an individual has Alzheimer's disease, the disease course is usually continuous in terms of experiencing symptoms, but the symptoms worsen over time. Family members experience little relief from the constant caregiving demands; they risk becoming physically and mentally exhausted as they need to take on new demands as the disease progresses. The progressive category is in contrast to the constant course category, where after an initial event, the disease course stabilizes, such as with spinal cord injury. The relapsing or episodic course, that can occur with illnesses such as asthma, involves vacillations between periods of stability and acute flare-ups. While family members receive a break from caregiving during periods of stability, they psychologically live with the uncertainty of when an acute crisis may occur. The demands of this living with impending danger, even within the periods of stability, can be emotionally strenuous for families (Rolland, 1987).

The outcome aspect of illness involves the likelihood that an illness will result in death and the extent to which it can abbreviate someone's life (Rolland, 1987). When family members first receive the diagnosis, what is the likelihood that the illness will result in death? This is a significant question as the expectation of death sets in motion anticipatory grieving in family members, and family members and the ill older adult are caught in the tension of wanting intimacy and trying to pull away from each other. The extreme emotions experienced in trying to deal with an impending death can lead to difficulties in getting the practical day-to-day tasks done. Further, if family members are already conceptualizing their older adult as buried and gone, they may exclude him from important family responsibilities (Rolland, 1994).

Incapacitation

Incapacitation refers to the degree of disability caused by the illness, and may involve impairment in cognition (e.g., from Alzheimer's disease), in senses (e.g., blindness), and in movement (e.g., rheumatoid arthritis or multiple sclerosis) (Rolland, 1994). The onset of the incapacitation (e.g., spinal cord injury) will determine when the greatest amount of adaptability needs to occur. As an example, incapacitation from a sudden spinal cord injury from a motorcycle accident is severe at onset and requires strong adaptability from the affected individual and family members from the outset of the injury. Other illnesses with a more progressive course toward incapacitation allow for individual and family adaptation to changes at a slower pace (Rolland, 1994).

Rolland (1994) noted one more important form of disability—that arising from social stigma. Whether an illness results in stigma due to facial or bodily disfigurement, such as severe burns, or stigma due to its association with a marginalized group, such as AIDS and individuals who are homosexual or intravenous drug users, stigma can be experienced as a huge handicap for those affected (Rolland, 1994). Even though AIDS does not carry the immediate death sentence that it once did, individuals aging with HIV/AIDS now worry about where they will live when they can no longer care for themselves (as we will discuss in later chapters).

Assessment and Intervention

Assessing and intervening with older adults experiencing transitions involves sophisticated and highly nuanced skills. The process involves digging deeper than the surface level of assessment and intervention. Assessment and intervention are related and are difficult to separate; for instance, by asking questions in assessment, the nurse or other professional is actually also intervening (Wright & Leahey, 2013). The following case study reveals the complexities of unraveling the complications stemming from transitions in an older adult's life.

Case Example

John is a 75-year-old man who was admitted to a mental health unit in a hospital in Houston, Texas. John has been diagnosed with depression and suicidal ideation. There have been several events that are related to his depression. First, John retired seven years ago. He loved his work and did not want to retire, but felt that he needed to look after his wife who was deteriorating with Alzheimer's disease. Second, John's wife Susan died six months ago. From the time he retired until the death of his wife, he spent most of his time caring for her. Initially, John's wife lived within their home. He stoically tried to keep her at home, but after several years caregiving, he needed to place her in a long-term care facility, for the following reasons: Not only was Susan voiding in the living room, she no longer recognized John. She also would leave the home when John was asleep and wander. Once, Susan was found wandering on a busy street, only scantily clad, in the dead of winter. John was frantic with worry. His physician was concerned: John's blood pressure was high, and now he needed medications to calm his frazzled nerves and to sleep. But when Susan entered a facility, John's caregiving did not stop. He would come daily to feed his wife. Even though he was not concerned about the care given at the facility, he felt that he could spend more time coaxing her to eat. In the years of caregiving for Susan, John lost most of his friends and social contacts. Initially, friends tried to keep in contact with John, but at times he would turn down their invitations because he was too tired. Also, John sensed that his friends really did not understand. They told him that he should "get on with his life," but John did not feel this was possible. He felt compelled to help Susan even when she did not recognize him or acknowledge his help.

The past six months after the death of Susan were a blur. John felt intense loneliness and lack of purpose. He did not know how to rekindle his prior friendships. John spent his days medicating his grief, loneliness, and boredom with alcohol. While the numbness was not particularly pleasant, John felt it was much better than feeling his pain. As a result of his pain and his attempts to deal with it, John began to become very depressed and even suicidal.

When on the mental health unit, the nurses and social worker began to work with John to examine the triggers of his depression. They agreed with John that the years of caregiving for Susan resulted in deep physical exhaustion that contributed to his depression. They also noted that John lost his sense of identity when he gave up his work and only seemed to recapture a sense of identity and purpose in life when he devoted himself wholeheartedly to Susan. After about one week on the unit, John began to develop trust in the staff, and made connections between his past experiences and his current depression. John told nursing and social work staff about the impact of the death of his mother when he was in his early fifties. John was temporarily working halfway across the country when his father phoned him to tell him that that his mother was ill.

John's father asked him to return, but he chose not to when his father stated that the illness did not appear to be too serious. John acknowledged that the unresolved grief and guilt of this situation has haunted him since, as his mother passed without him coming home. Also, John admitted that about a year after the death of his mother, he had a brief affair. Although he confessed this to Susan and they worked to rebuild their marriage and trust, John could never quite forgive himself. And, of great concern to him, his relationship with his son and daughter was strained, in part due to their knowledge of the affair, and in part due to misunderstandings caused by the stress of caregiving for Susan.

John's situation illustrates some of the concepts described within this chapter. Retirement, the loss of a spouse, social isolation, and loneliness can lead to profound loss, depression, and suicidal ideation in an older adult. Self-medicating with alcohol can exacerbate depression. Further, from a life course perspective, events from the past can have an acute impact on how older adults experience current transitions, even if they are not aware of the connections between the past and present. And, as will be explained shortly, some older adults have a significant need for forgiveness, from themselves, from others, and/or from God (Enright, 1996).

Assessment

Assessment of transitions, such as the death of a spouse, as well as depression related to that transition, necessitates a multifaceted approach. This approach entails examining the past, insofar as it relates to the present, as well as examining the present and possible future scenarios.

In working with John, nursing staff and the social worker examined past and current triggers of the depression and suicidal ideation. Through the questions asked of John, the professionals were able to ascertain that relatively current stressors included the exhaustion of caregiving and the death of his wife. In posing questions about his past experiences with grief, they found out that John had unresolved issues of grief and guilt related to his mother's death many years prior, as well related to the affair he had shortly after the death of his mother. By gently asking John whether these experiences contributed to his current experiences of grief, John was able to make the connection between past grief ("ghosts of the past") and his current grief. In essence, nurses and professionals were connecting the unresolved issues of John's past encounters with transitions to his present stressful experiences (Krause, 2007). This insight facilitated John's understanding of why he was unable to accept the advice of friends and family in getting additional help to care for Susan. It might also help John to connect past transitions with ones he will face in the future, assisting him in making healthy choices. With knowledge of the risk of suicide among older adults (Canadian Coalition for Seniors' Mental Health, 2009), professionals continually assessed John's level of depression and suicidal risk. This not only provided the staff a gauge with which to determine his progress, but also may have helped John understand the importance of self-monitoring when he returned home. Staff were also aware that examining past issues can be traumatic in and of itself, so they were cognizant to check in regularly with him to assess John's level of depression and suicidal ideation.

Understanding the importance of examining the reciprocal nature of the influence of the illness upon John and his ability to influence illness (Wright & Leahey, 2013; Wright, Watson, & Bell, 1996), nursing staff asked John to describe how depression has impinged upon his life. As a follow-up question, they asked him if there were things he did that influenced the impact of depression upon his life. For instance, on days where he had appointments or had to help a neighbor, did his feelings of depression lessen?

Professional staff on the mental health unit purposefully posed this question. They were aware that what John believes about the illness, including his ability to exert influence upon its impact in his life, carries significant weight in how he thinks and responds to the depression (Wright, Watson, & Bell, 1996).

While some nursing staff on the unit became frustrated by John's complaints of physical pain, others were particularly astute in listening for covert messages in John's conversation. For example, when John complained about a headache or back pain, they wondered if he was saying, "My head hurts, but I also hurt inside." Some of the nurses were aware that older adults may have more difficulty in admitting to mental distress.

Growing up in an era where emotional problems were not spoken of and where individuals were expected to "put up and shut up" about internal pain, many older adults incorporated a deep-seated belief that mental illness is shameful. Even though the stigma attached to mental illness has lessened somewhat in the twenty-first century, at the core of their being, many aging adults are unwilling to admit to mental distress (Connor et al., 2010). A number of the nurses on John's ward were not aware, however, that physical distress and pain can be linked to depression as the same neurotransmitters involved in mood (serotonin and norepinepherine) are also believed to be involved in pain (Marks et al., 2009).

The professionals on the mental health unit also explored John's support system (Wright & Leahey, 2013). Specifically, who did he have for support, both professional and family/friend/neighbor support? Who could he access for help on a regular basis and what kind of aid would that entail? The staff also explored John's beliefs about accepting help: *Does accepting help from others indicate weakness or an inability to cope?* Further, what are his coping methods and which methods were effective and which are not? Staff explored previous coping methods—besides drinking alcohol—to see if he had utilized healthy coping mechanisms in the past and could return to some of these. They also probed about John's past experiences with illness to understand how he might respond to depression in the future.

As John's depression started to lift and his suicidal ideation dissipated, staff assessed John's level of awareness regarding depression. Not only did this entail asking about his knowledge about the illness and medications, but also how he would be able to monitor himself in the future. Specifically, staff asked John how he would know when he was starting to become depressed again. What would he be feeling, doing, and thinking? They also asked who he would turn to if he noticed he was thinking, feeling, and behaving in ways that indicated his depression was back and worsening.

A key part of assessment also involved asking John about what gives him hope and meaning in life (Duggleby et al., 2012). This ties into the existential issues that some older adults face. Nurses asked John about what has given him hope in the past and what now gives him hope. The psychologist even asked John if positive meaning has come from the illness and death of Susan (Kim, Kjervik, Belyea, & Choi, 2011). They assessed what he can do activity-wise that will foster hope and a sense of purpose and meaning. They asked if John has engaged in volunteer work in the past and if this would give him structure and meaning in his life.

An important aspect of finding hope and meaning, as well as self-acceptance entails self-forgiveness (Ingersoll-Dayton & Krause, 2005). John was finding it difficult to forgive himself for not being present for his mother at her death and for having an affair about a year after the death of his mother. Unfortunately, as is often the case, professionals on the unit felt uncomfortable dealing with the spiritual issues and tried to avoid talking about forgiveness (Ramsay, 2008). What staff did not realize is that for some older adults, particularly those who espouse religious faith, emotional health and spiritual health are inextricably tied (Ramsay, 2008). Nursing staff, as well as John, were also unaware of the potential connection between John's unexpressed feelings of guilt and grief over missing the passing of his mother and the extramarital affair one year later. They did not realize that in the process of "shutting down" the grief and guilt felt over not being present for his mother's passing, John also emotionally shut down to others, such as his wife. This created a context within which he considered and engaged in a brief affair, when previously this kind of behavior was unthinkable to him (McGoldrick, 1993).

Interventions

As mentioned earlier, the very process of assessing through questioning is an intervention (Wright & Leahey, 2013). Questions are a powerful means to encourage older adults, such as John, to reflect upon their lives (Wright & Leahey, 2013), make connections between the past and present, and develop insight (McGoldrick, 1993). Insight allows older adults to make different choices about how they face future transitions and losses.

When John started to feel better and have increased concentration, staff took the opportunity to provide teaching on depression, medications, and the potential of relapse. To increase the likelihood that he could respond differently to future transitions, John needed to understand what depression is, how it can be treated, and how he can decrease the chances of ending up in hospital for depression in the future.

Although nursing and medical staff did not feel comfortable addressing John's spiritual issues, they referred him to the hospital chaplain. This chaplain, who was particularly astute at understanding the importance of self-forgiveness for physical, emotional, and spiritual health, worked with John to help him address this area. She understood that for some older adults, it is easier to grasp the concept of God's forgiveness, or the forgiveness of others, than self-forgiveness. Also, she grasped the notion that self-forgiveness involves reconciling differences between real and ideal self-schemas (views of how older adults perceive themselves) (Ingersoll-Dayton & Krause, 2005).

In her assessment of John's belief systems, the chaplain determined that John does not hold to a specific faith. Her practice was based upon the foundation that the *needs of the client* determine the intervention (Speck, 1998), and so she did not suggest that John seek solace from scriptures or seek God's forgiveness for help with self-forgiveness. Rather, she walked John through a process that examined his ability to understand his past regrets within the context of unresolved grief about his mother's death. Because John was not able to cognitively change his evaluation standards of himself, she focused on helping John to acknowledge this mistake and learn from it, as well as make reparations through a discussion with his son (Ingersoll-Dayton & Krause, 2005). She assisted John in recognizing that self-forgiveness does not mean condoning his previous behavior (Ramsay, 2008), but involves moving forward with new insight into the circumstances that resulted in his behavior and an honest acknowledgment of his efforts to live in a respectful manner toward others.

Although life review therapy was not offered by the occupational therapist on John's unit, nursing and social work staff informally engaged John in some life review. Life review is believed to be an effective intervention for older adults with depression (Chippendale & Bear-Lehman, 2012). Specifically, they asked John to review aspects of his life of which he is particularly proud, not just his regrets. The staff members were attempting to help John re-story his life in a balanced way, acknowledging his positive contributions to his wife, family, and the community; the purpose was to help him integrate the pieces of his life into the whole of self.

If a life review therapy/narrative therapy intervention had been offered on the unit, the occupational therapist might have worked with John to ask him to write about specific periods of his life or to write about different life themes in the presence of the occupational therapist. The writing could have occurred in individual sessions or within group sessions (Korte, Bohlmeijer, Cappeliez, Smit, & Westerhof, 2012). When writing about negative events, the occupational therapist could have helped participants like John integrate negative experiences into their lives in a meaningful way.

He could have posed questions that helped participants construct alternate stories about their negative experiences, such as how they coped through such events, what they learned, and what good came out of their respective situations. Participants would have been asked to link these written observations to their identity as persons and to future goals. They would also have been asked to write about positive memories; these memories might have been forgotten or subsumed under negative memories (Korte et al., 2012).

Nursing and other professional staff, such as the recreational therapist, engaged John in activities. Not only did this allow the recreational therapist to assess John's level of concentration and to assess how he interacted with others, but also to reintroduce John to the meaning and enjoyment of structured activities. As part of recreational therapy, John may have learned the importance and enjoyment of engaging in activities or hobbies, with the hope that those learnings would be transferred to John's home life.

Related to the importance of structured activities, nursing, social work, and recreational therapy staff suggested that John consider volunteer work. They mentioned to John that the importance of volunteer work goes far beyond providing structure and some social contact in his life. Older adults who are active in volunteer work experience self-reported better physical health (Lum & Lightfoot, 2005) and lower levels of depression (Musick & Wilson, 2003). Volunteer work is also associated with lower mortality rates for some older adults (Musick, Herzog, & House, 1999). Some older adults who volunteer even report benefits for their family members; namely, family members are less worried about them and also, family members benefit from the knowledge about information and resources that their older members gain (Morrow-Howell, Hong, & Tang, 2009). Further, an important aspect of volunteer work is that it can foster a sense of meaning and purpose in life and continued growth (Choi & Landeros, 2011).

Meaning and purpose is integral to personhood. Staff specifically suggested that John consider work that is meaningful to him, perhaps work that is related to social causes or areas of personal or professional strength. Ideally, this work would also link to his personal values or spiritual beliefs. In this way, his actions for the good of others would be congruent with, and indeed, an expression of, his beliefs and values (Choi & Landeros, 2011). The sense of "giving back"—with his new understanding of his real and ideal self —could also aid him in forgiving himself for incidents in his life that he had previously tried to forget. Volunteer work could be a form of empowerment that counteracts the losses he has experienced, as well as the loss of control he may be feeling in other avenues in life (Tang, Copeland, & Wexler, 2012).

Observing his enjoyment of reading, staff also proposed John consider educational pursuits as part of his need for continued growth (Choi & Landeros, 2011) and self-achievement (Cha, Seo, & Sok, 2012). Older adults may take courses, such as university classes or classes focused on activities such as dancing or exercise. Although educational pursuits may result in less significant benefits than volunteer opportunities, in one study, older adults still rated class-taking as valuable (Morrow-Howell, Kinnevy, & Mann, 1999). Presumably, how John chooses to express his sense of personhood—educational versus volunteer pursuits—will be based in part upon what he values and what opportunities are available in his community.

Toward the end of John's time on the unit, his psychiatrist suggested that John and his family members have a meeting with his nurse or the social worker on the unit. This was in part to assess family dynamics, including how John's son and daughter relate to him and each other. The professional would also be able to provide teaching about mental illness and supports that could be put into place to help John. However, the purpose of the meeting was also to examine how John and his children wanted their relationship to proceed. John has regretted the strained relationship and expressed the desire to explore with his children if they could resume some contact and what this contact would entail.

SUMMARY

Physical and mental health problems in advancing years may be considered a life transition, due to the multiplicity of changes that occur and the fact that the illness transition may cause other transitions, such as retirement or changes in living environments. Health and human service professionals who assess and intervene with older individuals need to consider not only these transitions, but also how these older clients have weathered previous transitions and the impact of these experiences on current transitions. Further, understanding that illness trajectories differ according to the progressive nature of an illness, or the eventuality of acute flare-ups within a progressive disease course, will help professionals recognize the enormous burden faced by older adults and their family members.

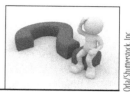

CRITICAL THINKING EXERCISES

▶ Think about an older adult you know, perhaps a grandparent, who has experienced the transition of a significant illness. How has that individual coped with the illness? What does he or she find most difficult and what strategies has the individual used to address the changes imposed by the illness? What kind of assistance has this individual found most helpful (from professionals and family or friends)?

▶ Reflecting again on the older adult that you know, how has he or she "made sense" of the illness transition? How does this individual express personhood, despite possible limitations of the illness?

INTERESTING WEBSITES

▶ Alzheimer's Association: http://www.alz.org/

▶ Alzheimer Society of Canada: http://www.alzheimer.ca/en

▶ Canadian Coalition for Seniors' Mental Health: http://www.ccsmh.ca/en/

▶ Heart and Stroke Foundation: http://www.heartandstroke.com/

▶ Substance Abuse and Mental Health Services Administration: http://www.samhsa.gov/

REFERENCES

Alzheimer Society of Canada. (2012). What is Alzheimer's disease? Retrieved November 20, 2014, from: www.alzheimer.ca/en/About-dementia/Alzheimer-s-disease

Alzheimer's Association. (2014). What is dementia? Retrieved November 15, 2014, from: http://www.alz.org/what-is-dementia.asp

American Heart Association. (2013). Statistical fact sheet: 2013 update: Older Americans and cardiovascular diseases. Retrieved December 15, 2014, from: http://www.heart.org/idc/groups/heart-public/@wcm/@sop/@smd/documents/downloadable/ucm_319574.pdf

American Psychiatric Association (APA). (2013). *The diagnostic and statistical manual of mental disorders (DSM V)*. Washington, DC: Author.

The Arthritis Society. (2015). Arthritis in Canada: Facts & figures. Retrieved November 8, 2015, from: www.arthritis.ca/page.aspx?pid=6239

Berryman, S. N., Jennings, J., Ragsdale, S., Lofton, T., Cooley Huff, D., et al. (2012). Beer's Criteria for potentially inappropriate medication use in older adults. *MedSurg Nursing, 21*(3), 129–132.

Boss, P. (1999). *Ambiguous loss: Learning to live with unresolved grief*. Cambridge: Harvard University Press.

Canada Safety Council. (2012, October). Drug safety for seniors. Retrieved February 10, 2015, from: http://canadasafetycouncil.org/node/1393

Canadian Coalition for Seniors' Mental Health. (2009). Depression in older adults: A guide for seniors and their families. Retrieved December 17, 2014, from: www.ccsmh.ca

Canadian Diabetes Association. (2015). Diabetes and you: Complications. Retrieved December 10, 2014, from: http://www.diabetes.ca/diabetes-and-you/complications/anxiety

Cassidy, K-L., & Rector, N. A. (2008). The silent geriatric giant: Anxiety disorders in late life. *Geriatrics & Aging, 11*(3), 150–156.

Centers for Disease Control and Prevention (CDC). (2010). Prescription drug use continues to increase: US prescription drug data for 2007–2008. Retrieved November 29, 2014, from: http://www.cdc.gov/nchs/data/databriefs/db42.pdf

Centers for Disease Control and Prevention (CDC). (2012). Suicide: Facts at a glance. Retrieved November 26, 2014, from: http://www.cdc.gov/violenceprevention/pdf/suicide_datasheet-a.pdf

Centers for Disease Control and Prevention (CDC). (2013). Chronic disease prevention and health promotion—Arthritis: Meeting the challenge of living well. Retrieved November 12, 2014, from: http://www.cdc.gov/chronicdisease/resources/publications/aag/arthritis.htm

Cha, N. H., Seo, E. J., & Sok, S. R. (2012). Factors influencing the successful aging of Korean older adults. *Contemporary Nurse, 41*(1), 78–87.

Chippendale, T., & Bear-Lehman, J. (2012). Effect of Life Review Writing on depressive symptoms in older adults: A randomized controlled trial. *American Journal of Occupational Therapy, 66*(4), 438–446. doi:10.5014/ajot.2012.004291

Choi, N., & Landeros, C. (2011). Wisdom from life's challenges: Qualitative interviews with low- and moderate-income older adults who were nominated as being wise. *Journal of Gerontological Social Work, 54*(6), 592–614. doi:10.1080/01634372.2011.585438

Cohen, D., & Eisdorfer, C. (2001). *The loss of self: A family resource for the care of Alzheimer's disease and related dementias* (Rev. ed.). New York: W. W. Norton.

Conwell, Y., Van Orden, K., & Caine, E. D. (2011). Suicide and older adults. *Psychiatric Clinics of North America, 34*(2), 451–468.

Connor, K. O., Copeland, V. C., Grote, N. K., Koeske, G., Rosen, D., et al. (2010). Mental health treatment seeking among older adults with depression: Impact of stigma and race. *American Journal of Geriatric Psychiatry, 18*(6), 531–543. doi:10.1097/JGP.0b013e3181cc0366

Duggleby, W., Hicks, D., Nekolaichuk, C., Holtslander, L., Williams, A., Chambers, T., & Eby, J. (2012). Hope, older adults, and chronic illness: A meta-synthesis of qualitative research. *Journal of Advanced Nursing, 68*(6), 1211–1223. doi: 10.1111/j.1365-2648.2011.05919.x

Ekstam, L., Tham, K., & Borell, L. (2011). Couples' approaches to changes in everyday life during the first year after stroke. *Scandinavian Journal of Occupational Therapy, 18*(1), 49–58. doi:10.3109/11038120903578791

Enright, R. D. (1996). Counseling within the forgiveness triad: On forgiving, receiving forgiveness, and self-forgiveness. *Counseling & Values, 40*(2), 107 ff.

Falk, H., Ekman, I., Anderson, R., Fu, M., & Granger, B. (2013). Older patients' experiences of heart failure—An integrative literature review. *Journal of Nursing Scholarship, 45*(3), 247–255. doi:10.1111/jnu.12025

Frankl, V. E. (2006). *Man's search for meaning.* Boston: Beacon Press.

Gammons, V., & Caswell, G. (2014). Older people and barriers to self-reporting of chronic pain. *British Journal of Nursing, 23*(5), 274–278.

George, S. R., & Thomas, S. P. (2010). Lived experience of diabetes among older, rural people. *Journal of Advanced Nursing, 66*(5), 1092–1100. doi:10.1111/j.1365-2648.2010.05278x

Gill, E. A., & Morgan, M. (2011). Home sweet home: Conceptualizing and coping with the challenges of aging and the move to a care facility. *Health Communication, 26* (4), 332–342. doi:10.1080/10410236.2010.551579

Grenier, S., Potvin, O., Hudon, C., Boyer, R., Preville, M., Desjardins, L., & Bherer, L. (2012). Twelve-month prevalence and correlates of subthreshold and threshold anxiety in community-dwelling older adults with cardiovascular disease. *Journal of Affective Disorders, 136*(3), 724–732. doi:10.1016/j.jad.2011.09.052

Health Canada. (2005). *Canadian Addiction Survey: A national survey of Canadians' use of alcohol and other drugs.* Ottawa: Health Canada.

Heart and Stroke Foundation of Canada. (2012). Retrieved February 10, 2015, from: http://www.heartandstroke.com/site/c.ikIQLcMWJtE/b.3483991/k.34 A8/Statistics.htm#heartdisease

Hirst, S. P., Lane, A. M., & Miller, C. A. (2015). *Miller's nursing for wellness in older adults (1st Canadian ed.).* Philadelphia: Lippincott Williams & Wilkins.

Huang, A. R., Mallet, L., Rochefort, C. M., Eguale, T., Buckeridge, D. L., & Tamblyn, R. (2012). Medication-related falls in the elderly. *Drugs & Aging, 29*(5), 359–376.

Ingersoll-Dayton, B., & Krause, N. (2005). Self-forgiveness: A component of mental health in later life. *Research on Aging, 27*(3), 267–289. doi:10.1177/0164027504274122

Jack, L., Airhihenbuwa, C., Namageyo-Funa, A., Owens, M., & Vinicor, F. (2004). The psychosocial aspects of diabetes care: Using collaborative care to manage older adults with diabetes. *Geriatrics, 59*(5), 26–32.

Jakobsson, U., Hallberg, I. R., & Westergren, A. (2004). Overall and health related quality of life among the oldest old in pain. *Quality of Life Research, 13*(1), 125–136.

Juurlink, D. N., Herrmann, N., Szalai, J. P., Kopp, A., & Redelmeier, D. A. (2004). Medical illness and the risk of suicide in the elderly. *Archives of Internal Medicine, 164*(11), 1179–1184.

Kim, S. H., Kjervik, D., Belyea, M., & Choi, E. S. (2011). Personal strength and finding meaning in conjugally bereaved older adults: A four-year prospective analysis. *Death Studies, 35*(3), 197–218. doi:10.1080/07481187.2010.518425

Korte, J., Bohlmeijer, E., Cappeliez, P., Smit, F., & Westerhof, G. (2012). Life review therapy for older adults with moderate depressive symptomatology: A pragmatic randomized controlled trial. *Psychological Medicine, 42*(6), 1163–1173. doi:10.1017/S0033291711002042

Krause, N. (2007). Evaluating the stress-buffering function of meaning in life among older people. *Journal of Aging and Health, 19*(5), 792–812. doi:10.1177/0898264307304390

Kuerbis, A., & Sacco, P. (2012). The impact of retirement on the drinking patterns of older adults. A review. *Addictive Behaviors, 37*(5), 587–595. doi:10.1016/j.addbeh.2012.01.022

Lum, T., & Lightfoot, E. (2005). The effects of volunteering on the physical and mental health of older people. *Research on Aging, 27*(1), 31–55. doi:10.1177/0164027504271349

Marks, D. M., Shah, M. J., Patkar, A. A., Masand, P. S., Park, G-Y., et al. (2009). Serotonin-Norepinepherine Reuptake Inhibitors for pain control: Premise and promise. *Current Neuropharmacology, 7*, 331–336.

McGoldrick, M. (1993). Echoes from the past: Helping families mourn their losses. In F. Walsh and M. McGoldrick (Eds.), *Living beyond loss: Death in the family* (pp. 50–78). New York: W. W. Norton.

McKenna, K., Liddle, J., Brown, A., Lee, K., & Gustafsson, L. (2009). Comparison of time use, role participation and life satisfaction of older people after stroke with a sample without stroke. *Australian Occupational Therapy Journal, 56*(3), 177–188. doi:10.1111/j.1440-1630.2007.00728.x

Ministry of Health and Long-Term Care. (2007). *Preventing and managing chronic disease: Ontario's framework.* Retrieved November 5, 2012, from: http://www.health.gov.on.ca/en/pro/programs/cdpm/pdf/framework_full.pdf

Morrow-Howell, N., Hong, S-I., & Tang, F. (2009). Who benefits from volunteering? Variations in perceived benefits. *The Gerontologist, 49*(1), 91–102. doi:10.1093/geront/gnp007

Morrow-Howell, N., Kinnevy, S., & Mann, M. (1999). The perceived benefits of participating in volunteer and educational activities. *Journal of Gerontological Social Work, 32*(2), 65–80. http://dx.doi.org/10.1300/J083v32n02_06

Musick, M. A., Herzog, A. R., & House, J. R. (1999). Volunteering and mortality among older adults: Findings from a national sample. *Journal of Gerontology: Social Sciences, 54B*(3), S173–S180. doi:10.1093/geronb/54B.3.173

Musick, M. A., & Wilson, J. (2003). Volunteering and depression: The role of psychological and social resources in different age groups. *Social Science & Medicine, 56*(2), 259–269.

National Institute of Health. (n.d.). Older adults and depression. Retrieved November 25, 2014, from: http://www.nimh.nih.gov/health/publications/older-adults-and-depression/index.shtml

National Institute of Medline Plus. (2011a). Chronic pain. Retrieved November 13, 2014, from: http://www.nlm.nih.gov/medlineplus/magazine/issues/spring11/articles/spring11pg5-6.html

National Institute of Health Medline Plus. (2011b). Seniors and chronic pain. Retrieved November 13, 2014, from: www.nlm.nih.gov/medlineplus/magazine/issues/fall11/articles/fall11pg15.html

National Institute on Alcohol Abuse and Alcoholism. (n.d.). Older adults. Retrieved December 15, 2014, from: http://www.niaaa.nih.gov/alcohol-health/special-populations-co-occurring-disorders/older-adults

Northcott, S., & Hilari, K. (2011). Why do people lose their friends after a stroke? *International Journal of Language & Communication Disorders, 46*(5), 524–534. doi:10.1111/j.1460-6984.2011.00079.x

Onubogu, U. D. (2014). Pain and depression in older adults with arthritis. *Orthopaedic Nursing, 33*(2), 102–108. doi:10.1097/NOR0000000000000035

Pickersgill, M. (2001). Grieving within a care home. *Nursing & Residential Care, 3*(12), 564–566.

Potvin, O., Forget, H., Grenier, S., Preville, M., & Hudon, C. (2011). Anxiety, depression, and 1-year incident cognitive impairment in community-dwelling older adults. *Journal of the American Geriatrics Society, 59*(8), 1421–1428. doi:10.1111/j.1532-5415.2011.03521.x

Poulsen, K., & Pachana, N. A. (2012). Depression and anxiety in older and middle-aged adults with diabetes. *Australian Psychologist, 47*(2), 90–97. doi:10.1111/j.1742-9544.2010.00020.x

Public Health Agency of Canada (PHAC). (2010). The Chief Public Officer's report on the state of public health in Canada in 2010. Retrieved November 25, 2014, from: http://www.phac-aspc.gc.ca/cphorsphc-respcacsp/2010/fr-rc/cphorsphc-respcacsp-06-eng.php

Public Health Agency of Canada (PHAC). (2014). Coroners' reports on suicide mortality in Montreal: Limitations and implications in suicide prevention strategies. Retrieved December 17, 2014, from: http://www.phac-aspc.gc.ca/publicat/cdic-mcbc/34-1/ar-04-eng.php

Ramsay, J. L. (2008). Forgiveness and healing in later life. *Generations, 32* (2), 51–54.

Reardon, C. (2012). The changing face of older adult substance abuse. *Social Work Today, 12*(1), 8.

Reynolds, S. L., Haley, W. E., & Kozlenko, N. (2008). The impact of depressive symptoms and chronic diseases on active life expectancy in older Americans. *American Journal of Geriatric Psychiatry, 16*(5), 425–432. doi:10.1097/JGP.0b013e31816ff32e

Rochon, P. A., Schmader, K. E., & Sokol, H. N. (2014). *Up to Date Wolters Kluwer Health: Drug prescribing for older adults.* Retrieved November 29, 2014, from: http://www.uptodate.com/contents/drug-prescribing-for-older-adults

Rolland, J. S. (1987). Chronic illness and the life cycle: A conceptual framework. *Family Process, 26*(2), 203–221. doi:10.1111/j.1545-5300.1987.00203.x

Rolland, J. S. (1993). Helping families with anticipatory loss. In F. Walsh & M. McGoldrick (Eds.), *Living beyond loss: Death in the family* (pp. 144–163). New York: W. W. Norton.

Rolland, J. S. (1994). *Families, illness, and disability: An integrative treatment model.* New York: Basic Books.

Rolland, J. S. (2005). Chronic illness and the family life cycle. In B. Carter & M. McGoldrick (Eds.), *The expanded family life cycle: Individual, family, and social perspectives* (3rd ed.; pp. 492–511). New York: Pearson.

SAMHSA (Substance Abuse and Mental Health Services Administration). (2009). Results from the 2009 National Survey on Drug Use and Health: Volume 1. Summary of National findings. Retrieved December 15, 2014, from: http://archive.samhsa.gov/data/NSDUH/2k9NSDUH/2k9Results.htm#3.1.1

SAMHSA. (2010). The TEDS report: Changing substance abuse patterns among older admissions: 1992 and 2008. Retrieved December 15, 2014, from: http://archive.samhsa.gov/data/NSDUH/2k9NSDUH/2k9Results.htm#3.1.1

Schulz, R., & Beach, S. (1999). Caregiving as a risk factor for mortality: The Caregiver Health Effects Study. *Journal of the American Medical Association, 282*(23), 2215–2219.

Scott, T., Mackenzie, C., Chipperfield, J. G., & Sareen, J. (2010). Mental health service use among Canadian older adults with anxiety disorders and clinically significant anxiety symptoms. *Aging & Mental Health, 14*(7), 790–800. doi:10.1080/13607861003713273

Smith, J. M. (2012). Portraits of loneliness: Emerging themes among community-dwelling older adults. *Journal of Psychosocial Nursing & Mental Health, 50*(4), 34–39. doi:10.3928/02793695-20120306-04

Speck, P. (1998). Spiritual issues in palliative care. In D. Doyle, G. W. C. Hanks & N. MacDonald (Eds.), *Oxford textbook of palliative medicine* (2nd ed.; pp. 805–814). Oxford: Oxford University Press.

Statistics Canada. (2010). *Healthy people, healthy places—82-229-X.* Author. Retrieved November 13, 2014, from: www.statcan.gc.ca/cgi-bin/IPS/display?cat_num=82-229-X

Tang, F., Copeland, V. C., & Wexler, S. (2012). Racial differences in volunteer engagement by older adults: An empowerment perspective. *Social Work Research, 36*(2), 89–100. doi:10.1093/swr/svs009

Turcotte, M., & Schellenberg, G. (2006). *A portrait of seniors in Canada.* Ottawa: Statistics Canada. Catalogue no. 89-519.

Weingarten, K. (2012). Sorrow: A therapist's reflection on the inevitable and the unknowable. *Family Process, 51*(4), 440–455. doi:10.1111/j.1545-5300.2012.01412.x

Wiklund, L. (2008). Existential aspects of living with addiction—Part 1: Meeting challenges. *Journal of Clinical Nursing, 17*(18), 2426–2434. doi:10.1111/j.1365-2707.2008.02356.x

World Health Organization (WHO). (2014). *Noncommunicable diseases: Country profiles 2014.* Retrieved November 12, 2014, from: http://apps.who.int/iris/bitstream/10665/128038/1/9789241507509_eng.pdf?ua=1

Wright, L. M., & Leahey, M. (2013). *Nurses and families: A guide to family assessment and intervention.* Philadelphia: FA Davis.

Wright, L. M., Watson, W. L., & Bell, J. M. (1996). *Beliefs: The heart of healing in families and illness.* New York: Basic Books.

CHAPTER 4

HOUSING TRANSITIONS

There is nothing more important than a good, safe, secure home.
(Rosalyn Carter, former American first lady)

Reflective Questions

- ▶ What residential options are available to older adults and what might influence their selection?
- ▶ What factors might influence the transition process for older adults who are changing settings?
- ▶ What interventions might be used to support the transition process for older adults and their families?

Redfoot and Gaberlavage (1991) wrote that "Housing . . . provides a secure and meaningful old age or magnifies the disability and isolation that too often accompany advanced years" (p. 35). Despite the need for secure housing, with advancing years transitions in housing do occur; some of these relocations can be very unsettling. Such moves may include relocating from one's own residence to another residence, moving from one institution to another, moving from one room in a facility to another, and relocating from one's own residence to an institution. For older adults, their life course journeys (e.g., employment positions, marriage, divorce, never married, retirement) influence their housing options in their later years. In addition, there are many factors, both positive and negative, that influence the relocation transition experience for the older adult, and the family.

In this chapter, we will describe the importance of home, explore some of the housing options that are available to older adults, discuss some of the theory and research that underlies our understanding of transitions (relocation), and identify interventions to promote positive adaptation to a new environment.

It is important to note that while there is a growing body of knowledge on the housing options of older adults, there is much that we do not yet know about the housing needs of older adults. For instance, the vast majority of research in this area is focused on urban populations. Yet, in Canada, 39.35% of older adults reside in rural settings (Turcotte & Schellenberg, 2007). As of 2007, seniors in the United States made up 7.5 million of the 50 million people living in rural areas (Rural Assistance Center, 2002–2014). Older adults in rural areas may have limited options for relocation when needed and may need placement in a long-term care facility in a town or city miles away from home. There are also other sub-populations of older adults that are more vulnerable than the general population of older adults to relocation issues, such as those living with AIDS. Their housing needs are largely unstudied. An exception is the work of Furlotte, Schwartz, Koornstra, and Naster (2012). They examined the housing experiences of 11 older adults living with HIV/AIDS and reported that participants were concerned about being accepted into retirement homes and long-term care, experienced barriers to accessing subsidized housing, and a few had been homeless. Participants experienced confusion and concern about their future housing prospects.

Another vulnerable sub-population of older adults is those aging with developmental disabilities. These older adults, in essence, may "fall between the cracks" within the housing sector for aging individuals. If they are placed in residential living, such as a group home, staff may not know how to address health problems, including dementias that present in some older adults with Down syndrome.

If they enter into long-term care, staff may not know how to address communication difficulties that may be due to their developmental disabilities. Also, older residents in a long-term care facility may not know how to connect with the adult who is admitted with a developmental disability, as this individual will probably be significantly younger (possibly in their 50s or early 60s) than them.

The importance of safe housing cannot be overstated. Housing is the means by which individuals can take care of their health and their families (Lane, Hirst, & Reed, 2013). The significance of housing has been demonstrated in a housing project for severely mentally ill individuals within the

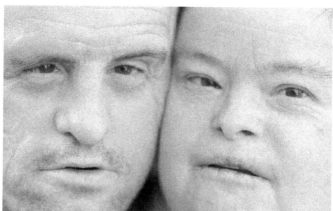

Marcel Jancovic/Shutterstock, Inc.

United States called the *Housing First* project. Historically, significantly mentally ill individuals only obtained housing when they had shown improvement in symptoms due to compliance with their treatment programs (medications, etc.). The rationale for this protocol was the notion that the severely mentally ill could only maintain housing when they were mentally well (Tsemberis, Moran, Shinn, Asmussen, & Shern, 2003). Thus, some mentally ill individuals chose to remain on the streets. However, the Housing First project rejects the assumption that the mentally ill must first comply with a treatment program prior to receiving housing. This program considers housing a basic human right (Tsemberis et al., 2003), and thus, individuals can access housing without adherence to a treatment program.

This program and approach has been demonstrated to be effective. In a longitudinal study, 225 individuals with mental illness were randomly assigned to receive housing based upon mental health treatment and sobriety (control group), and the other half received immediate housing with no conditions regarding treatment (experimental group) (Tsemberis, Gulcur, & Nakae, 2004). Over a two-year period, individuals in the Housing First set (the experimental group) accessed housing sooner and remained securely housed. The participants in the Housing First group stated that they felt more in control of their lives. Interestingly, there were no differences between the control and experimental groups in regard to the use of substances or in symptoms of mental illness (Tsemberis et al., 2004).

From the example of Housing First, it is evident that housing is crucial for individuals to maintain health and stability. We propose that just as housing provides the basis for those with severe mental illness to maintain health and stability, so secure housing should be available for *all* older adults, regardless of health or financial status (Lane et al., 2013).

The Concept of Home

The Oxford dictionary defines *home* both as a place of origin and as a goal or destination. Hollander (1991) documented that the Germanic words for home, *heim, ham, heem*, are derived from the Indo-European *kei*, meaning lying down and something dear or beloved. The implication of his work is that the *home* is a place to lay down one's head; it is also a place that evokes warm emotions.

Sir Edward Coke (1552–1634), English jurist and politician, said, "The home to everyone is to him his castle and fortress, as well his defence against injury and violence, as for his repose" (Brainy Quote, 2015). Home provides basic shelter and security, and is the place where one belongs. The meaning of *home*, however, extends far deeper than a physical location, or even the autonomy and safety that the physical building affords. The meaning of *home* takes on an ethereal quality. In an interesting study, Gillsjo and Schwartz-Barcott (2011) interviewed three older women about their understanding of *home*, including a description of it, the location of home, and what home means to them. Two of the women were currently living within their own residences in the community and one had just moved into a residential facility. The women spoke of home as a place, as involving cherished relationships, and as including experiences and memories. Two women discussed multiple homes, including their anticipated homes in heaven. The authors suggested the importance of health care professionals recognizing that for older individuals, home is more than a building: it is the very center of their lives (Gillsjo & Schwartz-Barcott, 2011). "The ache for home lives in all of us, the safe place where we can go and not be questioned" (Maya Angelou, Brainy Quotes, 2015); perhaps that ache is even greater, the older one becomes.

The meaning of home differs between individuals and may vary between those with and without cognitive impairment. The multifaceted understanding of *home* is recognized by health and human service professionals who work with older adults experiencing dementia. Some individuals with dementia may frequently repeat the sentence "I want to go home." This raises questions as to the meaning of home for those with dementia. Does this mean the home of their childhood, as dementia usually robs more of the short-term memory than long-term memory? Does this mean that the older adult wants to leave the hospital or the long-term care facility and return to his or her previous place of residence? Or, does this individual just want to feel safe and comfortable? Despite the fact that we may not know what individuals with dementia mean when they frequently ask to go home, it is clear that the construct of home involves much more than a building; it is imbued with feelings of security and warmth and belonging.

Whatever meaning is ascribed to the concept of *home*, for some aging individuals, this meaning includes the presence of pets, including cats and dogs. Pets can provide companionship within the home, a sense of security, emotional support, and a reason to get up in the morning. We know of individuals who have had pets, lost them (through death), and afterward noticed a strange phenomenon. These individuals reported feeling like there was no reason to come home; nobody (their pet) was waiting for them. The home felt empty, and hence so did the person living there. Because of this, at a certain point, these individuals bought another dog or cat so that the feeling of warmth and being welcomed within the home would return. There are also other benefits to pet ownership. Aging adults who regularly walk their dogs show increased levels of exercise and fitness (Parker-Pope, 2009; Thorpe et al., 2006). They also may experience an increased sense of *home* within their neighborhoods when walking their dogs; individuals will readily stop to pet their dog, talk about the animal, and exchange pleasantries (Cangelosi & Sorrell, 2010). While some contest the benefits of pet influence upon the psychological health of older adults, a number of therapists acknowledge the therapeutic value of pets upon the mental health of individuals (Imber-Black, 2009; Walsh, 2009). The powerful attachment that older adults have to pets may be illustrated by older adults' unwillingness to leave their homes during wide-scale disasters without their pets (Torgusen & Kosberg, 2006). Within Chapter 8 (Future Directions) we will offer suggestions regarding the presence of dogs and cats within assisted living facilities, as well as in long-term care.

Just as the concept of home is imbued with meaning, so the notion of *leaving home* is loaded with significance. Aminzadeh, Dalziel, Molnar, and Garcia (2009) explored the perspectives of individuals with dementia regarding their meanings and experiences associated with imminent relocation to a care facility. A qualitative design was employed, which involved in-depth interviews with 16 individuals with dementia at their homes two months prior to relocation. Participants viewed relocation to a facility as a major residential change and life transition requiring significant adaptive efforts. The experience of leaving their current home to move into a new one had profound personal meaning for them. The researchers noted that the participants recognized that relocation symbolized the end of an era and that life, as they once knew it, would be changed. Participants also spoke about how relocation signaled the downward decline of aging and meant that they would reside in a more dependent and structured environment. Of note, some participants also mentioned how they were survivors and could use their coping skills to make the best of the situation. This is significant, as the *home* can be representative of security and self-identity (Aminzadeh et al., 2009). By drawing on the metaphor of "survivor," these aging individuals with dementia were expressing that even though their identity within their home may be left behind, they would still carry some identity as survivors into the new setting. Presumably, their identity as survivors would carry them through the initial adjustment period in the care facility.

Ideally, a home should provide the highest possible level of independence, function, and comfort. Many older adults prefer to remain in their own homes and *age in place*, rather than relocate, particularly to institutional living (Ewen, Hahn, Erickson, & Krout, 2014). The ability to age in place depends on appropriate support for changing physical and psychosocial needs, so the older adult can stay where he wants to be. In order to support continued aging in place, basic home care services may be provided and/or the individual can purchase services from a private health care agency.

Within developed countries, home care services may include assessment, case management, professional nursing, rehabilitation therapy, social work, and personal care. Services are based on assessed unmet needs for short-term or long-term care and may include end-of-life care. Home care also provides assessments for applications to designated assisted living sites, facility-based respite care and long-term care. Assessment is of special importance since each situation is unique and therefore requires a review of the functional capacity of the older adult and individual health status. Services may be provided on a daily or intermittent basis, according to the needs of the older adult. In the provision of such services, good communication strategies are needed to ensure that all members of the health care team, and the client's family, are aware of the older adult's needs and progress toward identified goals. Chappell, Havens, Hollander, Miller, and McWilliam (2004) found that home care is significantly less expensive than long-term care, even when informal caregivers' (e.g., family members) time is valued at either minimum or replacement wage.

Global Perspective

Within a larger societal context, *age-friendly communities* are places that actively value, involve, and support older adults, both active and frail, with infrastructure and services that effectively accommodate their changing needs. Within this context, there is a global initiative to develop age-friendly communities and increase opportunities to age in place (Geller, 2015). An *age-friendly* community is one that provides opportunities for people to age in place by making resources available for day-to-day living. It means, for example, that grocery stores, pharmacies, transportation services, health care facilities, community centers, and religious buildings are within easy reach of and accessible to older adults. The implication is that older adults can continue to live in and contribute to their community. It also means that services are available when needed, such as home-delivered meals. In other words, the community is one in which older adults may live with dignity and independence.

Through the World Health Organization (WHO), 33 cities, including four in Canada, have implemented and evaluated age-friendly principles. While Portland, Oregon, was the only city in the United States to participate in WHO's original study in 2007, other American cities, such as New York, have since implemented age-friendly measures.[1] As a direct result of the positive response to the original 2007 study, WHO has created a global network of age-friendly communities (WHO, 2007). In Canada, the Age-Friendly Communities Initiative, based on WHO program principles, is led by the Public Health Agency of Canada (PHAC) in collaboration with other federal, provincial, territorial, and non-government partners. At the provincial level, British Columbia, Manitoba, Nova Scotia, and Quebec have Age-Friendly Community programs (PHAC, 2008). Several municipalities beyond these provinces have both formally and informally adopted age-friendly principles by assessing their communities and designing interventions to enhance the ability of older adults to remain in their own homes and familiar environment.

Why are age-friendly communities or cities necessary? It is estimated by the year 2030 two thirds of the population (worldwide) will live in urban areas. Additionally, within cities in higher income countries, it is projected that approximately one quarter of the population will be 60 years of age

---

1. Currently in New York, there are over 1 million citizens over 65 years of age. It is estimated that by 2030, that number will increase by 50%. See AgeFriendlyNYC (New York Academy of Medicine, n.d.).

or older (McGarry, 2012). The sheer numbers of the older adult population justify the need to make communities more amenable and accessible to older adults. Second, another reason why age-friendly communities are necessary is because the current physical layout and structure of most cities works against the older population, particularly those who are frail or who cannot drive. Many decades ago (up to 100 years ago), residential areas were moved away from commercial (urban) areas in order to deal with the congestion of people and unsanitary conditions; people moved to the *suburbs*. This was done by city policies and zoning regulations (Scharlach, 2009). This meant that families grew up in residential communities away from the overcrowding of the inner city, but were geographically removed from many stores and services. For younger families who are healthy and have access to cars, this has and still does work well. However, within the twenty-first century, there is the recognition that older adults are compromised by this type of city structure, particularly those who cannot drive or for whom the bus system does not work well (Kennedy, 2010). Third, housing structures were built in the past, and are still currently constructed in the present, for younger people; they are not designed for aging individuals (Scharlach, 2009). For instance, many houses have multiple stairs; some stairways may be quite steep. Aging individuals may have difficulty navigating these stairs. With a basic understanding of the principles of age-friendly communities, we will now discuss current housing options for older adults within developed countries.

Housing Options in Later Life

Some aging adults, by choice or by need, move from one type of residence to another. The term that we used earlier in this chapter was *relocation*. Residential options range along a continuum from remaining in one's home to: retirement communities; shared housing with family members, friends, or others; residential care communities such as assisted living settings; and for those with most needs, long-term care facilities (such as nursing homes and auxiliary hospitals). There are many different types of housing. The terms used to describe the various types depend upon geographic location. Generally, all housing options can be categorized into one of three main categories: independent living options, supportive housing, and health care facilities.

A great deal of work has been done on the housing options for older adults, but far less research has been conducted on what influences the decision-making process. In examining the housing choices of older Canadians, Perks and Haan (2010) identified that social support characteristics are the strongest predictors of dwelling type; this means that older adults choose their residence type primarily on the basis of their social needs and wants, rather than on their economic resources or even their health needs.

While a number of housing options exist for those with sufficient finances, not all older adults have such resources. Strohschein's (2012) study was designed to investigate characteristics of seniors in the Canadian population who were involuntary stayers and to assess the associations with health. *Involuntary stayers* are older adults who want to relocate, but are unable to due to finances or other situations. Data from the 1994 Canadian National Population Health Survey, with the sample restricted to those 65 and older ($N = 2551$), was used. Almost 1 in 10 older adults was identified as an involuntary stayer. Those older with few socioeconomic resources, poor health, greater need for assistance, and low social involvement were more likely to identify as involuntary stayers. Furthermore, those older adults who were involuntary stayers reported significantly more distress and had greater odds of low self-rated health than their peers. This study brings into visibility older adults who are unable to move from their present location despite their desire to do so. In spite of the current emphasis on "aging in place," this study identifies that not all aging adults want to remain in their current location.

A lack of financial resources may not only lead to older adults remaining in a current living situation which is undesirable (involuntary stayers), but can also lead to relocating into accommodation which is not necessarily ideal for seniors. For instance, Lewinson and Morgan (2014) found that limited finances resulted in some seniors living in extended-stay budget hotels. While the aging individuals appreciated some features of these budget hotels, such as surveillance safety and supportive amenities, they felt significant stress over other features of these hotels, such as poor air quality, unsanitary surroundings, neglected property management, disruptive guests, and restrictive policies. While extended-stay budget hotels were one way to deal with their housing needs with limited finances, this choice provided limited satisfaction.

Independent Living Options

Independent living describes any housing arrangement in which the older adult maintains control over the environment. It may describe the home that an older adult has lived in for most or even all of his life. Or it may be used to describe a housing facility with the same goal (of maximizing independence), that is exclusively for older adults, generally those aged 55 and over. With respect to the latter distinction, housing options vary widely, from apartment-style living to freestanding homes. Other terms associated with independent living include *retirement communities, retirement homes, senior housing,* and *senior apartments.*

With the aging of the baby boomer generation, architects, engineers, and builders are focusing on home designs that adjust to the changes that may accompany aging. Their goal is to enable older adults to stay in their homes safely even if they experience illness and functional decline. These new designs are marketed as *transgenerational* or *universal* designs and can benefit everyone, not just older adults. Designs and modifications may include fittings in the bathroom, walk-in bathtubs, wider hallways, remote-controlled devices for lights, raised counter tops, and adjustable-height sinks. These kinds of modifications facilitate independent living longer for older adults or individuals with disabilities.

Social Housing

Social housing is also often referred to as *subsidized housing* or *public housing*. Subsidized housing encompasses all types of housing in which the government provides some type of subsidy or rent assistance. In most situations, the subsidy ensures that the older adult does not spend more than 30% of personal income on rent. Social housing is an important option for older adults who are experiencing poverty or significantly restricted incomes. While social housing fills an important niche in housing options for older adults, depending upon the city, the demand for this option can be high, resulting in older adults being placed on long waitlists to access it.

Life Lease Arrangements

A *life lease* is an arrangement where the older adult purchases the *right to occupy* a housing unit and to use the common facilities, usually until he or she dies or moves. The major market for life lease arrangements are adults aged 55 and older. This arrangement means that older adults can move into smaller and usually more affordable housing. At any time, the aging individual can decide to transfer this right of occupancy back to another qualifying purchaser, either directly or by way of the sponsor organization, depending upon the lease contract arrangements. In this way, older adults earn a return on their investment similar to the return on the sale of their own home. Usually, the lease requires a single upfront payment as well as monthly fees for management and maintenance of the property and yard.

Adult Lifestyle Communities

Adult lifestyle communities are also known as retirement communities or 55-plus communities. Housing is usually condominium style—in a tower, townhouses, or semi-detached homes. The units are designed for the newly retired adult and the community often includes recreation facilities (e.g., golf course, tennis courts, a swimming pool). Some of these communities are gated and may have security. Many have age requirements.

While little research has been conducted on age-restricted housing, there are a few exceptions. In one study (Crisp, Windsor, Anstey, & Butterworth, 2013) the researchers examined factors that influenced older Australians to move into a retirement village, and detractors from this kind of accommodation. They found that seniors were attracted to outdoor living areas, support to maintain their autonomy, and close proximity to medical facilities. They were less impressed by luxury features, such as pools. Similarly, Bekhet, Zauszniewski, and Nakhla (2009) studied reasons why older Americans move to retirement communities. They found that older adults reported factors that *pushed* them into moving, such as their failing health, or that of their spouse, the need to reduce their responsibilities, previous accommodations closed, as well as loneliness. These triggers for moving were viewed as negative. Factors that *pulled* older adults to move into retirement communities, and as such were viewed more positively, included familiarity with the facility, security, and joining friends.

Supportive Housing

Shared housing

Shared housing among adult children and their older relatives is a preferred choice for some older adults. The sharing may relieve the economic burdens of maintaining a home after widowhood or retirement on a fixed income. Cultural influences predict the frequency of multigenerational residences. In Canada, about half of multigenerational households are headed by immigrants; the majority of them are of Asian origin. Among Asians and South Asians living in Canada, shared housing is often an expectation (Kaida, Moyser, & Park, 2009). While citing U.S. census data,

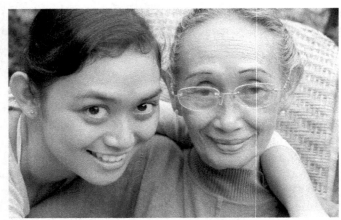

Keene and Batson (2010) provided an overview of multigenerational families, citing that among these households, the largest group consists of adult
householders, their children, and their grandchildren, comprising about
65% of these multigenerational families (or 2.6 million families). In these
multigenerational families, the householder is the grandparent; an adult
child and his or her children have moved in with the grandparent. Other
family configurations are those in which a parent or parent-in-law lives
with the householder and his or her children; this accounts for about one
third of multigenerational households or 1.3 million households. In these
multigenerational families, the householder is the adult child with whom
the aging parent lives, in addition to dependent children that may still be
living within the home.

Relocating from one's own home to the home of an adult child can have
many benefits, but without adequate preparation it can also be stressful for
both the family and the older adult. Older adults and adult children need
to negotiate the new shared living arrangement in terms of roles (who does
what?), a balance between togetherness and privacy, joint or single social
gatherings, and even parenting. For instance, the older adult may not want
to be "parented" by her children; also, an adult child may not appreciate the
aging individual parenting his children (grandchildren of the aging adult).
Being able to navigate close proximity between the generations takes flexibility on the part of all involved, as well as a sense of humor!

A variation of shared housing has long existed in what has become
known as *granny flats*. These may be apartments added to existing homes
or the construction of small housing units on family property with privacy;

these too involve the sharing of time and resources. These arrangements allow families to be close enough to be of assistance if needed, but to remain separate from their older member. For some families, the private apartment or suite satisfies the need for privacy in the midst of togetherness.

A variety of other shared intergenerational housing options have emerged in the community over the last few decades. Small home residences that offer independent or supportive housing may not have the extensive amenities of a multi-unit complex, but they can provide a home-like atmosphere and personal touches. Increasingly, older homeowners are expanding or opening their homes to several "guests." Accommodations may range from an individual suite to a bedroom in a shared residence with the homeowner. Most often these situations provide some level of support to ensure the older adult stays safe, but housing "guests" are mainly there to provide companionship and socializing for the older adult in a family-like setting. Living with an older adult frees up some additional finances for the family, as well as affords the benefits of the senior's presence and wisdom; the guests provide company, safety, and a home environment for the aging individual.

A variation of this theme is when an older adult opens up the family home for a younger generation—for example, a university or college student. Often this will appeal to older adults who can care for themselves without outside assistance but who live alone and are struggling with isolation, lack of stimulation, and have concerns for personal well-being should they have an accident with no one around. The student may provide help with snow shoveling or the garden in return for a minimal amount of rent. There are many such programs scattered throughout North America, the United Kingdom, Europe, and Australia; for example, there are approximately 100 homesharing programs throughout the United States (Steinisch, 2007). The purpose of the match-up is for the mutual benefit of the older adult and the younger adult. The young adult lives for very little cost in the home of an older adult and provides agreed-upon services, and the older adult not only has services provided for free, but also enjoys greater safety with the student living in the home. Proponents of these programs suggest that they delay institutionalization (Fox, 2010); the safety of having another individual in the home, as well as the services they can provide, delays the need to move to more supervised levels of care. Regardless of whether these arrangements delay institutionalization, they provide a solution for older adults who want to remain in their homes, but are lonely, desire some social contact with another, or perhaps want the safety of having another person within their home.

Assisted Living Facilities

As adults age, there is a tendency to simplify living space and lifestyles. Assisted living is a housing option for older adults who want or need help with some of the activities of daily living (e.g., cooking meals, getting up to the bathroom in the middle of the night, keeping house, and traveling to appointments), but also want and can maintain some independence. Perkins, Ball, Whittington, and Hollingsworth's (2012) study involved a synthesis of findings from three qualitative grounded theory studies that addressed aspects of autonomy in assisted living facilities. They found that older adults, living in these facilities, viewed autonomy as an expression of the self that is uniquely defined by each older adult and is based upon personal experiences and environmental and social contexts.

Assisted living is the fastest growing type of housing option for older adults in the United States (Stevenson & Grabowski, 2010). These facilities are designed for older adults who do not need care in a long-term care facility, but who need more support than is available in shared housing. This type of facility is known by different names across the continent, including assisted living, retirement homes, seniors' residences, personal care homes, retirement residences, residential care, board and care, congregate care, and sheltered housing.

In general, assisted living is a residential type facility, ranging from converted homes to apartment buildings. Assisted living facilities are often operated by for-profit corporations or by not-for-profit organizations. In countries such as the United States and Canada, they are not part of the formal health care system and costs are not covered through regional health insurance. Older adults are tenants who pay fees for accommodation and for any health care purchased. Most of these facilities offer two or three meals per day, light weekly housekeeping and laundry services, as well as provide optional social activities. Many facilities have transportation services and Internet access. Some have exercise facilities, movie theaters, pharmacies, and hair dressing services. Some provide apartment-style living with scaled-down kitchens, while others provide rooms. In some, an older adult may need to share a room. The housing unit is adjusted to meet the needs of the older individual, for example, grab bars in the bathroom, call-for-help lights, or low kitchen cabinets. Most facilities have a group dining area and common areas for social and recreational activities.

Within assisted living facilities, resident councils are often encouraged for older adults to provide support systems for each other; one example is where a resident council creates a system in which older adults check on one another the first thing each morning. Older adults may sit on the councils and, depending upon the facility, the council may determine some policies for that facility. Resident councils offer older adults a greater sense of control and influence upon their living environment and hence, some aging individuals value and enjoy taking part in this opportunity.

Many older adults and their families prefer assisted living facilities to long-term care because they are more homelike and offer more opportunities for control, independence, and privacy. Because some facilities have a health care professional on staff, or may contract out to the local community health center for services, older adults can still receive care and yet function somewhat independently. However, many older adults may have long-term health care needs associated with chronic illnesses, and with time they may require more care than the facility is able to provide. Or, if a sudden health crisis or accident occurs, older adults may be transported to hospital and then be transferred to long-term care. Bellantonio and colleagues (2008) examined whether an interprofessional team intervention minimized unanticipated transitions out of an assisted living facility for persons with dementia. Such unanticipated transitions included permanent relocation to a long-term care facility, emergency department visits, and acute care hospitalization. They found that falls were the primary reason for a transition. While the intervention reduced the risk of unanticipated transitions, the results were not statistically significant. Interestingly, however, is that more men than women experienced an unanticipated transition. The researchers suggested several explanations as to why this occurs. For instance, men enter facilities with a greater number of co-morbidities (other concurrent illnesses). Moreover, men are more likely to have Parkinson's disease or Lewy body disease, which are more commonly associated with gait and balance disorders. In addition, men with dementia may have more support to remain at home than women (because women tend to live longer than men and hence provide care for their husbands) and thus may delay relocation longer than women; when they do enter into long-term care, they have a higher level of disability (Bellatonio et al., 2008).

Health Care Facilities

Long-term care facilities

Long-term care facilities are a purpose-built congregate care option for individuals with complex, sometimes unpredictable medical needs, who require 24-hour on-site registered nurse care and/or treatment. These facilities may be called nursing homes, long-term care facilities, auxiliary hospitals, special care homes, or personal care homes. When used appropriately, long-term care fills an important need for older adults and their families. A significant portion of long-term residents are 85 years or older (Turcotte & Schellenberg, 2007; United States Census Bureau, 2011). There are more than twice as many women than men residing in long-term care facilities. In part, this is because women live longer than men (on average) and thus may reach their oldest-old years (85 years of age and older) and require the care provided by such facilities.

One of the main reasons to move to a long-term care facility is the inability to perform activities of daily living (ADLs), and most very elderly adults require significant assistance with ADLs and instrumental activities of daily living because of physical disabilities. Another reason older adults enter into long-term care is due to the presence of cognitive impairment. More than two thirds of the residents in long-term care facilities are cognitively impaired. The incidence of dementias increases significantly as individuals age (as noted in Chapter 2) and so these vulnerable, older adults require the assistance with ADLs. So whether for physical disabilities or for cognitive impairment, these very elderly adults require the type of assistance found in long-term care.

There is another side to the decision-making about relocating an older adult to long-term care, however. The health of the major caregiver and lack of assistance also plays a role in the decision to place an older adult into a nursing home. For example, when the primary caregiver experiences cardiac problems, or is depressed, family members may decide that placement is necessary. Also, when family relationships are deteriorating because of the behaviors of the older adult (related to dementia), or the primary caregiver cannot obtain help from family members, then the placement process may activated (Chang & Schneider, 2010).

While older adults relocate, as needed, into long-term care facilities (from less restrictive to more supervised settings), on occasion, older individuals may relocate from a *more* restrictive environment to a *less* restrictive environment. This sometimes occurs when a family removes an elder from a long-term care facility and brings the individual home to live with them. As a unique twist on the usual movement from an assisted living facility into long-term care, Hutchings and colleagues (2011) reported on the relocation of older adults with dementia from long-term care to an assisted living facility. They interviewed 10 family members of eight older adults about their experiences of the relocation. They reported that the client-centered care resulted in positive outcomes for both the older adults and their family members. The older adults and their family members were more contented with the assisted living placement, appreciated the privacy offered by the new environment, and some family members suggested that their older family member experienced improvement in their functional abilities (Hutchings et al., 2011). We should note that this kind of reversal in the level of care (from more restrictive to less restrictive) is rare.

Hospice

The term *hospice* refers to more than just a site of care; hospice is also a philosophy of care. Palliative care offered within stand-alone hospices, or within designated units in long-term care facilities and hospitals, offers services to help relieve suffering and improve quality of life for people with a life-limiting illness, as well as to those grieving the impending death of a loved one.[2] Making the transition to hospice care can be difficult for individuals and their families. This type of housing arrangement—and philosophy of care—will be discussed in length within Chapter 6 and touched upon in Chapter 8.

Theory and Research That Underlies Our Understanding of Transitions

The Decision to Relocate

As individuals age and their family situation changes (e.g., children leave home), and their physical status changes, a relocation from the family home is often considered. And, for most people, relocation is a major decision. Older adults in urban areas may find that they are living in unfamiliar areas because the neighborhood around them has now changed. For example, some older adults may have originally settled in an area that was settled by people of the same ethnic background. Over time, the ethnic composition may have changed and thus the sense of shared culture and background may be lost. For adults in rural areas, the geographic distance and lack of supportive services may lead to serious consequences, especially if they are functionally impaired.

---

2. There are differences in understanding the terms *hospice* and *palliative care*. These concepts will be defined more clearly within Chapter 6.

Often physical or mental health influences the decision to relocate. For instance, Leland and colleagues (2011) examined the relationship between the occurrence of falls and the expectations older adults have about making future residential moves. They found that older adults who had fallen had a much greater probability of considering relocation. It seems that when there is tangible evidence of failing health, older adults become more open to the notion of moving. Extreme frailty, and thus an inability to cope with living alone, may also influence the decision to relocate. Sometimes, older adults decide to relocate due to loneliness; they believe that living with others will be preferable to living in solitude (Heppenstall, Keeling, Hanger, & Wilkinson, 2014).

Demographic or contextual factors can also influence the decision to relocate. Hence, factors such as gender, age, household income, geographical location, driving status, the appropriateness of the current home to meet the older adult's needs, as well as unmet heavy cleaning needs can significantly influence the decision to relocate (Weeks, Keefe, & MacDonald, 2012). Older adults with lower incomes may be less likely to consider relocation, because they have fewer affordable options. Elders who are having difficulty with heavy cleaning in their current residence may be more motivated to relocate (Weeks et al., 2012).

As with many transitions, there are both potential negative and positive outcomes to moving residences. Overall, research indicates that relocation is associated with increased morbidity and mortality. However, there is research that suggests that relocation does not always result in serious effects on mental or physical health. For instance, Capezuti, Boltz, Renz, Hoffman, and Norman (2006) examined the physical and mental health characteristics of 120 residents three months following their involuntary transfer from one long-term care facility to another. While there was a statistically significant increase in the number of residents who fell during the post-transfer (76.9%) compared to the pre-transfer (51.2%) period, overall, there were few changes noted. Residents did not demonstrate any other significant physical or mental health changes during the three months following the transfer, when compared with their pre-transfer status. Similar findings were reported by Walker, Curry, and Hogstel (2007). They interviewed eight long-term care facility residents and eight assisted living facility residents 2–10 weeks after admission, when symptoms of relocation stress are most likely to appear. Findings from these studies indicate that the incidence of relocation stress may be overestimated.

Despite the research of Capezuti and colleagues (2006), and others, suggesting the adaptability of older adults who are involuntarily transferred, the bulk of research suggests that individuals are better able to meet the challenges of relocation if they have a sense of control over the circumstances and have the confidence to carry out the needed activities associated with a move. Self-efficacy, defined as the individual's judgment about being able to perform a particular activity, may be an important variable in positive adjustment to relocation. The Self-Efficacy Relocation Scale (SERS), developed by Rossen and Gruber (2007), can be used to assess self-efficacy in individuals who are relocating, identify potential pre-relocation adjustment issues, and guide interventions to promote positive relocation outcomes.

Relocation Trauma

A variety of terms have been used to describe the results of relocation: *relocation trauma, relocation shock, translocation shock,* and *transfer trauma. Relocation trauma* describes a stressful move from one environment to another. If you have moved from one city to another, you will understand the stress of this transition. It takes time to adjust to any move. During a move, an older adult may have less personal energy available than a younger adult to cope with the stress of the move. Not only do aging individuals have less energy than younger individuals, older adults may be already using a considerable amount of energy to cope with some of the chronic conditions with which they are suffering, such as chronic obstructive pulmonary disease or the residual effects of a cardiovascular accident. If an acute condition (whether a flare-up of a chronic disease, or an acute experience of the flu) requires additional coping strategies, then the older adult may find that his coping skills have been exhausted. This may make the move seem insurmountable. Thus the transition from one setting to another may be termed *relocation trauma.*

Relocation is a stressor, and sometimes a crisis, for the older adult and the family. Relocation to a long-term care facility is one of the more stressful kinds of relocations and one that many older adults dread. The dramatic change in both physical and social demands as a result of long-term care placement has been widely discussed in the literature as a life stress event for older adults. Accordingly, researchers have attempted to untangle the challenges older adults encounter in making the transition from home on the "outside" to life in a long-term care facility. Researchers have identified that older adults experience feelings of abandonment, a lack of privacy within the long-term care facility, and decreased opportunities for contact with family and friends. These different losses experienced when transitioning into long-term care cause much suffering for these older adults. Not only do new residents need to learn to adjust to the public nature of living in long-term care, but they need to adjust to the restrictions imposed by institutional rules and regulations. "I've always been the boss, and now I'm being told what to do!" said one man whose transition to long-term care was described by him as being a shock.[3] And, they have to adapt to the close proximity of sick and confused people; they may feel that it is only a matter of time before they end up in a similar condition as their very ill co-residents. "I just have to keep moving!" said this same gentleman as he ambulated with his walker, glancing at someone in a wheelchair. With the stresses involved in moving into long-term care facilities, it is no wonder that the term *relocation stress syndrome* is sometimes used within health care literature. Relocation stress syndrome is a nursing diagnosis characterized by symptoms such as anxiety, confusion, hopelessness, and loneliness. It usually occurs in older adults shortly after moving from a private residence into long-term care (Walker et al., 2007).

Consequences of Relocation: Health Decline

Some researchers have theorized about the reasons behind the decline in health status of some older adults who have been relocated. Their theories can be divided into three main categories: the older adult (patient/client), facility effects, and the transfer effects. Research on the effects on older adults has focused on their direct experience of the relocation. Hypotheses have changed over time as researchers attempt to ferret out what factors lead to health decline. One hypothesis is that those who are relocated are more ill compared to those who are not relocated; thus, the illness itself is the reason for the transfer. The underlying assumption of this hypothesis is that the relocation did not cause illness, but rather the illness in essence caused the relocation.

Another theory addressing the impact of relocation upon older adults is the stress hypothesis. This hypothesis focuses on the stress experienced by new residents due to the lack of personal control experienced when being relocated and after the move. The stress of relocation can then lead to health decline (Ewen & Kinney, 2013; Walker et al., 2007).

The effect of facilities upon older adults is another category of theories examining the impact of relocation upon seniors. Within this category, the

---

3. As a side note, this elderly gentleman adjusted more easily to months on a hospital ward, because there he had the hope of getting better and going home. When that lengthy hospitalization resulted in transfer into long-term care, that hope was extinguished.

underlying premise is that a decline in the health of a resident may be due to the lack of "fit" between the older adult and new facility. The new facility must be able to handle the medical requirements of the transfer patient, especially if it is possible that his health status could decline upon transfer. For instance, can a facility handle issues related to a mental illness of the older adult, or can the facility manage issues related to an older adult's extreme obesity (Lane, 2007)? It has been documented that those older patients who experience an easy adjustment to their new environment fare better than patients who have a difficult transition.

The transition theory category focuses on the impact of the transfer upon older adults, specifically, the varying levels of care and support received by older adults through the transfer. The underlying hypothesis in this theory is that the quality of transfer differs between older adults; there are varying levels of care at facilities, and some provide better individualized care and attention than others. How well individuals are received and helped in the transition then impacts how well they transition to a new facility (Walker et al., 2007).

It is also important to remember that the characteristics of the transfer itself can influence the impact relocation has on older adults. Thorough preparation by all members of the health care team can contribute to the success of the relocation. Preparation for the physical transfer involves anticipating and allowing for adequate time for necessary preparations to be put into place. (Sometimes transfers are so rushed that important details to be communicated between health care professionals may be missed). It involves preparing the older adult emotionally for the change, and providing a meaningful "send-off" as he leaves one home for another. One hospice, when transferring a resident to a long-term care facility or to home, has a card signed by staff, and opportunity for staff and family to say goodbye over a cup of tea.[4] Research has highlighted the importance of proper patient monitoring and being sufficiently prepared for adverse events as being essential to making a patient transfer successful.

Transitions Within and Between Health Care Facilities and Home

Relocation transitions can have negative physical and psychological effects on all clients/patients, regardless of age and type of facility. These effects

---

4. Though transfers *out* of a palliative care setting are not the norm, they do happen. Sometimes the condition of a terminally ill person can stabilize, and their health care needs can be then met at home or within long-term care.

are more pronounced in those over 80 years, particularly those who are frail. Acute care patients and long-term care residents are at an elevated mortality risk when they are relocated. Studies examining the effect of transferring (relocating) different patient groups between institutions have found that transferred patients were at an elevated mortality risk between 1.99 and 3.76 times greater than those patients who were not transferred (Robinson, 2002). Contradictory studies that have not found an increased mortality risk for transferred patients often have methodological problems. Some of the methodological concerns include small sample sizes, inadequate statistical power, and a lack of control groups.

Evidence from the United States indicates that transfers between care settings are frequent in the last few months of life but may produce little improvement in symptom or pain control (Van den Block, Deschepper, Bilsen, Van Casteren, & Deliens, 2007). Hanratty and colleagues' (2012) study was designed to explore the experiences of older adults as they moved between places of care near the end of their lives. They interviewed 30 adults between the ages of 69 and 93 years of age who had been identified by their physicians as being in the last year of their lives. The research participants described the difficulties they faced in transfers between facilities. They described institutional processes that included little flexibility for patients, being released out of hospital before they felt prepared, feeling unheard by health care professionals and care that, at times, lacked dignity (for instance, when false teeth were lost). The older adults who were interviewed also mentioned professionals who were very responsive to their needs. Clearly, the need to provide not just safe transfers, but also transfers that recognize the needs of those being relocated, is critical to ailing older adults.

Not only can transitions be difficult between facilities, transitions between units within the *same* facility can be precarious for older adults. When patients are transferred from one unit to another, there can be adverse events, such as medication errors and falls (Blay, Duffield, & Gallagher, 2012). These adverse events have greater impact upon older patients than their younger counterparts, due to physiological issues. After a medication error, an older adult may experience confusion or delirium and take months to become cognitively lucid. The need to minimize the number of unit to unit transfers during a single hospitalization is key; reduced moves within a hospitalization is associated with more consistent nursing care, fewer adverse incidents (e.g., health care associated infections, falls, and medication errors), shorter hospital stays, and lower overall costs (Kanak et al., 2008).

Although many older adults are thrilled to transition from hospital to home, the transition can be challenging and fraught with surprises for aging adults (Fabbre, Buffington, Altfeld, Shier, & Golden, 2011). The transition from hospital to home can carry risks, especially for older adults who have multiple health concerns (Naylor & Keating, 2008). In addition to experiencing medication errors, a poor transition may result in placement into a long-term care facility, increased caregiver burden, and increased health costs (Coleman, Parry, Chalmers, & Min, 2006). Lower income seniors may encounter difficulties accessing care when home from hospital, but may be too ashamed to admit this to professionals (Kangovi et al., 2014). Awareness of these consequences has grown substantially in the past decade among health care providers, administrators, and third-party insurers. Several randomized control trials have studied the effectiveness of specific interventions to enhance the transition process, including the use of nurse-led case management programs (Chow & Wong, 2014).

Long-term care facility placement

Although there is a body of literature addressing older adults' post-placement challenges, less is known about the actual *process* of how these older adults handle these challenges and adjust after long-term care facility placement. The transition, the *relocation*, into a long-term care facility is a common and significant event for older adults. And as noted within this chapter, the transition to long-term care can be very difficult for older adults. In 1963, the first study on the effects of relocation from one long-term care facility to another roused much attention with its findings that a high mortality rate was associated with the move (Aldrich & Mendkoff, 1963). And yet, over the years, we have realized that the picture is not as bleak as perhaps revealed in the aforementioned study; there can be benefits of admission. Quinn and colleagues (2009) examined the influence of admission upon procedures related to diabetes mellitus for residents with dementia in 59 Maryland long-term care facilities. Results indicated that these newly admitted residents experienced higher levels of monitoring procedures (such as fasting glucose level testing) in the year after admission than they had experienced in the year before admission. The implication is that the policies of the facility may have contributed to resident health through regular monitoring (Quinn et al., 2009). Other researchers have documented psychological benefits in the form of increased friendships (Wolff, 2013) and reduction in psychiatric symptoms (Bakker et al., 2011). And it must be noted that since the early 1960s, much work has been done in long-term care to raise the level of care for residents.

What do older adults experience when transitioning to long-term care? Generally speaking, the initial transition period is the most difficult. Older adults may experience sadness, anger, loneliness, betrayal, and fear (Brandburg, 2007; Heliker & Scholler-Jaquish, 2006; Wiersma, 2010). During the first six to eight weeks, they may feel overwhelmed, homeless (Heliker & Scholler-Jaquish, 2006), and in a state of disorganization (Brooke, 1989). However, as noted by researchers, many older adults move toward acceptance during the first year. For instance, Wilson (1997) interviewed newly admitted older adults 24 hours after admission, every second day for two weeks post admission and one month after admission. She postulated that the transition into a long-term care facility involved three phases: overwhelmed phase, adjustment phase, and initial acceptance phase (Wilson, 1997). Similarly, Lee, Woo, and Mackenzie (2002) reported that Hong Kong Chinese residents went through four stages in adjusting to long-term care and trying to regain some semblance of normalcy in their lives: orienting, normalizing, rationalizing, and stabilizing. While Johnson and Bibbo (2014) reported that individuals moving into a long-term care facility did not consider it to be a home, they actively changed their attitudes toward it in order to adjust. The implication is that while the initial transition to long-term care can be traumatic, aging adults may adapt to this new setting and regain their stability.

The Family Lens

There is consensus within the literature that placing a loved one into a long-term care facility is a painful and stressful experience for many family members (Park, Butcher, & Maas, 2004). The decision to place a loved one has long been considered one of the most difficult decisions that family members will make and can be truly gut-wrenching. Indeed, most caregivers prefer to take care of their family members with chronic conditions at home and regard the long-term care facility placement as the last resort.

When placing an older adult, family members may experience very strong, yet ambivalent emotions, including sadness, grief, guilt, anxiety, and relief (Kao, Travis, & Acton, 2004; Reuss, Dupois, & Whitfield, 2005). Relocation experiences are perceived more negatively when family members feel that they have had to make the placement decision on their own (with little support from professionals) (Davies & Nolan, 2003), and when they believe staff members lack compassion or empathy toward their situation (Strang, Dupuis-Blanchard, Donaldson, Nordstrom, & Thompson, 2006). It is important to note that placement of an older adult may decrease some stress, and yet magnify other stresses. For instance, Garity (2006) reported that family carers experienced relief from the physical exhaustion of caregiving, yet the emotional burden of placement, including guilt and worry for the future, continued for some despite admission of an older member to a long-term care facility.

We also believe that a cultural lens needs to be applied to the relocation experience. Specifically, what precipitating events tend to lead to placement of elders from various ethnicities, such as Asian older adults? This is a particularly salient question, as in the past, Asian families were less likely to place their older adults. In one study, Chinese family caregivers (living in Taiwan) began to consider placement when their older members displayed disturbing, destructive, or risky behaviors (Chang & Schneider, 2010). The aforementioned study examined placement decisions in relation to Asian Chinese within an overseas context; however, studies that examine the relationship of housing and ethnic minorities living *within* Canada are sparse. As an exception, Weeks and LeBlanc (2010) examined the housing concerns of Aboriginal elders and older adults from visible minorities. Aboriginal individuals are considered one of the most poorly housed groups within Canada (Weeks & LeBlanc, 2010). The researchers concluded that many minority older adults (including those who are Aboriginal, have disabilities such as intellectual disabilities, or are from another ethnic minority) have many concerns: the costs of housing (including renting); the possibility of relocating due to an inability to afford their current housing; the inappropriateness of their current location (e.g., house too small, heating problems, not enough bedrooms, difficulty in using stairs, lack of security related to power outages); a lack of housing options, in particular, low-cost housing options (long waiting lists); and the importance of cultural appropriateness. For instance, older Aboriginal adults and those from other ethnic minorities felt that they were not accepted in the dominant culture of their neighborhoods (Weeks & LeBlanc, 2010). Cultural concerns impact all housing transitions, including long-term care placement.

Family members need considerable support when an older person moves into a long-term care facility. In particular, family members desire emotional support and good communication with the staff caring for their older members (Davies, 2005; Strang et al., 2006). We cannot stress the importance of emotional support enough; no matter how extenuating the circumstances, or how rational the placement decision is, family members often feel that they have in some way failed the older adult. And this sense of failure leads to guilt and much grief.

Interventions to Promote Positive Transition Experiences

In order to facilitate positive transition experiences, conversations with the older adult (and possibly family members) should take place to explore what type of housing option is most suitable. Knowledge of the various kinds of housing options is vital, especially for aging adults who are vulnerable, including those from different ethnicities, impoverished individuals, and those with significant physical or mental illness or disability.

For example, if it is determined that an appropriate option is assisted living, then it is important to get a written outline of what services are or are not available from the facility. The older adult will also want to inquire into the staffing, security features, exit processes (e.g., if an individual's health deteriorates, can she access staff to assist her, or is she obligated to move out of the residence?). She will also want to know specific details about the size of the suite, how many bedrooms there are, and other particulars, so that she knows what belongings she can bring from her current home.

In order to assist older adults with relocation decisions and adjustment, health and human service professionals should be aware of resources available to the older person, assess the older adult's relocation needs, individualize a realistic relocation plan, promote coping while making a relocation decision, assist with pre-move preparation, and facilitate continuity of care. After relocation, health and human service professionals should: tailor interventions to the older adult's values and preferences; promote the individual's sense of control, autonomy, and mastery; provide social support and activities; promote coping with relocation; orient the person to the new surroundings; maintain continuity of care; and ensure that physical and psychosocial needs are met. And, research has indicated that the timing of the decision-making is also an important factor to consider; the move to retirement living needs to happen "before it's too late" (Walker & McNamara, 2013, p. 448). All in all, no small feat!

Thinking About Shared Housing

Health and human service professionals should be familiar with the variety of housing options in their communities and be knowledgeable about the rights of tenants in assisted living facilities, low cost seniors' complexes, or other facilities. They may also have to answer questions from family members when it is suggested that an older adult move into the home of an adult child. This can feel uncomfortable for the professional, particularly if the older adult and family members disagree on the course of action. The following questions may guide the conversation.

FIGURE 1   Thinking about adding an older family member to one's home.

Questions that might be asked of family members and the older adult:

- What are the needs of the new household member and of the family?
- Where will space be provided for the new member?
- What space will be provided for the older member?
- How will the new member be included in existing family patterns?
- How will responsibilities be shared?
- What resources in the community will assist in the adjustment?
- Is the environment safe for the new member?
- How will family life change with the older member?
- How does each family member feel about the addition of the new member?
- What are the differences in the routines of the new member and the current household pattern?
- What are the older person's expectations?
- Will there be a change in household roles and responsibilities?
- Will the older member be making a contribution to household expenses?

Addressing these questions *prior* to older adults moving into family members' homes may prevent uncomfortable conversations *after* the move has taken place.

Improving Transitions Across the Continuum of Care

Health and human service professionals in hospitals, the community, and long-term care facilities frequently care for older adults who have experienced relocation. They therefore have a responsibility to help older adults and their family members to understand the impact of relocation and to help facilitate the adjustment to this transition. The first issue to address in any move is whether it is necessary and whether it will provide the least restrictive lifestyle appropriate for the individual. For older adults who are not functioning or are not safe within their homes, health and human service professionals may need to refer their clients to home care for an assessment to determine the level of placement required. Home care professionals can then place these individuals on a wait list, if placement is deemed appropriate. Additional professional interventions include the need to assess the impact of relocation and determine how to mitigate any negative reactions. This can involve providing information to aging adults and their family members, as well as extending emotional support. As will be discussed in Chapters 6 and 7, this may also involve "standing with" family members as they try to make sense of how to relate to the aging individual, as well as their siblings, as they navigate this transition.

It is important that health and human service professionals recognize the complexity of the health care needs of older adults and are aware that aging individuals often require care in multiple settings across the continuum. Thus, they experience multiple care transitions. Care transition refers to movement of patients from one health care practitioner or setting to another as their condition and care needs change. Transitional care requires that health and human service professionals utilize a set of clinical and communication interventions to facilitate the moves of older adults from one care setting to another. To illustrate, an older adult may be treated by a family practitioner, hospitalized and treated by a nurse practitioner, discharged home or to an assisted living facility, where the family practitioner may or may not continue to follow her. (Many health care providers practice in only one setting and are not familiar with the specific requirements of other settings.) As a result, there are often significant misunderstandings and criticism of care in the different settings across the continuum.

In order to address the typical complexity of care transitions experienced by older adults, intervention strategies have been developed. In a review of the literature, four well-developed transitional care intervention strategies were located. The Transitional Care Model (Naylor et al., 2010), Project RED [Re-Engineered hospital Discharge] (Jack et al., 2009), the Care Transitions Intervention (Coleman, Parry, Chalmers, & Min, 2006;

Coleman et al., 2004) and BOOST [Better Outcomes for Older adults through Safe Transitions] (Society of Hospital Medicine, 2011) all serve the hospitalized older adult population with a goal of decreasing readmissions, while maintaining a high level of patient satisfaction. Secondary goals common to all the programs include increasing the patient's ability to self-manage health care.

There are several programmatic differences among these transition programs. Some programs are limited to hospital-based interventions and contact, whereas others follow the patient into the post-discharge environment. Another difference is the professional identified to provide the interventions. The Transitional Care Model and the Care Transitions Intervention provide advance practice nurses and nurse transition coaches to coordinate and provide the interventions both in hospital and after discharge. Home visits and follow-up phone calls are used by both these programs to provide education on disease management and to reinforce adherence to care plans. In contrast, Project RED and BOOST focus on interprofessional hospital care teams to implement the intervention.

Not all transitional care models utilize nurses, however. Watkins, Hall, and Kring (2012) reported on the results of a study designed to evaluate a transitional care model using a social worker navigator for at-risk older adults being discharged from hospital to home. The purpose of their study was to evaluate the effectiveness of an innovative hospital to home transition program that used a social worker navigator who identified frail elders at risk for readmission (further hospitalizations) during their current hospitalization and followed them into their home environments. The navigator focused not only on health-related needs but also on instrumental activities of daily living (IADLs) to ensure a successful transition; for example, the navigator may have worked with an individual in helping them to plan a ride to the bank, so that this frail elder could manage his finances. Their results demonstrated the importance of extending social support and health education into the home after discharge from hospital. The navigator reinforced medical management and connected participants to appropriate community resources in order to remain safe at home.

When the Transition Is to a Long-Term Care Facility

Nolan and colleagues (1996) proposed a four-stage typology that describes how admission to a long-term care facility occurs (the process). The typology ranges from an ideal type of admission into long-term care to a less desirable kind of admission. The best kind of admission process is termed a *positive choice.* This occurs when an admission is planned and the older member is fully involved in the discussion and decision-making process. The second type of admission is the *rationalized alternative.* This is the most frequent form of admission. While there is less choice on the part of the older adult, the aging individual is still able to create and sustain a perception that the admission is legitimate and/or reversible. The third type of admission is the *discredited option.* This type starts as a positive choice or rationalized alternative but after admission, the resident finds that the situation is not as was expected. For instance, she may have expected a private room but, upon admission, finds that this is not possible. The *fait accompli* is the worst-case scenario where virtually all the basic conditions for an acceptable move are absent. The older adult did not anticipate the move, others may have made the decision, and there was no opportunity to explore alternatives and prepare emotionally for the move (Nolan et al., 1996). When at all possible, health and human service professionals, as well as family members, should aim to facilitate transitions to long-term care facilities that fall within the positive choice category (Nolan et al., 1996), whereby aging adults are involved in the process of decision-making.

Unfortunately, it is not always possible to involve older adults in the decision-making process. However, on a more pragmatic level, there are simple interventions that health and human service professionals can do to promote positive adaptation to relocation to a long-term care facility. For instance, on the first day of the move for the older adult, stimulation and the introduction of new activities and people should be limited. The older adult can be oriented to the environment slowly, so that he can incorporate new ideas and routines gradually and at a pace that he feels comfortable with. Specifically, on the first day, limit introductions to only those key people and places that are necessary; for an aging individual just admitted to a facility, the only important place to be orientated to might be the dining room. Health and human service professionals can seek out ways to help the older adult make connections between the old environment and the new one. The more familiar the older adult is with the new environment, the easier the transition will be.

It is important to note that family also require support during any relocation, but most noticeably when an older member is admitted into long-term care. Sussman and Dupuis (2012) noted that when families were not given the opportunity before the move to emotionally accept the placement decision, they tended to experience more adjustment issues in the period following admission. This bears witness to the fact that health and human service professionals work with two clients—the older adult and the family.

SUMMARY

Within this chapter we have provided an overview of the housing options available to older adults. Basic guidelines for the housing of older adults includes facilitating as much personal decision-making as possible, selecting the least restrictive environment, and providing support for older adults and family members prior to the transition, during the transition, and after the relocation. Long-term care facilities and other health care housing options for older adults are currently undergoing major changes, and these changes are likely to continue well into this century. We suggest that changes need to continue in order to facilitate appropriate housing for older adults, particularly those who are most vulnerable. Some suggested changes will be offered in Chapter 8 (Future Directions).

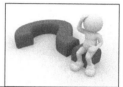

CRITICAL THINKING EXERCISES

- ▶ Ask an older family member what items within the home are significant and why. Consider what items you might select from your own personal environment if you were entering an assisted living facility or a long-term care environment.

- ▶ In your clinical experience, what settings have you encountered? Explore with colleagues how the environment might influence the older adult, his or her family, and your own professional role.

- ▶ Design your ideal home, recognizing that aging brings physical, functional, psychological, spiritual, and other changes.

INTERESTING WEBSITES

- ▶ Canada Housing and Mortgage Association: https://www.cmhc-schl.gc.ca/en/inpr/bude/hoolca/

- ▶ Service Canada: http://www.servicecanada.gc.ca/eng/about/publication/bundling_seniors/index.shtml

- ▶ US Department of Housing and Urban Development, Information for Seniors: http://portal.hud.gov/hudportal/HUD?src=/topics/information_for_senior_citizens

► Medicare.gov—Your Guide To Choosing a Nursing Home or Other Long-term Care: https://www.medicare.gov/Pubs/pdf/02174.pdf

REFERENCES

Aldrich, C., & Mendkoff, E. (1963). Relocation of the aged and disabled: A mortality study. *Journal of the American Geriatrics Society, 11*, 185–194.

Aminzadeh, F., Dalziel, W. B., Molnar, F. J., & Garcia., L. J. (2009). Symbolic meaning of relocation to a residential care facility for persons with dementia, *Aging and Mental Health, 13*(3), 487–496. doi:10.1080/13607860802607314

Bakker, T. J., Duivenvoorden, H. J., van der Lee, J., Rikkert, M. G., Beekman, A. T., & Ribbe, M. W. (2011). Integrative psychotherapeutic nursing home program to reduce multiple psychiatric symptoms of cognitively impaired patients and caregiver burden: Randomized controlled trial. *American Journal of Geriatric Psychiatry, 19*(6), 507–520. doi:10.1097/JGP.0b013e3181eafdc6

Bekhet, A. K., Zauszniewski, J. A., & Nakhla, W. E. (2009). Reasons for relocation to retirement communities: A qualitative study. *Western Journal of Nursing Research, 31*(4), 426–479. doi:10.1177/0193945909332009

Bellantonio, S., Kenny, A. M., Fortinsky, R., Kleppinger, A., Robison, J., Gruman, C., Kulldorff, M., & Trella, P. (2008). Efficacy of a geriatric team intervention for residents in dementia-specific assisted living facilities: Effect on unanticipated transition. *Journal of the American Geriatrics Society, 56*(3), 523–528. doi:10.1111/j.1532-5415.2007.01591.x

Blay, N., Duffield, C. M., & Gallagher, R. (2012). Patient transfers in Australia: Implications for nursing workload and patient outcomes. *Journal of Nursing Management, 20*, 302–310. doi:10.1111/j.1365-2834.2011.01279.x

Brandburg, G. L. (2007). Making the transition to nursing home life: A framework to help older adults adapt to the long-term care environment. *Journal of Gerontological Nursing, 33*(6), 50–56.

Brainy Quote. (2015). Retrieved December 9, 2014, from: www.brainyquote.com

Brooke, V. (1989). How elders adjust. *Geriatric Nursing, 10*(2), 66–68.

Cangelosi, P. R., & Sorrell, J. M. (2010). Walking for therapy with man's best friend. *Journal of Psychosocial Nursing & Mental Health Services, 48*(3), 19–22.

Capezuti, E., Boltz, M., Renz, S., Hoffman, D., & Norman, R. G. (2006). Nursing home involuntary relocation: Clinical outcomes and perceptions of residents and families. *Journal of the American Medical Directors Association, 7*(8), 486–492. doi:http://dx.doi.org/10.1016/j.jamda.2006.02.011

Chang, Y. P., & Schneider, J. K. (2010). Decision-making process of continuing care facility placement among Chinese family caregivers. *Perspectives in Psychiatric Care, 46*(2), 108–117. doi:10.1111/j.1744-6163.2010.00246.x

Chappell, N. L., Havens, B., Hollander, M., Miller, J. A., & McWilliam, C. (2004). Comparative costs of home care and residential care. *The Gerontologist, 44*(3), 389–400. doi:10.1093/geront/44.3.389

Chow, S. K. Y., & Wong, F. K. Y. (2014). A randomized controlled trial of a nurse-led case management programme for hospital-discharged older adults with co-morbidities, *Journal of Advanced Nursing, 70*(10), 2257–2271. doi:10.1111/jan.12375

Coleman, E. A., Parry, C., Chalmers, S., & Min, S. J. (2006). The care transitions intervention: Results of a randomized controlled trial. *Archives of Internal Medicine, 166*(17), 1822–1828. doi:10.1001/archinte.166.17.1822

Coleman, E. A., Smith, J. D., Frank, J., Min, S., Parry, C., & Kramer, A. M. (2004). Preparing patients and caregivers to participate in care delivered across settings: The Care Transitions Intervention. *Journal of the American Geriatrics Society, 52*(11), 1817–1825.

Crisp, D., Windsor, T. D., Anstey, K., & Butterworth, P. (2013). What are older adults seeking? Factors encouraging or discouraging retirement village living. *Australasian Journal on Ageing, 32*(3), 163–170. doi:10.1111/j.1741-6612.2012.00623.x

Davies, S. (2005). Meleis' theory of nursing transitions and relatives' experiences of nursing home entry. *Journal of Advanced Nursing, 52*(6), 658–671. doi:10.1111/j.1365-2648.2005.03637.x

Davies, S., & Nolan, M. (2003). Making the best of things: Relatives' experiences of decisions about care-home entry. *Ageing & Society, 23*(4), 429–450. doi:http://dx.doi.org/10.1017/S0144686X03001259

Ewen, H. H., Hahn, S. J., Erickson, M. A., & Krout, J. A. (2014). Aging in place or relocation? Plans of community-dwelling older adults. *Journal of Housing for the Elderly, 28*(3), 288–309. doi:10.1080/02763893.2014.930366

Ewen, H. H., & Kinney, J. (2013). Application of the model of allostasis to older women's relocation to senior housing. *Biological Research for Nursing.* Retrieved December 29, 2014, from: http://brn.sagepub.com/content/early/2013/01/28/1099800412474682 doi:10.1177/1099800412474682

Fabbre, V. D., Buffington, A., Altfeld, S. J., Shier, G. E., & Golden, R. L. (2011). Social work and transitions of care: Observations from an intervention for older adults. *Journal of Gerontological Social Work, 54*(6), 617–625. doi:10.1080/01634372.2011.589100

Fox, A. (2010). HomeShare—An intergenerational solution to housing and support needs. *Housing, Care and Support, 13*(3), 21–26. http://dx.doi.org/10.5042/hcs.2010.0707

Furlotte, C., Schwartz, K., Koornstra, J. J., & Naster, R. (2012). Got a room for me? Housing experiences of older adults living with HIV/AIDS in Ottawa. *Canadian Journal on Aging, 31*(1), 37–48. doi:http://dx.doi.org/10.1017/S0714980811000584

Garity, J. (2006). Caring for a family member with Alzheimer's disease: Coping with caregiver burden post-nursing home placement. *Journal of Gerontological Nursing, 32*(4), 39–48.

Geller, L. (2015). Age-friendly communities. *The Canadian Nurse, 111*(1), 23–27.

Gillsjo, C., & Schwartz-Barcott, D. (2011). A concept analysis of home and its meaning in the lives of three older adults. *International Journal of Older People Nursing, 6*(1), 4–12. doi:10.1111/j.1748-3743.2010.00207.x

Hanratty, B., Holmes, L., Lowson, E., Grande, G., Addington-Hall, J., Payne, S., & Seymour, J. (2012). Older adults' experiences of transitions between care settings at the end of life in England: A qualitative interview study. *Journal of Pain and Symptom Management, 44*(1), 75–83. doi:10.1016/j. jpainsymman.2011.08.0

Heliker, D. M., & Scholler-Jaquish, A. (2006). Transition of new residents: Basing practice on residents' perspective. *Journal of Gerontological Nursing, 32*(9), 34–42.

Heppenstall, C. P., Keeling, S., Hanger, H. C., & Wilkinson, T. J. (2014). Perceived factors which shape decision-making around time of residential care admission in older adults: A qualitative study. *Australasian Journal on Ageing, 33*(1), 9–13. doi:10.1111/j.1741- 6612.2012.00644x

Hollander, J. (1991). The idea of a home: A kind of space. *Social Research, 58*(1), 31–49.

Hutchings, D., Wells, J. L., O'Brien, K., Wells, C., Alteen, A. M., & Cake, L. J. (2011). From institution to 'home': Family perspectives on a unique relocation process. *Canadian Journal on Aging, 30*(2), 223–232. doi:http://dx.doi. org/10.1017/S0714980811000043

Imber-Black, E. (2009). Snuggles, my cotherapist, and other animal tales in life and therapy. *Family Process, 48*(4), 459–461. doi:10.1111/j.1545-5300.2009.01295.x

Jack, B. W., Chetty, V. K., Anthony, D., Greenwald, J. L., Sanchez, G. M., Johnson, A. E., & Culpepper, L. (2009). A reengineered hospital discharge program to decrease rehospitalisation: A randomized trial. *Annals of Internal Medicine, 150*(3), 178–187.

Johnson, R. A., & Bibbo, J. (2014). Relocation decisions and constructing the meaning of home: A phenomenological study of the transition into a nursing home. *Journal of Aging Studies, 30*, 56–63.

Kaida, L., Moyser, M., & Park, S. Y. (2009). Cultural preferences and economic constraints:The living arrangements of elderly Canadians. *Canadian Journal on Aging 28*(4), 303–313. doi:http://dx.doi.org/10.1017/S0714980809990146

Kanak, M., Titler, M., Shever, L., Fei, Q., Dochterman, J., & Picone, D. M. (2008). The effects of hospitalization on multiple units. *Applied Nursing Research, 21*(1), 15–22. http://dx.doi.org.ezproxy.lib.ucalgary.ca/10.1016/j.apnr.2006.07.001

Kangovi, S., Levy, K., Barg, F. K., Carter, T., Long, & Grande, D. (2014). Perspectives of older adults of low socioeconomic status on the post-hospital transition, *Journal of Health Care for the Poor and Underserved, 25*(2), 746–756 | 10.1353/hpu.2014.0111

Kao, H. F., Travis, S. S., & Acton, G. J. (2004). Relocation to a long-term care facility: Workingwith patients and families before, during and after. *Journal of Psychosocial Nursing &Mental Health Services, 42*(3), 10–16.

Keene, J. R., & Batson, C. D. (2010). Under one roof: A review of research on intergenerational coresidence and multigenerational households in the United States. *Sociology Compass, 4*(8), 642–657. doi:10.1111/j.1751-9020.2010.00306.x

Kennedy, C. (2010). The city of 2050—An age-friendly, vibrant, intergenerational community. *Generations, 34*(3), 70–75.

Lane, A. M. (2007). *The social organization of placement in geriatric mental health.* Unpublished doctoral dissertation, University of Calgary.

Lane, A. M., Hirst, S. P., & Reed, M. B. (2013). Housing options for North American older adults with HIV/AIDS. *Indian Journal of Gerontology, 27*(1), 55–68.

Lee, D. T. F., Woo, J., & Mackenzie, A. E. (2002). The cultural context of adjusting to nursing home life: Chinese elders' perspectives. *The Gerontologist, 42*(5), 667–675. doi:10.1093/geront/42.5.667

Leland, N., Porell, F., & Murphy, S. L. (2011). Does fall history influence residential adjustment? *Gerontologist, 51*(2), 190–200. doi:10.1093/geront/gng086

Lewinson, T., & Morgan, K. (2014). Living in extended-stay hotels: Older residents' perceptions of satisfying and stressful environmental conditions. *Journal of Housing for the Elderly, 28*(3), 243–267. doi:10.1080/02763893.2014.899540

McGarry, P. (2012). Good places to grow old: Age-friendly cities in Europe. *Journal of Intergenerational Relationships, 10*(2), 201–204. doi:10.1080/15350770.2012.672123

Naylor, M. D., Brooten, D., Campbell, R., Jacobsen, B. S., Mezey, M. D., Pauly, M. D., & Swartz, S. J. (2010). Comprehensive discharge planning and follow-up of hospitalized elders: A randomized clinical trial. *Journal of the American Geriatric Society, 281*(7), 613–620. doi:10.1001/jama.281.7.613.

Naylor, M., & Keating, N. (2008). Transitional care: Moving patients from one care setting to another. *American Journal of Nursing, 108*(9 Suppl), 58–63. doi:10.1097/01.NAJ.0000336420.34946.3a

New York Academy of Medicine (-). AgeFriendlyNYC. Retrieved December 9, 2014, from: http://www.nyam.org/agefriendlynyc/

Nolan, M., Walker, G., Nolan, J., Williams, S., Poland, F., Curran, M., & Kent, B. C. (1996). Entry to care: Positive choices or fait accompli? Developing a more proactive nursing response to the needs of older people and their carers. *Journal of Advanced Nursing, 24*(2), 265–274. doi:10.1046/j.1365-2648.1996.01966.x

Oxford dictionary. (2015). Retrieved February 10, 2015, from: www.oed.com

Park, M., Butcher, H. K., & Maas, M. L. (2004). A thematic analysis of Korean family caregivers' experience in making the decision to place a family member with dementia in a long-term care facility. *Research in Nursing & Health, 27*(5), 345–356. doi:10.1002/nur.20031

Parker-Pope, T. (2009, December 14). The best walking partner: Man vs. dog. *The New York Times.* Retrieved February 10, 2015, from: http://well.blogs. nytimes.com/2009/12/14/the-best-walking-partner-man-vs-dog/?_r=0

Perkins, M. M., Ball, M. M., Whittington, F. J., & Hollingsworth, C. (2012). Relational autonomy in assisted living: A focus on diverse care settings for older adults. *Journal of Aging Studies, 26*(2), 214–225.

Perks, T., & Haan, M. (2010). The dwelling-type choices of older Canadians and future housing demands: An investigation using the aging and social support survey (GSS16). *Canadian Journal on Aging, 29*(3), 445–463. doi:http:// dx.doi.org/10.1017/S0714980810000413

Public Health Agency of Canada (PHAC). (2008). *Age-friendly communities.* Retrieved February 10, 2015, from: www.phac-aspc.gc.ca/seniors-aines/afc-caa-eng.php

Quinn, C. C., Gruber-Baldini, A. L., Port, C. L., May, C., Stuart, B., Hebel, J. R., Zimmerman, S., Burton, L., Zuckerman, I. H., Fahlman, C., & Magaziner, J. (2009). The role of nursing home admission and dementia status on care for diabetes mellitus. *Journal of the American Geriatrics Society, 57*(9), 1628–1633. doi:10.1111/j.1532-5415.2009.02382.x

Redfoot, D., & Gaberlavage, G. (1991). Housing for older Americans: Sustaining the dream. *Generations, 15*(3), 35–38.

Reuss, G., Dupuis, S. L., & Whitfield, K. (2005). Understanding the experience of moving a loved one to a long-term care facility. *Journal of Gerontological Social Work, 46*(1), 17–46. doi:10.1300/J083v46n01_03

Robinson, V. (2002). *A brief literature review of the effects of relocation on the elderly.* Prepared for The Hospital Employee Union of British Columbia.

Rossen, E. K., & Gruber, K. J. (2007). Development and psychometric testing of the Relocation Self-Efficacy Scale. *Nursing Research, 56*(4), 244–251. doi:10.1097/01.NNR.0000280609.16244.de

Rural Assistance Center. (2002–2014). Rural aging. Retrieved December 9, 2014, from: www.raconline.org/topics/aging

Scharlach, A. E. (2009). Creating age-friendly communities. *Generations, 33*(2), 5–10.

Society of Hospital Medicine. (2011). Project BOOST: Better outcomes for older adults through safe transitions. Retrieved February 6, 2015, from: www. hospitalmedicine.org/AM/Template.cfm?Section=Home&Template=/CM/ HTMLDisplay.cfm&ContentID=27577

Steinisch, M. (2007). Senior homesharing a win-win. Retrieved February 6, 2015, from: http://hffo.cuna.org/36473/article/1802/html

Stevenson, D. G., & Grabowski, D. C. (2010). Sizing up the market for assisted living. *Health Affairs, 29*(1), 35–43. doi:10.1377/hlthaff.2009.0527

Strang, V., Dupuis-Blanchard, S., Donaldson, C., Nordstrom, M., & Thompson, B. (2006). Family caregivers and transitions to long term care. *Clinical Nursing Research, 15*(1), 27–45. doi:10.1177/1054773805282356

Strohschein, L. (2012). I want to move, but cannot: Characteristics of involuntary stayers and associations with health among Canadian seniors. *Journal of Aging and Health, 24*(5), 735–751. doi:10.1177/0898264311432312

Sussman, T., & Dupuis, S. (2012). Supporting a relative's move into long-term care: Starting point shapes family members' experiences. *Canadian Journal on Aging, 31*(4), 395–410. doi:10.1017/S0714980812000384

Thorpe, R. J., Simonsick, E. M., Brach, J. S., Ayonayon, H., Satterfield, S., Harris, T. B., Garcia, M., & Kritchevsky, S. B. (2006). Dog ownership, walking behavior, and maintained mobility in late life. *Journal of the American Geriatrics Society, 54*, 1419–1424. doi:10.1111/j.1532-5415.2006.00856.x

Torgusen, B. L., & Kosberg, J. I. (2006). Assisting older victims of disaster: Roles and responsibilities for social workers. *Journal of Gerontological Social Work, 47* (1/2), 27–44. doi: 10.1300/J083v47n01_04

Tsemberis, S. J., Gulcur, L., & Nakae, M. (2004). Housing First, consumer choice, and harm reduction for homeless individuals with a dual diagnosis. *American Journal of Public Health, 94*(4), 651–656.

Tsemberis, S. J., Moran, L., Shinn, M., Asmussen, S. M., & Shern, D. L. (2003). Consumer preference programs for individuals who are homeless and have psychiatric disabilities: A drop-in center and a supported housing program. *American Journal of Community Psychology, 32*(3/4), 305–317. doi:10.1023/B.AJCP.0000004750.66957.bf

Turcotte, M., & Schellenberg, G. (2007). *A portrait of seniors in Canada, 2006.* (Statistics Canada Catalogue, No. 89-519-XIE). Ottawa, ON: Statistics Canada.

United States Census Bureau (2011). Census Bureau releases comprehensive analysis of fast-growing 90- and old population. Retrieved January 29, 2015, from: http://www.census.gov/newsroom/releases/archives/aging_population/cb11-194.html

Van den Block, L., Deschepper, R., Bilsen, J., Van Casteren, V., & Deliens, L. (2007). Transitions between care settings at the end of life in Belgium. *Journal of the American Medical Association, 298*(14), 1638–1639.

Walker, C. A., Curry, L. A., & Hogstel, M. A. (2007). Relocation stress syndrome in older adults transitioning from home to a long-term care facility: Myth or reality? *Journal of Psychosocial Nursing Mental Health Service, 45*(1), 38–45.

Walker, E., & McNamara, B. (2013). Relocating to retirement living: An occupational perspective on successful transitions. *Australian Occupational Therapy Journal, 60*, 445–453. doi:10.1111/1440-1630.12038

Walsh, F. (2009). Human-animal bonds 1: The relational significance of companion animals. *Family Process, 48*(4), 462–480. doi:10.1111/j.1545-5300.2009.01296.x

Watkins, L., Hall, C., & Kring, D. (2012). Hospital to home: A transition program for frail older adults. *Professional Care Management, 17(3)*, 117–123. doi:10.1097/NCM.0b013e318243d6a7

Weeks, L. E., Keefe, J., & MacDonald, D. J. (2012). Factors predicting relocation among older adults. *Journal of Housing for the Elderly, 26*(4), 355–371. doi: 10.1080/02763893.2011.653099

Weeks, L. E., & LeBlanc, K. (2010). Housing concerns of vulnerable older Canadians. *Canadian Journal on Aging, 29*(3), 333–348. doi:http://dx.doi.org/10.1017/S0714980810000310

Wiersma, E. C. (2010). Life around . . . : staff's perceptions of residents' adjustment into long-term care. *Canadian Journal on Aging, 29*(3), 425-434. doi:http://dx.doi.org/10.1017/S0714980810000401

Wilson, S. A. (1997). The transition to nursing homelife: A comparison of planned and unplanned admissions. *Journal of Advanced Nursing, 26*(5), 864–871. doi:10.1046/j.1365–2648.1997.00636.x

Wolff, F. C. (2013). Well-being of elderly people living in nursing homes: The benefits of friendship. *KYKLOS, 66(1)*, 153–171.

World Health Organization (WHO). (2007). Global age-friendly cities: A guide. Retrieved February 5, 2013, from: http://www.who.int/ageing/publications/Global_age_friendly_cities_Guide_English.pdf

CHAPTER 5

EXISTENTIAL TRANSITIONS

*To be human is to keep rattling the bars
of the cage of existence, hollering, "What's it all for?"*
(Robert Fulghum, American Author)[1]

Reflective Questions

- ► How is a sense of personhood developed?
- ► How do life's changes affect that sense of self?
- ► How can personhood remain intact through the transitions of old age?
- ► What can health and human service professionals do to validate personhood in each older adult with whom they work?

What does the term *existential* mean? In its most basic definition, *existential* refers to that which deals with existence (Free Online Dictionary, 2015). However, in its operational form, *existential* usually refers to issues about meaning and purpose in life and is intricately tied into individuals' sense of self or personhood. As Robert Fulghum noted in the quote

---

1. Quoted in Poor and Poirrier (2001, p. 113).

above, most humans cry out at some point, even at many occasions in their lives, "What is this all about?" To try to address these essential questions about the meaning in life, many individuals seek to find meaning and purpose in activities, goals, and values. For some, an inability to find meaning can lead to great emotional distress and even lead to actions that nullify personhood—suicide (Hunter, 2007–2008; Moore, 1997).

The "bars of the cage of existence," or issues of meaning and purpose, become more pronounced as one gets older (Dwyer, Nordenfelt, & Ternestedt, 2008). The "I," the sense of personhood, which was likely once built upon a foundation of occupation, family, and friends, becomes threatened with the passing of years, retirement, and death of family members, as well as the final transition: death.

Within this chapter we will discuss personhood, briefly exploring the formation of a sense of personhood. Primarily, we grapple with what *existential* means and focus upon the existential transitions of aging. We address interventions within the family and health care system that help maintain that sense of personhood. Further, we encourage health and human service providers to do their own existential work. Finally, we allude to ethical issues that will become pressing as our population ages (see also Chapter 8). It is our goal that, for the reader, the bars of the cage of existence will be rattled: *"What's it all for?"* (Fulghum).

Development of Personhood

Definition

What is personhood? In its most basic form, *personhood* can be defined as "the state or condition of being a person" (Free Online Dictionary, 2015). This can be understood to primarily reflect the physicality of an individual. However, *personhood* means much more: meaningful self-expression, self-determination, conscience, empathy, passion, and an individual's values (Hirst, Lane, & Reed, 2013). Although Gress and Bahr distinguish between "person" and personhood, stating that *person* refers to the totality of one's being and that *personhood* describes the lifelong growth of that multifaceted being (1984, p. 20), the literature tends not to split these two concepts, and so we purposefully have kept the two together.

In spiritual/religious terms, the ethereal part of the person is termed *soul* or *spirit*.[2] A person's spirit is his "energy and power" (May, 1982, p. 7), "the essence of self" (Ley, 1992, p. 209). Power (2006) deemed personhood and spirit to be synonymous. It is what it means to be truly human—so often expressed by family members as they are standing around the bedside of a loved one who has just passed: "She's gone now; the body is just the shell."

The terms *existential* and *spiritual* are used consistently throughout this chapter. They are related in that both refer to the experience of an individual—"felt" in the inner being and observable by others. They are typically used in the context of life meaning and purpose; hence the existential and spiritual often come to the fore in times of transition. The two terms differ in that *existential* has the connotation of being "observable" and "objective" (Merriam-Webster Online Thesaurus, 2015); *spiritual* tends to be understood as being subjective. The expression of the spiritual may be understood to be a response to that which is existential.[3] While having different nuances, *existential* and *spiritual* are inextricably tied to the experience of personhood.

Initial Formation of Personhood

When a baby enters the world, he comes with a specific set of needs. The person within that 7-pound bundle of joy demands to be fed, changed, and comforted. While in utero, the fetus had all his needs met; he was warmed and sheltered, he was fed, and his bodily functions were taken care of by his mother's body. But birth into this world—a harrowing journey in and of itself—now means that his basic requirements are not automatically fulfilled. He is apart from his mother and part of a larger system that may, or may not, meet his needs. The vulnerability of the little one, coupled with his lack of ability to communicate on an adult level, leads to the piercing expression of need: crying.

It is in these early days of development that an infant learns that he is distinct; he is not his parent or the environment around him. A sense of

2. Jewish and Christian theologians will often distinguish between soul and spirit; soul being understood to be the "source of human genuineness, depth, emotion" (Walsh, 2009, p. 6), with the spirit being the "image of God" within (Genesis 1:27). See Walsh (2009), for a succinct distinction between the two terms. (For the purpose of this text, soul and spirit will be used interchangeably, as they are overlapping constructs, and this seems to be the common usage today.)

3. It could be argued that the *effects* of spirituality are demonstrable. For example, the altruistic work done by Mother Teresa and Mahatma Gandhi had a very spiritual motivation.

personhood is in its early stages. He recognizes that he is dependent upon others for his survival. His understanding of the world as safe or not safe (or somewhere in-between) begins to be formed. If his physical needs are taken care of, and if he is held and cuddled and cooed to, he will grow. The *soul's* requirements—including touch, emotional stimulation, hearing one's name spoken in love, for example—have been highlighted in the literature repeatedly, beginning with Bowlby's seminal pamphlet, *Maternal Deprivation.*[4] Cuddling by parents, or a consistent parent substitute, leads to physical and psychological health (Ainsworth, 1967; Attachment Parenting International, 1994–2014; Bowlby, 1999; Coila, 2015). The baby *attaches* on a visceral level to his significant others. From this secure place of connection, he is able to explore his limited world safely, returning to the parents for comfort regularly. This prepares him to form later attachments with the outer world.

Lifelong Development of Personhood

From this basis of security —"I am!" "I matter!"—comes a greater understanding of who one is in relation to others. A child begins to understand who he is—gender, abilities, passions, and self-determination. He begins to form ideas about what he would like to do in the world—what will bring him meaning—based upon his interests and talents. And, if the development of personhood is healthy, this child will understand that he *is* in a world where others *are*. While "I" matters, "thou" matters too![5] Hence the moral development of the child begins.

In early childhood, a child functions with primarily an external locus of moral control. "Don't!" says the parent as a child puts his hand on the hot stove. As children grow older, this external locus needs to shift to an internal one. The home, school, and community (and sometimes a faith community) give guidance to aid in this process. "How must Billy have felt when you hit him?" External rules gradually are replaced by internal

---

4. *Maternal Deprivation* was written for the World Health Organization, at the request of the United Nations, and based upon Bowlby's observations of orphaned children following World War II. This began what later was, through much more research, Bowlby's "attachment theory." *Maternal Deprivation* is available in print today in the book *Child Care and the Growth of Love*. See reference list (Bowlby, 1953).
5. Martin Buber's (1958) construct of "I-thou" relationship will be referred to throughout the chapter. When used to refer to this construct, the words will be italicized.

motivations of respect for others, the welfare of the community, and other considerations. The development of empathy is vital.[6]

The healthy sense of self recognizes that both *I* and *thou* have inherent value. Buber spoke of this relationship as being of subject to subject. A person, out of his own sense of self, *relates to* another—the *thou*. Thou can be other human beings and it can be God (*the eternal Thou*, terms Buber). The respectful relationship is mutual and leads to growth in each party. Personhood involves the continual development of self over a lifetime (Gress & Bahr, 1984; Hirst et al., 2013).

Within Buber's (1958) construct, the *using of* others is termed *I—it—* from subject to object. This is a malformation of the human personality. Relationships are characterized by exploitation and control. The *I* lacks conscience, empathy, and concern for others. Rather than relate to others in a healthy manner, people are treated as commodities to be used. "Where there is no empathy . . . the seeds of violence are there" (Cram, 2003, pp. 56, 61).

While the basic sense of personhood is formed early in life (Ainsworth & Bowlby, 1991), throughout the human journey, there will be significant shaping of the human soul. Transitional milestones, such as marriage or the birth of a child, will change an individual's identity and role. These milestones will stretch the inner capacities of soul—to which any parent awake at 2 a.m., walking the floor with an infant with colic, will attest. The development of these inner capacities is often referred to as *character* and *maturity*—essential in the lifelong growth of personhood. The parent is able to look beyond his or her own needs to an extent greater than imagined—setting aside personal "rights" to look after the welfare of another. Qualities such as *hope* and *resilience*, highlighted in this text, are developed in these stretching experiences.

---

6. Moral development—essential to a healthy sense of self—is not automatic with chronological age. Kohlberg's Stages of Moral Development, Levels 1 and 2 (Preconventional Morality and Conventional Morality) elucidate a morality that is based (in Level 1) in a fear of punishment or (in Level 2) upon an obedience to outer authority, regardless of whether it is moral. While an internal locus of motivation, based upon universal principles of justice and respect (Level III: Postconventional Morality, Stage 6: Universal Principles, on Kohlberg's Scale) is a preferable guide for behavior, laws provide an essential external protection for the physicality of personhood. (See the reference list at the end of the chapter for Munsey, 1980.) Martin Luther King Jr. wryly noted "It may be true that the law cannot make a man love me . . . But . . . it keeps him from lynching me, and I think that's pretty important also" (1962).

Cognitively, a person's existential/spiritual views will develop through-out his or her life (Hood, Spilka, Hunsberger, & Gorusch, 2003; Walsh, 2009; Worthington, 1989). A fully developed person will mature morally and spiritually over time; she will process life, consciously revising and being revised by ideas and experiences. As part of her existential work, she will integrate her experiences and beliefs. If her beliefs and experiences do not align, the sharp discrepancies will lead to cognitive and spiritual dissonance. In times of transition, the "bigger questions" will be asked:

▶ Who am I?
▶ What is this all for?
▶ Will I make it?
▶ What do I *really* believe?
▶ Is there an afterlife?

A person's philosophy, or paradigm, has a major impact on how she copes throughout life and particularly, in the transitions of older adulthood.

Spirituality and Personhood

Man lives in three dimensions: the somatic,
the mental and the spiritual. The spiritual dimension
cannot be ignored, for it is what makes us human

(Frankl, 1986, pp. xv–xvi).

As alluded to earlier in the chapter, the noncorporeal aspects of personhood often are captured by the words *soul* and *spirit*. Using this terminology, then, the life of the human spirit—personhood—is expressed through a person's spirituality. The expression of spirit is all about finding meaning and making meaning in the world; it is about inner wholeness (Walsh, 1999, pp. 3, 4) and connection with others (Walsh, 1999; Weingarten, 1999)—*I-thou* relationships.

Spirituality and religion are not synonymous. The differences have been highlighted by a number of researchers (Anandarajah & Hight, 2001; Benner Carson & Koenig, 2004; Hawley, 1993; McKernan, 2005; Wright,

2005) and may be summarized as follows: Religious faith tends to involve a group of people (community) with a codified set of beliefs; it involves codes of conduct and has incorporated into it standard rituals and practices for the transitions of life. Spirituality tends to be more private in nature, with widely varying individual beliefs, containing aspects common to all religions: kindness, charity, and so on. It involves "an awareness of relationships with all creation, an appreciation of presence and purpose that includes a sense of meaning" (VandeCreek & Burton, 2001, p. 82). The practice of religion is one way of conceptualizing and expressing one's spirituality (Benner Carson & Koenig, 2004; Hamilton, 1998; Mount, 1993). From this perspective, religious practice is one aspect of the expression of spirit, or personhood. "Religion, at its best, provides a home for the nourishment and development of the spiritual life" (Wright, 2005, p. 5).

The question is often asked: "Can a person be spiritual, without being religious?" Based upon the aforementioned criteria, most certainly. An individual can have an internal system of beliefs and ideals (a worldview, a philosophy), practicing those principles in day-to-day life, without ever setting foot into a religious institution. Reciprocally, "Can an individual be religious, without being spiritual?" Again, yes. An individual can practice a religion without ever meaningfully integrating those beliefs into personhood. His religious commitment to a set of ideals may not be adequately internalized, integrated into his soul.[7] As the expression of the spirit is about meaning, profound transcendent experiences of joy and awe happen to those who practice religious faith and those who do not (VandeCreek & Burton, 2001).

To summarize, personhood encompasses much more than the physical; it also involves those intangible elements of being. A person's essence and philosophy are expressed through her spirituality. The characteristics of well-developed personhood—such as maturity, hope, and resilience— are the tools an individual uses to survive, even thrive, when the transitions of older adulthood challenge the very core of the being. Older adulthood can whittle away at a sense of person; conversely, the sense of person can continue to grow, leaving a lasting legacy to those who follow.

---

7. Gordon Allport (1967) distinguished between extrinsic religion and religion that is intrinsic. Extrinsic faith is characterized by what religion can do for an individual, such as church attendance for the purpose of providing social or business contacts. Intrinsic religion is faith that is internalized—integrated into one's being, "lived" from the inside out. See Allport and Ross (1967).

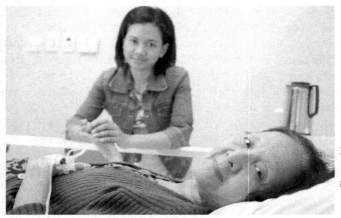

Existential Transitions in Older Adults

Integrity Versus Despair

Erik Erikson, a psychologist and psychoanalyst, delineated stages of psychosocial development for individuals across the lifespan (Erikson, 1982). For older adults, attaining integrity (instead of despair) refers to the process of older adults reviewing their lives and deriving a sense of meaning and achievement (Thomas & Cohen, 2006). If aging individuals review their lives and come to the conclusion that their lives were meaningless and futile, they will often feel great emptiness and despair. For many, however, the life review process can be profoundly affirming. "My life has been meaningful!" *I*, in relation to *thou* (and perhaps *Thou*), have made a difference!

Informally, family members listening to stories from their older adults are providing opportunities for life review. As has been explicated throughout this text, the challenges of our fast-paced lifestyle, of geographical distances, of institutionalized care (rather than elders living in the home of adult children) have reduced the occasions for this type of interaction. While these sociological realities have impoverished the elderly, depriving them of doing the work to achieve *integrity*, many would say that the generations that follow them are losing out as well (Byock, 1997).

Moving From "Doing" to "Being"

Thus far in this text we have enumerated the numerous transitions of old age. *Loss* is one word that captures what so many older adults feel as they move from being active to less active, to being cared for rather than caring for others, from being a *thou* in relationships to feeling like an *it*. As individuals, and as a society, we value ourselves and others on the basis of the contribution made, not on the inherent worth of humanity.

This feeling of lack of worth—*within* the older adult population and *toward* the older adult population—is a phenomenon found in developed countries. In some ancient societies and eastern countries, old age—with all of its transitions—is venerated. An older adult has a position of influence and respect and is often physically situated in the midst of the family, irrespective of physical or psychological capacities. The older an individual grows, the more respect that may be received; the older adult becomes the "patriarch" or "matriarch" of the family—not because of what he or she can do, but because of who he or she was and is currently. That person's identity is firmly situated within the family construct: "*I am* because *we are*" described African theologian John Mbiti (quoted in Walsh, 2009, p. 24; italics ours).

The term *ageism*—referring to discrimination against the elderly—originated with Butler (1969). Ageism is widespread within our society, impacting older adults in the western world in the areas of work, health care, and sometimes even within the family setting, with elder neglect/abuse. Within the realm of work, discrimination of older adults is widespread (Caldwell & Caldwell, 2010). Dennis and Thomas (2007) reported that most complaints regarding age-related prejudice in the workplace are dismissed without action. Within health care, ageism is understood to negatively impact the care, as well as the well-being of the elderly patient (Reyna, Goodwin, & Ferrari, 2007). Within the media, as well as within some religious circles (Caldwell & Caldwell, 2010), youth—with physicality and sexuality being prominent—are venerated. The virtues of aging—wisdom, experience, and honor—are not. This social construct of aging "does not allow the paradoxes of later life: aging is a source of wisdom *and* suffering, spiritual growth *and* physical decline, honor *and* vulnerability" (Stoneking, 2003, p. 70, italics hers). The older adult can feel like an *it*, rather than a *thou.*

How does an individual value self when her capacities have declined? How is personhood maintained, even enhanced? First, it is vital that an individual, and her loved ones, prepare for the transitions of her old age

(Kind, 2010). This preparation can come gradually, if the losses of aging come one at a time; and it will involve medical decisions, lifestyle choices, and financial options. For instance, the individual who begins to develop plans and hobbies for retirement will be better prepared to face the changes of this particular transition. Such plans need to be specific to the person herself and must be personally meaningful. While traveling may be soul-enriching to one, it may not be to another. Over time these plans continue to be revised as needs change. If an older adult can no longer run due to arthritis, then taking to the pool for exercise can nourish both body and soul.

It is not simply the tangible preparations for change that are important, but also the soul preparations. It is well-documented in the literature that during the changes of mid- to later life, people wrestle with the issues of life's meaning (Erikson, Erikson, & Kivnick, 1986; Walsh, 2009). Past experience with significant transitions, coupled with the necessary spiritual work to develop inner resources (such as resilience) to negotiate these transitions, pay dividends. Wilma was a palliative care patient; in my work with her, I (MBR) wondered if she possessed the resources needed to face into her death. She continued to resist the obvious physical transitions occurring as her demise neared; she was "dressed to the nines" in her hospital bed. In her struggle to face into her imminent passing, she wrestled with despair; her sense of personhood—her very being—was being threatened. I asked her about the tools she had used in the past to get her through difficult times. A lengthy silence ensued. Upon reflection, she could not identify one coping skill: "Perhaps I've had too easy a life!" she proclaimed. In Wilma's situation, the blessings of an "easy" life did not help her address existential issues as she faced death.

In popular psychology and in palliative care, the construct of *human being* vs. *human doing* is often referred to (Byock, 1997; Hemfelt, Minirth, & Meier, 1991). For the human *being*, self-worth resides within; what he achieves in life comes from the security of his own personhood. For the human *doing*, worth must consistently be proven to the self and to the world through ongoing achievement. This is necessary to prop up a fragile sense of self. When achieving—with its internal and external rewards—is no longer possible, a critical point in personhood is encountered. For the individual facing such an existential crisis, deep spiritual work needs to occur. This labor involves the understanding of recognizing personal losses, accepting that what could be done before is no longer possible, grasping that he or she still has value, and tapping into deep spiritual resources that will allow that revelation in the soul to take hold. In our North American culture that eschews illness and denies death, this process can seem morbid. Byock (1997) spoke of Douglas, a relatively young man facing into his death. The following quote captures his journey of diminished capacities and yet the maintenance, even growth, of personhood. Douglas moved from a *human doing* to a *human being* through the crisis of cancer.

In accepting his sadness, Douglas reconnected with parts of himself that were threatened by his impending demise . . .
By acknowledging his losses, he had, paradoxically, become more whole. The exhilaration he expressed typifies the experience of personal growth, the sense of mastery, in a changed life situation (pp. 79–80).

For the aged person living alone, this existential transition from doing to being can be very difficult. The philosophical foundation of the value of human life is essential. Suicide rates among older adults are significant; the World Health Organization reports that globally, the highest rates are in those 70 years and older (WHO, 2014).[8] Diminishing physical, mental, and emotional capacities may lead to what Holocaust survivor Frankl (2006) called "an existential vacuum" (p. 106): a state of inner emptiness, a void within self. The loss of a partner, a change in social roles (through retirement, for example), and social isolation add to that sense of emptiness and are considered to be risk factors for suicide (American Association of Suicidology, 2015). The initial formation of personhood, as well as the existential work done throughout life, girds the older adult through losses of capacity, a spouse, poor health, retirement, social isolation. The inner resources of maturity, resilience, and patience are tools to access this foundation and rest upon it.

But as the infant described at the beginning of the chapter is vulnerable, so the older adult is vulnerable. He needs family and community to reinforce that sense of personhood as he navigates the transitions. Just as the infant required more than simply physical care, so the older adult needs "soul care" to thrive. This involves time and attention from adult children

---

8. Older Caucasian men in both the United States and Canada have the highest rates of suicide in terms of population groups (Centers for Disease Control, 2012; Public Health Agency of Canada—PHAC, 2010).

or other relatives—a challenge in our fast-paced society (Hirst et al., 2013). It involves meaningful connection with family members and community.

In this *sandwich generation*, few things conjure more guilt in adult children than the message that aging parents have increased needs. The sense of responsibility can be overwhelming (Kind, 2010) and can lead to existential crises in family members (MacMillan, Peden, Hopkinson, & Hycha, 2000). That "What about my dreams for the future?" and "What does this all mean?" are questions agonized over by older adults in transition is readily understood. However, it is often not acknowledged that their family members may face the same crisis of meaning.[9] The bars on the cages of their existence are rattled, too.

Dr. Ira Byock (1997), a well-known palliative care physician, encouraged family members to face into the challenge, and he openly spoke of the *family's need* to care for their loved one. While the transitioning older adult needs physical and emotional attention, *the family needs to give this.* Through caregiving, family members can grow in personhood; they have the opportunity do their own existential work. Caregiving can be spiritually enriching for both the older adult receiving care and the family that care for him (Walsh, 2009).

Meaning is often found in unexpected places. The transitioning older adult needs his family—and his family needs him! Embraced for millennia by eastern societies, this existential understanding is slowly being acknowledged in North America. The perception of meaning in the older adult's life is inextricably tied to self-acceptance (Hughes & Peake, 2002), as well as the acceptance of others.

Resolving Inner Conflicts

Throughout a person's life, there will be questions of meaning. A paradigm that sufficed in one's 20s may no longer be adequate later on, as life's experiences challenge previously held beliefs. As a goal of being human is the integration of beliefs with life experiences, there will be times of inner tension. Frankl (2006) articulated this eloquently when he stated that mental health is based upon some inner tension:

---

9. Bioethicist Viki Kind used the term *care-grieving* to describe some of the struggles that adult children of dying parents experience. Besides the putting aside of work, hobbies, etc., to care for an elderly parent, these adult children experience anticipatory grief. The "I don't know if I can handle this" response—very common in family members—produces a great deal of guilt (Kind, 2010, pp. 105–107). Normalizing these feelings to families can be profoundly helpful. (More will be discussed on *care-grieving* in Chapter 6.)

. . . the tension between what one has already achieved and what one still ought to accomplish, or the gap between what one is and what one should become. Such a tension is inherent in the human-being and therefore is indispensable to mental well-being (pp. 104–105).

The recognition of this tension and the existential work to resolve it is a sign of soul health. For many people, however, this inner tension is ignored in the business and busyness of life. The bigger existential issues of life purpose and growth can get silenced in the routines of daily living. Sometimes these issues are submerged until older adulthood, when the many transitions impinge upon personhood, and these unresolved inner conflicts rise to the surface.

The details of these inner conflicts can be many—however, they often center on a severance of relationship, of connection (Weingarten, 1999)—with self, with others, and with the Transcendent. This brokenness can be buried in guilt and shame. A sense of regret is how these disconnections usually manifest themselves; the "should haves, could haves, would haves" can haunt.

Disconnection with self

In the challenges of daily life, and often in the course of a lifetime, a person can become disconnected with her soul, her essence, her passion. The job that puts food on the table can be mind-numbing and soul-crushing. It is not always possible to do what we want to do, to grow in every aspect of our lives. Over the course of time, however, a person may become very detached from who she really is. One woman captured this beautifully: "I feel like I am on the outside of the glass, looking in at life. I don't know who I am."

For the older adult, this may be particularly pronounced. The mother and grandmother who put aside all her dreams to focus on her children and then her grandchildren may feel that she has never realized her own dreams. She may no longer know what she wants and what she needs. The transitions of her adult children (such as moving out of geographic proximity for the sake of employment, taking the grandchildren with them) may thrust her into a crisis of being—a crisis that has opportunity for growth.

Here, she may go back to the interests of her pre-children days—beginning to paint again, or pursuing the university degree she never attained.

In studies examining life regrets in older adults, some of the common regrets, besides ruptures in relationships, often involve decisions regarding work, such as not taking risks at work or making the most of opportunities, as well as not pursuing more education (Timmer, Westerhof, & Dittmann-Kohli, 2005). As some of these regrets involve decisions that were time specific (e.g., work decisions), it becomes difficult to resolve these regrets; an older adult cannot return to young adulthood and choose a different career, for example. However, as will be described in greater length in Chapter 8, there are options for some older adults who regret not getting a university degree.

Further, ways in which to address lifetime regrets can be very individual and creative. A family story speaks of this. My (MBR) spouse had a grandmother who fulfilled the role of wife, grandmother, churchgoer, and volunteer faithfully. She dressed in somber hues and lived within the defined parameters of her roles for decades. When she was in 80s, her spouse passed; she grieved the loss greatly. However, she knew that she still had living to do; so she learned to drive, took a helicopter trip, listened to rock music, and dressed in vivid colors! She tapped in to who she really was—affirming personhood—and then enjoyed her*self*!

Disconnection with others

Severed relationships can cause profound dis-ease within the human spirit. The transitions of older adulthood—such as the loss of friends due to death—bring this dis-ease to the surface. The older adult may have more time on his hands, but fewer friends (due to death or relocation). He may regret the loss of relationships that were dropped due to busyness or conflict. On a deeper level, he may be re-evaluating his priorities; although work previously took priority, now that he is retired he may be rethinking what is most important to him. "What was it all for?" he may be thinking and saying.

Disconnection with God

Many individuals wrestle, in their older adult years, with faith that has been lost, or, at least, "set aside." Disappointment with organized religion, the inability to bring together previously held beliefs with difficult life experiences, and—sometimes—a life that has gone "too smoothly" (to need a power greater than self), all can lead to this sense of disconnection with the Divine.

When the transitions of older adulthood occur, many find their inner resources insufficient, and (re)turn to a religious expression of spirituality (Balboni et al., 2013; Milardo Floriani, 1999; Hamilton, 1998; Satterly, 2001; Speck, 1998; VandeCreek & Burton, 2001). Some seek out new experiences in religion and/or spirituality (Speck, 1998). In years of experience as a palliative care chaplain (MBR), I observed that more people tend to return to the spirituality, faith, or rituals of their childhood.[10] In one case, a Sikh gentleman came to Canada, got married here, and had a family. His wife was a Christian, and so he attended church with her and their children for many years. In his dying, he requested Sikh rituals—a return to the religious expression of his youth—as well as a church funeral.[11]

North American researchers are not surprised by this phenomenon. Religion is understood to be culturally present and accessible. For example, a 2011 Gallup poll indicated that 92% of Americans believe in God or a universal spirit (Newport, 2011); sociologist Reginald Bibby (2012) noted that for two in three Canadians, religious and spiritual beliefs are important.[12] What about in very secular societies? la Cour (2008) studied religious and spiritual expression among those admitted to Danish hospitals. For those with less severe or short-term issues, little or no change was noted in religious and spiritual expression. But severity of illness was correlated with greater expression of spiritual and religious activity among patients, despite the fact that religion is less culturally present there. The existential crisis of severe illness prompted a (re)connection to spiritual and religious expression.

---

10. See "Anne's garden: A journey of the human spirit" for a powerful example of one woman's spiritual journey back to the symbols of her youth (Hall, McCarney, Hamilton, Robertson, & Yates-Fraser, 1996).

11. Along the same lines, Carol Milardo Floriani, RN, spoke of a Cambodian man who converted to Christianity during his life in the United States. In his dying, he needed to reconnect with his Buddhist roots/practices, and so the spiritual care he received was both Christian and Buddhist (see Milardo Floriani, 1999).

12. While spiritual beliefs and practices are still significant to North Americans, regular attendance at religious institutions tends to be lower. Canadian sociologist Reginald Bibby (2012) reported that while one in two Canadians engage in a religious or spiritual practice at least once a month, only 30% of Canadians attend a religious institution *once a month*. In the United States, *weekly* religious service attendance has been estimated to be between 40–50% by Gallup polls and Barna reports, staying relatively consistent throughout the first decade of the new millennium. However, a number of sources dispute this figure, saying that people in the United States overestimate church attendance. See The Barna Group (2009) and ReligiousTolerance.org (1999–2007). The data would seem to reveal significant personal spiritual practices in both countries, with less institutional involvement in religion. It is interesting to note the cultural differences between Canada and the United States, as well. This data suggests that Canada could be considered to be a more secular nation than the United States.

The ties that support and that bind:
The place of religious faith in dealing with inner conflicts

As has been emphasized throughout this chapter, religious expression is one form of the expression of the spirit. As a subset of spirituality, it is about having and making meaning in the world. Much has been said about its benefits in difficult life transitions. "When (one) stands on the firm ground of religious belief, there can be no objection to making use of the therapeutic effect of his religious convictions and thereby drawing upon his spiritual resources," said Frankl (2006, p. 119). People of faith often attach a "higher meaning" to their crises, which takes away the sense of randomness that calamity can bring. "If a man knows the wherefore of his existence, then the manner of it can take care of itself . . ." stated German philosopher Nietzsche (1911, p. 2).[13] Frankl (2006), springboarding off of this concept, spoke of the necessity of a higher purpose for those imprisoned in World War II.

We had to learn ourselves, and, furthermore we had to teach the despairing men, that it *did not matter what we expected from life, but rather what life expected of us. (p. 77, italics his)*

For some, in the concentration camps, this meant living for family members. For others, it meant choosing to honor a power greater than the Nazis—God. Religious faith brought meaning to sacrifice (Frankl, 2006). "Faith fuels the resilient spirit," stated Walsh (2009, p. 24).

Although the example of meaning in concentration camps may seem extreme, it is almost a "meta-example" for all existential crises—including the deep inner conflicts that occur within older adults. For instance, many people in older adulthood experience regret over life choices. "If I could do it all over again . . ." is a common theme. The "what if's" and "if only's" torment the sensitive soul. Within the major religious traditions are vehicles for obtaining forgiveness for these regrets. Rituals designed to communi-

13. This statement has been frequently quoted, many times in a slightly different fashion. When Frankl (2006) used this quote, he gave credit to Nietzsche, and phrased it this way: "He who has a *why* to live for can bear with almost any *how*" (p. 76, italics his).

cate God's forgiveness for wrongdoing, facilitate reconciliation between self and others, as well as reconnect with self can bring freedom from these regrets. Many people, during times of transition, will find meaning in these rituals, to "mark" that time and place—a physical action signifying a deep spiritual transaction. The teachings of religion and accompanying rituals can bring great peace (Walsh, 2009).

Although the ties of religion can support, they can also bind. In times of formation or transition, the belief system of an individual may not be appropriate or adequate for her circumstances, and thoughtlessly applied "truths" by others or self can be very damaging (la Cour, 2008; Purcell, 2008; Walsh, 2009). Rather than providing meaning and allowing the individual to incorporate the experience into her being—cognitively and spiritually—the belief system can tie her up, causing profound anguish of personhood, of spirit.

Dying individuals sometimes connect physical illness to sin, God's judgment, or bad karma. If an individual rigorously applies such theology to her circumstances, she will suffer profoundly. Many people, representing a good number of the world's major religions, have expressed such inner dissonance when trying to come to grips spiritually with why they, or their loved ones, are terminally ill. Letting go of the faith system upon which they have built their identity, their personhood, would be untenable, but believing what others have told them and what doctrines may have been emphasized within their faith tradition is equally so. This results in a double bind! Identity, religious faith, and family relationships can all be threatened.[14] For some, their future is in jeopardy, as they fear hell (Egan & Prud'homme Brisson, 2006). This is a crisis that is multifaceted and profoundly existential. Others thoughtlessly applying these types of beliefs to vulnerable souls (the young, the old, and everyone in-between) has been understood by Purcell (2008) to be "spiritual abuse" and "spiritual terrorism."

---

14. One situation stands out in my (MBR) experience. A man was dying of cancer. The family belief in faith healing—as a sign of God's favor—was so strong that any outcome other than total restoration of health meant that this fellow was not a Christian. The mother of this man feared that if her son were not healed, he was not a Christian and he would go to hell. (And then she would not see him again.) The father of the terminally ill man believed so strongly in physical healing that he said that his wife (the dying man's mother) must be keeping the healing away with her "unbelief." Because of her unbelief, she was not considered to be a Christian by her own husband. In the death of her son, this mother—because of the belief system to which the family adhered—stood to lose her son physically (to death), her faith (her husband no longer believed she was a Christian and she feared she was not), and the reunion of her family in heaven—if either her son or she herself were not Christians!

Religious faith can be a tremendous resource for older adults in coping with transitions. With deep conviction (from the depths of her soul!) one dear elderly lady experiencing major life transitions said, "My faith and prayer—they anchor me." At times, however, it can complicate matters; dealing with this internal dissonance, from a professional perspective, will be touched upon later in this chapter. A guiding principle in this discussion is explicated beautifully by the twentieth-century theologian, William Barclay:

The real test of religion is, does it make wings to lift a man up or a dead weight to drag him down? Is a man helped by his religion, or is he haunted by it? Does it carry him, or does he carry it?"
(Barclay, in Blue, 1998, p. 86).

Resolving External Conflicts

As individuals age or approach death, there may be a need to repair damaged relationships with others, especially estranged family members. Older adults may seek to make contact with family members, ask forgiveness, and to some degree, restore the damaged relationship (McSherry, 2011). Or, some older adults may want to express to their loved ones how much they have loved them and what they have meant. This is part of the unfinished business of aging and dying and may bring meaning to individuals' lives as they approach death.

Significant repair of relationships may not be possible. As one adult child said, "He left our lives. An 'I'm sorry' won't restore all those years we lost." The dying patient's children did see him once before his death. After this meeting, the palliative man said, "Sometimes it's just too late." There was no intervention that could erase the past. But what was significant, meaningful to both the dying father and his son, was the opportunity to say "I love you." Knowing one is loved is a basic need of personhood, and, even in a limited way such as this family's tenuous reunion, can bring a dying individual some peace and grieving adult children a measure of solace.

Facing Into an Unknown Future

Facing into an unknown future involves anticipating further physical decline and possible cognitive decline. Research reveals that some older adults fear memory loss (Corner & Bond, 2004; Dark-Freudeman, West, & Viverito, 2006). Older adults recognize "the bigger picture," that bodily decline ultimately leads to death. Although younger adults have greater fears about death than older adults, aging individuals still experience fear about death (Cicirelli, 2001; Arnup, 2013). Fears can be related to fear of the dying process (Cicirelli, 2001); specifically, older adults may fear that they will experience overwhelming pain in the death process (Arnup, 2013). This is common. With the palliative medications available today, that fear is generally unfounded (Byock, 1997).[15] But an elderly adult facing into her death may remember the passings of her parents, perhaps in her living room, in profound pain. She carries these memories into her own process. Loss of control is another fear; being unable to toilet oneself, loss of "dignity" with the effects of medication, and losing the ability to make one's own decisions can factor in. In one study examining religious faith, fear of death, and advance care planning among chronically ill older adults, religious faith, as well as fear of death, was associated with advance care planning (living will) (Dobbs, Emmett, Hammarth, & Daaleman, 2012). It could be that these older adults feared the death *process*, rather than actual death, and that a completed living will enhanced feelings of control in this transition.

As discussed earlier, religious belief can be a great comfort; it can, however, complicate matters. Individuals may fear the coming afterlife (Egan & Prud'homme Brisson, 2006). Dying people often ask, "What's it like on the other side?" Others request assurance that life does not end with the death of the physical body (Turesky & Schultz, 2010). They, or family members, express the need to know that personhood does not end with physical death; the hope of a reunion on "the other side" predominates. From a palliative perspective, stories of *death bed phenomena* abound;[16] I (MBR) will, from time to time, share what I have observed, to bring some peace to those afraid that personhood ends at death, or of what may lie beyond.

At times this anxiety about life after death is a deep-seated fear of hell (Egan & Prud'homme Brisson, 2006). A terminally ill person may have not

---

15. Dr. Ira Byock (1997) said, "Physical suffering can *always* be alleviated" (p. xiv, italics his). But whether physical suffering can be totally eradicated is debatable. Palliative care makes an enormous difference in a dying person's end-of-life, but it does not mean that one will not experience physical symptoms at all. This topic will be discussed more in Chapter 6.

16. There are many published stories of near death experiences. And, popular today, are stories of those who have been declared clinically dead who have "come back" and shared their experiences of the after-life. This would validate North America's interest in the spiritual. It also speaks much of the human "need" that personhood not be extinguished at death. This subject will be discussed more in Chapter 6.

practiced the religion in which she was raised during her adult years. As mentioned earlier, when death approaches, people can reflect back upon the faith system in which they were raised; it is often "programmed onto the hard drive" of their souls. If this system and respected people within it have emphasized punishment for wrongdoing, great fear can result. For some, the rituals of that background are enough to alleviate the trepidation. For example, a significant number of people who were raised Roman Catholic and are no longer practicing their faith will request a priest and the Sacrament of the Sick in their dying. Sometimes, more than this is needed. Conscious of respecting all people's faith systems, it can be helpful for the spiritual care provider to gently work *with* an individual's personal theology that is "damning" (pun intended). If there is a theology of sin, it follows that there also be a theology of atonement/forgiveness from God and others—within the same faith system. To utilize one (forgiveness) to counteract the other (sin) can be helpful.[17]

Unfortunately, some have been raised with the stated or implied idea that "nothing is good enough." This is spiritual pain (caused by deep, internal shame), rather than religious pain (caused by guilt) (Satterly, 2001); an individual feels that his true self will be known by God, and that he (personhood) will be found lacking.

In such situations, a ritual is often not sufficient, as rituals tend to address guilt, rather than shame. Discussion about this shame and a counteracting of this, *within the person's paradigm,* can be beneficial; shame is counteracted by unconditional love (Satterly, 2001). These are waters for a chaplain trained in palliative care to wade into (Benner Carson & Koenig, 2004; Coates, 1995; Koenig, 2001; Sulmasy, 2006)! For faith systems unfamiliar to the health care chaplains, a clergyperson from within the faith system can also be invaluable (Benner Carson & Koenig, 2004; Coates, 1995).

Legacy

Older adults often feel a need to leave a legacy. Legacy refers to the act(s) of leaving something behind for others after death (Hunter, 2007–2008). It is a tangible way of remembering the individual who has passed; while this person is physically gone, some aspect of him carries on. Legacies may be

---

17. For instance, a chaplain can stress to the suffering older adult the love of and forgiveness from God, to balance off the heavy emphasis upon sin. Rituals—such as prayer—can be utilized to bring forgiveness into the equation, to bring spiritual relief.

very personal and specific to individuals;[18] the common theme in legacies is that they bring meaning to life. Legacies can involve material objects, such as bequeathing personal belongings to the next generation. They can also be symbolic, in that persons may attach their names to things that will remain long after death. Legacies can also be related to values, in that individuals pass on their own beliefs and values to others (Hunter, 2007–2008).

For example, one woman, in her dying, was very concerned that her grandson be baptized. This was a value of hers, not her daughter's (the mother of the child). As this woman was dying, her daughter organized the baptism of her child in the palliative care facility, so that her terminally ill mom could be present. This was truly a gift to her mom, so that she could pass in peace. ("Now every one of my family members is in the fold!" this older woman exclaimed.) For this dying woman, the legacy she wanted to pass along to her children and grandchildren was her faith and the values and rituals associated with it. Her adult daughter recognized this, and, in essence, "received" this gift from her mom on behalf of herself and her son by having this young boy baptized.

When materials are passed on to family members, such as a dining room table or rings, the purpose behind the objects are more than material or monetary. Older adults often pass on these objects in hope that the recipient values the furniture or jewelry because they elicit memories about family members, and perhaps signify characteristics of the older adults, such as strength or resilience (Hinck, 2007).

Individuals can also pass down the legacy of knowledge. They may teach skills and provide knowledge about gardening to their children, who then enjoy the benefits of gardening in their adulthood, and can pass this on to their children. Not only does the activity provide a sense of enjoyment and productivity in the present, but there is the connection with the past (their parents' legacy) and hopefully, with the future through their children (Heliker, Chadwick, & O'Connell, 2001).

---

18. Generally, legacies reflect what one has had in life. Occasionally, a legacy reflects what has been *missing* in an older adult's life. One woman, who had grown up in poverty and lived "hand to mouth" all her life, left a certain amount of cash to each grandchild. Because she had always been lacking in financial resources (a lifelong source of shame and grief for her), she wanted to be remembered by her grandchildren as someone who gave to them the material resources she possessed. It is quite likely that this legacy was more reflective of what was important to *her* than to her grandchildren, as each came from homes that were well-off financially. However, it was an important part of her end-of-life work.

Interventions to Address Existential Issues in Older Adults

Interventions with older adults involve working with them in one or more of the following areas, as needed by the elderly person to validate personhood, helping the individual to reconnect with self, others, and (possibly) the Transcendent; aid the elder to recognize and (if necessary) re-establish meaning and purpose in life; help to restore hope; and assist the older adult in dealing with regrets, including doing the work of forgiveness. As such the following interventions target these various aspects of existential issues.

The Ministry of Presence

Not simply a "skill" or an intervention, the *ministry of presence* is about whom the health or human service professional is and how he is with people. Benner Carson and Koenig (2004) used the term *ministry* in terms of professional ministry, as they spoke of spiritual care in health care settings. However, the term can and should be understood more broadly. *Ministry* can also mean "vehicle," "agency," and "instrument" (Merriam-Webster Online Thesaurus, 2015). The health or human service professional is a vehicle, an agent, an instrument of presence for the older adult and his family. It is less about *doing* to and more about *being* with the older adult and his or her family (Heyse-Moore, 1996).

Benner Carson and Koenig (2004) explained what this ministry of presence involves: active listening, empathy, being vulnerable, humble,[19] and committed to the family one is working with. These characteristics and skills are explicated more fully in the interventions listed below. They are highlighted here to emphasize that they are not simply what is done *to* or *for* a family; they flow *out of* who the nurse, chaplain, or other health or human service professional *is*. Her spirit "touches the spirit" of the person being cared for (Thompson O'Maille & Kasayka, 2005, p. 64): the *I–thou* relationship. Those who have faced life-threatening illness or death themselves (and their family members) know which professional is simply practicing what is required of her and those from whom this presence flows. "You can tell she really cares," said one woman, of a physician that had seen her and her husband through one health crisis after another. "You just know." In this context, there is a *ministry* in a spiritual sense—from what-

---

19. Pittroff (2013) used the lovely term "the humbled expert" to refer to health care professionals who provide such ministry of presence.

ever professional is providing the care; her care comes with the scent of the sacred, and those who catch a whiff of that fragrance are ministered to!

Establish Rapport and a Trusting Relationship

For some, the existential issues surrounding aging, physical decline, dying, and death are very personal and private. Therefore, in order for health and human service professionals to gain access to such concerns, a trusting relationship needs to be developed with older adults (Benner Carson & Koenig, 2004; Pittroff, 2013; Ryan, 2005). This involves genuine interest in older clients, patient listening to their concerns, and an acknowledgment that aging, dying, and death encompass more than just the body, but also pertains to individuals' entire lives and the meanings they attribute to the transitions (Ryan, 2005). It involves addressing concrete tasks of older adults (Egan & Prud'homme Brisson, 2006); perhaps the requests focus upon small, but significant concerns (e.g., contacting the pharmacy, helping to do something in a senior's home) that demonstrate to older adults the level of care professionals have toward all areas in their lives.

Validating Personhood

Regardless of age, human beings need to feel a sense of value and worth as human beings. This sense of worth and dignity is essential to good mental health and quality of life. However, the process of aging, particularly if there is significant pain and physical disability, may preclude some from

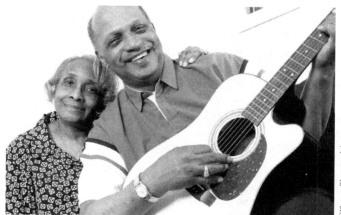

GWImages/Shutterstock, Inc.

engaging in the very activities that enhance their sense of personhood and worth. The work of health and human service professionals in recognizing and validating personhood in older adults involves valuing individuals for their inherent worth and demonstrating that valuing, as well as tailoring interventions to the level of functioning of the older adults.

Encouraging older adults to talk about what they did and who they were in the past is a first step. Before these elderly people needed extra care in the home, transitioned to long-term care, or became residents within a hospice setting, they were agents of meaning and change within the world. They raised families, labored within the workforce, coached soccer teams, and were active members of Block Watch (for example). These activities revealed both abilities and character qualities that can be affirmed and brought (to some degree) into the present. One gentleman, for whom painting had been a passion, was encouraged to have family members bring in some of his paintings into the hospice; these adorned the walls of his room. Although he could no longer paint large masterpieces, he still enjoyed "dabbling," and the volunteer artist at this hospice would paint together with him in one of the quiet spaces within the facility. Here, he was able to practice his craft (on a smaller scale), talk about his work with someone who had similar interest and talent (the volunteer artist), and enjoy the community's appreciation for his work. What begun as conversation about what a patient had liked to do in the past was really about valuing personhood; this led to him being able to express that same passion of his spirit within a different context: the hospice.

Within a hospice setting, the typical rules of institutions can be relaxed and valued attachments and activities are commonly made possible. Pets are allowed to visit; residents may be able to imbibe (with physician awareness), and guests are accommodated.[20] The purpose is to affirm that which has brought meaning, purpose, and comfort to a resident.

The palliative experience of older adults and their family members tends to be shorter in length than the long-term care experience. Hence, the gentleman in the aforementioned example was only able to paint for a short period of time before he was physically no longer able to engage in these person-affirming activities. Staff could and did continue to validate his personhood through conversation (including speaking about the pictures on the wall), and treating him and his family with respect.

---

20. Boundaries, of course, must be respected; policies are in place and procedures followed so that the experience of all residents and family members, as well as staff members, is safe and positive.

Living within a long-term care facility can pose challenges for self-expression, in part because of the numbers of older adults residing on units, as well as the duration of time the older adult spends within the institution. Certainly, in the past, being institutionalized could be demoralizing; the longer a person lived within the institution, the more challenging it was to maintain personhood (Goffman, 1961). However, there is a movement within long-term care to shift toward a culture that values personhood and that recognizes that the older adult was and is unique and brings a lifetime of experiences and memories to the community. The valuing of the personhood of residents needs to be a primary concern of administrators and staff (Hirst et al., 2013). Getting to know the residents is elemental. Knowing a resident's name, and calling him by the title he prefers, is essential; so is a supportive and respectful tone of voice (Hirst et al., 2013). Meaningful decision-making for older adults in long-term care facilities, such as bath times and bedtimes, affirms personhood (Crandall, White, Schuldheis, & Talerico, 2007).

Gently Assess for Spiritual Distress

What is spiritual distress and how does it manifest itself? As has been affirmed in this chapter, the spirit is the essence of a person; it is the core of his being. Hence, spiritual distress is a deep, existential distress and it can be evidenced in many ways: by pain that cannot be controlled by medication (Milardo Floriani, 1999; Kuhl, 2003); insomnia; withdrawal, or isolation from spiritual support systems; conflict with family members and friends and/or support staff; anxiety; mistrust of family and physicians; breathlessness; depression; guilt; hopelessness; fear/dread; and feelings of failure in life (Hay, 1989; Heyse-Moore, 1996). For this desperate state, the founder of the modern hospice movement, Dame Cicely Saunders, coined the term "total pain" (Mount, 1993, p. 28).

Some of the above criteria could be deemed psychosocial. The distinction between psychosocial pain and that which is classified as spiritual is often a matter of degree. A high level of this type of discomfort is deemed to be spiritual pain. *Why me, God? Where will this illness lead? What is the meaning to my suffering?* These questions are asked by those who define themselves as being spiritual and/or religious and those who do not, and they evidence spiritual distress (Coates, 1995; Downing, 2003). Queries and symptoms such as these are evidence that the spirit, the essence of self, has been threatened; a person has become "estranged" from who he really is (Heyse-Moore, 1996, p. 308).

Egan and Prud'homme Brisson (2006) examined outreach nurses' perceptions of the spiritual needs of older adults who were housebound. These nurses discussed the difficulties faced by older adults who are unable to get out and about, including emotional and spiritual distress. They described how some of their older clients experience anger, guilt (and desired forgiveness), feelings of abandonment, and fear. The nurses stressed the need for spiritual needs to be addressed cautiously, and only after trust had been established with older adults. Usually, they waited for older adults to suggest their desire to discuss spiritual distress. The nurses expressed concern that they do not force their beliefs upon their elderly clients, and neither do they want to make older adults feel like they have to discuss spiritual issues. Possible ways of broaching spiritual issues included offering help with completing advanced directives or asking older adults if they would like a referral to clergy (Egan & Prud'homme Brisson, 2006).

Within a health care facility, nurses and social workers can and do informally assess for spiritual distress. A referral to a chaplain typically follows.

Address Meaning and Purpose in Life

For human beings, meaning in life is absolutely essential to quality of life. Not only is having meaning in life linked to better physical health (Krause, 2004, 2009) and mental health (Fry, 2000; Reker, 1997), and believed to counterbalance stressors in some older adults (Krause, 2007), it is also associated with lower death rates (Krause, 2009). As individuals age, meaning in life may evolve and change to incorporate life's experiences (Moore, Metcalf, & Schow, 2006). Sadly, for some older adults, their sense of meaning and purpose dwindles as they get older, stop working, and face the deaths of family members, spouses, and friends. The work of professionals involves, in part, helping aging adults review their lives and come to a sense of *integrity*, rather than *despair.*

Meaning and purpose in life can be addressed by health and human service professionals in a number of ways. First, professionals can ask older clients directly, "What gives you meaning and purpose in life?" and "What gave you meaning in life in the past?" The purpose of this is to assess whether the older individual feels a sense of meaning and purpose now. If so, the professional can tap into this by asking follow-up questions about how often older adults engage in meaning-making activities and if there are any hindrances or barriers to these activities. For example, an older adult who loves to read but is having trouble seeing pages can be informed of where to access large-print books, as well as books on tape. Or, a senior who finds church services essential to his spirituality and sense of meaning in life can be encouraged to contact a nearby church to ask if a parishioner would be willing to transport him to services, if he is no longer able to drive. If an older adult states that she has no meaning or purpose in life, the professional can inquire about what gave her meaning in the past. The professional can then explore with the older client possible ways to re-establish that sense of meaning. Unfortunately, as mentioned in the previous example of Wilma, if older adults have not engaged in some struggle and development of meaning earlier on in their lives, they may experience greater problems in wrestling with meaning in advanced age.[21] Some formal ways of re-establishing meaning—alluded to a number of times in this chapter—are listed below.

Engage in life review and reminiscence

Older adults often engage in reminiscing and reviewing their lives (Butler, 1963). However, as a means of helping older adults address issues of meaning and purpose in life, professionals may embark upon a structured process of life review with their aging clients. The purpose of life review is to help older adults to reflect upon their past lives, accept the past, and successfully integrate the past with the present. Older adults can be asked questions about who they are as individuals and how they have lived their lives (Lewis, 2001). Life review is noted to help older adults with symptoms of depression (Chippendale & Bear-Lehman, 2012; Korte, Bohlmeijer, Cappeliez, Smit, & Westerhof, 2012) and to improve self-esteem and confidence (Chiang, Lu, Chu, Chang, & Chou, 2008).

Life review may involve a very structured group program, such as the Life Review Group Program developed by Butler (1963) and Haight (1988). This program involves topical discussions over an eight-week period, including discussions on childhood, adolescence, the participant's family and job, the participant's friends, the most significant thing the participant has accomplished in life, a summary of the life review and an integration of life events (Chiang et al., 2008).

Life review may also occur in a more informal manner, whereby nurses, chaplains, or other professionals can ask older adults questions that lead them to reflect upon the events of their lives. They may be asked to

---

21. Moore et al. (2006) eloquently addressed the role of growing through adversity and what this brings to the older adult in her last days. Coming through adversity early in life was positively correlated with being able to handle the challenges of old age.

describe an obstacle in their life and how they overcame this obstacle, as well as the skills they utilized to tackle the problem (Jenko, Gonzalez, & Seymour, 2007). They can be asked about what they have achieved in their lives and what they most enjoyed. Nurses, social workers, chaplains, and other professionals can inquire about what older adults would like to leave with their family and how they wish to be remembered by others (Jenko et al., 2007).

Reminiscence

Reminiscence therapy is similar to life review; however, some believe that it is a less active process than life review (Haight, 1988). The purpose of reminiscence therapy is to assist older adults to resolve conflicts from the past (Bohlmeijer, Valenkamp, Westerhof, Smit, & Cuijpers, 2005) and involves the process of thinking or telling others about their past lives (Cappeliez, O'Rourke, & Chaudhury, 2005; Westerhof, Bohlmeijer, & Webster, 2010). Reminiscence therapy can take various forms. For example, on some hospital units, a recreational therapist will conduct a reminiscence group once a week where older adults can attend. The therapist may show a particular item from the past, such as an old-fashioned chamber pot, which becomes a springboard upon which older adults can reflect upon their pasts and share stories with each other. For older adults with dementia, reminiscence can be particularly meaningful because they can still remember and talk knowledgeably about events, circumstances, and objects of the past. Thus, it can also bolster a sense of mastery and competence.

Like life review, there are variations in how reminiscence therapy can be conducted. For example, one kind of reminiscence therapy is entitled "Searching for the Meaning in Life" (Bohlmeijer et al., 2005). This form of creative reminiscence does not rely as heavily upon orally reviewing life, and hence, may be effective for those who prefer nonverbal forms of self-expression. Also, this form of reminiscence relies upon metaphors and creative ways of representing life; this taps into creativity and self-expression. This form of reminiscence involves 12 sessions that focus on topics such as friendships and houses in which older participants have lived (Bohlmeijer et al., 2005).

Another form of reminiscence therapy, spiritual reminiscence, involves telling life stories with importance placed upon meaning; it is based upon the underlying assumption that individuals have a spiritual dimension (MacKinlay & Trevitt, 2010). Older adults are guided to talk about what gives them meaning in life and what has brought joy, sadness, or other feelings. Within this form of spiritual reminiscence, six themes are discussed: ultimate meaning, adults' responses to meaning, self-sufficiency/vulnerability, provisional life meanings/final meaning, relationship/isolation, and hope/despair. This approach is viewed as being an effective way to engage older adults with dementia (MacKinlay & Trevitt, 2010).

Reminiscence therapy can also be undertaken in a directed, yet solitary fashion. Older adults can be asked to write about their lives. This may be particularly effective for older adults within long-term care facilities, where staff may have limited time to talk with residents (Elford et al., 2005). This exercise allows the older adult to reflect upon his life, and to pass along to loved one stories and information in written form that can be part of his legacy to family members. In one case, I (MBR) was privileged to read some of the history of a dying woman. She had lost family members in a fire as a young girl; it was a trauma that was rarely spoken of. In her last weeks, she passed along to her children her written reminiscences; it helped her to integrate pieces of her life and to express memories; she felt a sense of pride in what she had come through (difficulties) and what she had accomplished. And it gave her adult children a priceless legacy. They learned about their mother, coming to understand her and how she lived her life, on a much deeper level.

A caution is in order, however. While reminiscence therapy is believed to be effective in helping older adults in alleviating symptoms of depression and in achieving a sense of meaning, it may not be helpful in all circumstances (Cappeliez et al., 2005). For instance, reminiscence focused on the loss of significant individuals, especially for older adults who have the tendency to ruminate, may actually cause psychological distress (Korte, Cappeliez, Bohlmeijer, & Westerhof, 2012). Also, reminiscence for the purpose of relieving boredom may not be effective (Cappeliez et al., 2005; Westerhof et al., 2010).

Recommend activities that foster meaning

Activities can foster meaning for people, including older adults. Activities that tie into enjoyment and even spiritual qualities enhance meaning. For instance, some older adults enjoy horticulture. They may view gardening as a spiritual experience where they feel close to the earth or God; for them, gardening is a healing and nurturing experience (Heliker et al., 2001). Not only does gardening connect older adults to the earth and to their spiritual dimension, it may also bring back pleasant memories of the past, when perhaps a parent taught them how to garden. When taking part in a gar-

dening program with others, loneliness may be ameliorated and life satisfaction increased (Tse, 2010).

Other activities that are known to cultivate meaning include taking
educational courses and volunteering (as discussed in Chapter 3). Taking
educational courses may address and in some ways, rectify, regrets from
the past, where older adults wished they had pursued interests in art or
writing, or where they may deal with their disappointment at not having
attended university. As will be addressed in Chapter 8, volunteer work can
be extremely therapeutic and meaningful for older adults. Volunteer work
with vulnerable individuals (such as with troubled youth) may bring richness; here, the wisdom acquired through the years can be shared and make
a great difference. If an aging person is no longer able to perform strenuous activities, he may find great meaning in assisting in an organization
representing a cause that he values. Many older adults are not able to do
overseas work, but they assist in sending out correspondence or in checking
items donated for organizations that provide relief for the suffering in other
parts of the world. Not only does volunteer work provide the opportunity to
make a vital contribution to those in need and increase social contact with
others who share a common passion, it also offers structure to everyday life.

Instilling Hope

As mentioned in Chapter 2, it can be very difficult to move some older
adults toward hope, especially if they have lost the aspects of their lives that
give them hope, such as family members, friends, work, and health. What
is hope? Hope has been defined as:

> *a multidimensional dynamic of life force characterized by a
> confident yet uncertain expectation of achieving a future good which,
> to the hoping person, is realistically possible and personally significant.*
> (Dufault & Martocchio, 1985, p. 380)

Hope changes as people age. Individuals may hope for great wealth when
they are younger, or hope for a rewarding career in a particular field, but as
they age they realize that they will probably never see these dreams come
to fruition. As such, older adults will then need to refine and redefine that
for which they hope.

Within the literature, hope has often been examined in relation to young or middle-aged adults with chronic illness and to those who have been diagnosed with cancer. As well, hope has been explored in and for individuals who are dying. However, there is a growing body of literature examining hope in older adults. We applaud the recognition that hope may be different for aging adults than for younger adults. For example, hope in younger and middle-aged adults often pertains to goals and sought after achievements (Herth & Cutcliffe, 2002). *What* older adults hope for is most likely different than their younger counterparts, as energy levels, health, and work opportunities often change as they age. Also, what relatively healthy older adults hope for may be very different than for terminally ill individuals. For individuals who are dying, hope may be placed in achieving a peaceful death or making amends with family members. While aging adults who are not actively dying may wish for the same, a peaceful death is still in the future. They need to find hope in the present and sustain hope for the future prior to death. And for some, this is not easy.

Assessing hope in older adults involves asking them directly, "What gives you hope?" and "What causes you to lose hope?" Health and human service professionals can assess for factors that promote hope in aging adults. Herth (1993) examined hope in older adults residing in the community and those living within institutional settings. For younger–old adults who were healthy and still living within their homes, they hoped for continued health, the ability to travel, and comfort. The hopes of older residents (over 80 years of age) within institutional settings varied from those who still lived independently. These very aged individuals placed their hopes upon family members or upon life after death (Herth, 1993).

Dunne (2001) used the construct of "faith, hope, and love"[22] for encapsulating the needs of the dying, as well as sources of meaning for them. We suggest that this construct can apply to older adults who are not dying, as well. Regarding hope, Dunne spoke of "images and raw experiences" that give people hope (2001, p. 26). Practically speaking, this involves experiences of beauty, of nature, and of relationship. From a spiritual perspective, these things connect people with transcendence, with *life*. For those in their homes, as well as institutionalized older adults, this may involve regular visits from significant people in their lives; it may mean sitting outside,

---

22. Dunne (2001) mentioned that typically these three terms are used religiously (i.e., as a quotation from the New Testament, 1 Corinthians, 13th chapter). He stated that this can be broadened to mean the following: *faith* means the commitments that the older adult has fulfilled in his or her life. *Hope* will be explained in the paragraphs following. And *love* means (possibly) love for God, and, certainly, love for others.

enjoying the sun and breeze; it may mean a glass of wine to the individual who really enjoys that. Meaning is squeezed out of life, wherever it is! Hope is both a need and a source of meaning.

The motto of Dame Cicely Saunders was "live until you die"; this is the philosophy of palliative care. Hence, people's sources of meaning are met, in some form, as best can be possible. This is hope in the short term: hope for a visit by a staff member or loved one, anticipated time outside in a restful garden, music being played in the common room across the hall, the contemplative exercise of watching the birds at the feeder outside of one's window—these things both engender hope and bring meaning.

Professionals should also be aware of factors that dampen hope. For example, in Herth's work (1993), older adults listed the following factors that impede hope: others, significant fatigue, uncontrollable pain and suffering, and impaired cognition. Some of these factors may not be able to be mitigated; however, health and human service professionals may be able to intervene in relation to teaching about fatigue levels, as well as assessing and treating pain. If older adults are better able to manage fatigue and pain, they may experience greater hope and enjoyment in life.

In working with aging individuals to instill hope, it is vital that the object of hope is realistic. It probably is not reasonable for an older adult, who has never exercised, to hope to run a full marathon. However, if hope is tailored to the senior's fitness level, and thus involves increasing exercise to a level that is manageable (and approved by the individual's physician), then this goal can provide hope and purpose and also be attainable.

Examine and Attend to the Internal Dialogue of Older Adults

I've developed a new philosophy . . .
I'm only going to dread one day at a time
(Charles Schulz, *Brainy Quotes,* 2015).

Charlie Brown's statement is both humorous and heartbreaking. It brings us humor, because we can relate, on some level, to the stresses that would cause us to dread some things in life (and Charlie Brown was honest enough to admit it). It is also heartbreaking, because there are people who truly do dread each day. And sometimes these people do not openly express such dread; rather, they live with an internal conversation that is fearful and punishing. It robs them of joy and meaning in life. The elderly are not exempt from this; and with the losses and stresses of growing old, they may be particularly vulnerable.

One way in which older adults can attend to a sense of meaning in life relates to monitoring their internal dialogue. Internal dialogue refers to how individuals talk to themselves about various situations. In one study researchers interviewed 12 older residents living in Swedish nursing homes about their views on dignity (Dwyer et al., 2008). Based upon their initial findings, the researchers then interviewed in-depth 3 of the 12 women. Dwyer and colleagues (2008) discovered that the inner dialogue of the older individuals helped create meaning in their situations, despite physical disabilities. The researchers' description of inner dialogue was more than just cognitive reframing, or cognitive appraisal. It involved recognizing personal strengths and drawing upon meaning from the past in the present. For instance, one woman would spend much time in her room looking at pictures of her family; this focus did not involve morbid rumination of how things were better in the past. Rather, the older woman pondered, with pride, her roles as wife, mother, and grandmother in the past and how she still felt valued and prized by her family now, even if she did not see her family often (Dwyer et al., 2008).

Another woman, who was blind at the time of the interview, revealed inner dialogue that reflected her ability to accept both the good and the bad in life. She used the metaphor of a fighter to describe how she had faced difficulties in the past and the present. She stressed how her sharp cognitive abilities provide her meaning and allow her to compensate for the loss of eyesight. She took great pride in keeping on top of social issues and readily engaged others in conversations about women's rights and class disparities (Dwyer et al., 2008). Both of these women demonstrated an ability to bring meaning, derived from relationships, passions, or strengths, from the past into the present, despite significant physical deficits. Although these women were not coached or counseled by professionals about how to manage their internal lives in such a fashion, this could be an avenue for some professionals to explore.

Address Issues of Forgiveness

Nurses, social workers, chaplains, and other professionals should be attuned to the possibility that older adults desire to either extend or receive forgiveness. Extending forgiveness has been understood to be a developmental step along the lifespan, with older adults being more likely to forgive than younger people (Allemand, Steiner, & Hill, 2013). Forgiveness can be extended to another in person or simply from within the older adult's soul.

Receiving forgiveness can be more problematic, as there typically is an interaction that needs to happen (between the *I–thou*, or the *I–Thou*). This can pose practical challenges. However, the benefits of receiving forgiveness outweigh those challenges, as when an older adult feels the need for forgiveness, this can impact his quality of life, as well as his sense of meaning and purpose. An aging individual may look back over his life and feel a need for forgiveness from God, from others, or from himself (Allemand et al., 2013). And of the three possible sources for forgiveness—God, others, or the self—forgiveness of the self may be the most difficult to achieve (Enright, 1996).

Why is forgiveness important? Generally speaking, issues surrounding forgiveness—the ability to forgive others and feel forgiven—are associated with better physical and mental health (Ingersoll-Dayton, Torges, & Krause, 2010; Lawler et al., 2005; Toussaint, Williams, Musick, & Everson-Rose, 2008). Also, the act of forgiveness is associated with meaning in life. Those who perceive their lives to be filled with meaning and purpose are more apt to forgive others (Hantman & Cohen, 2010). Hence it would seem that the relationship is reciprocal: a sense of meaning in life may lead to a greater willingness of older adults to forgive others; similarly, being able to forgive the self and others may also enhance meaning in life.

For many professionals (except, perhaps chaplains), the idea of assessing whether older individuals have a need for forgiveness seems foreign, and even intrusive. After all, not all aging individuals experience pressing spiritual needs or distress (Milligan, 2011). While most professionals will not routinely assess this area, they can listen carefully to the stories of older adults as they talk about the present and reflect on the past. Similarly, when engaging older adults in reminiscence therapy or life review, particularly if the purpose is to tap into the meaning older adults ascribe to their lives, issues of regrets about previous relationships, as well as the desire for forgiveness, may emerge (Gunther, 2008).

When engaged in life review or reminiscence therapy, older adults might spontaneously recall incidents of the past. As they talk through an incident, they might have a moment when they see the occurrence in a different light. In that moment, they may think or say, "Now I know why (a person) did that to me . . . Now I understand." Especially if years have passed since an offense and through the years they experienced similar situations that may have contributed to their understanding of the behavior of someone who hurt them, they may now respond with empathy and understanding and discover that the anger is gone. This construct is termed "deferred empathy" (Gunther, 2008) and may assist older adults to move toward forgiveness. We do not mean to imply that forgiveness is easy or natural for older adults. The act of attaining or granting forgiveness is extremely complex (Hayward & Krause, 2013), and older adults can agonize over this. Regrets about how they treated others, how they were hurt by others, or questions about whether God can forgive them can result in great anguish and torment of the soul. We also recognize that some hold misunderstandings about what the act of forgiveness entails. While forgiveness involves a letting go of the right to think, feel, and behave negatively toward someone, it does not necessarily involve trust. For example, a person can forgive a former partner who acted violently toward her, but she does not necessarily need to enter into a relationship again with this person. The ex-partner may not be trustworthy and hence, it would be unwise to make herself vulnerable to this individual (Enright, 1996).

Forgiveness issues are very personal and there is always the potential that older adults—vulnerable individuals—may be wounded by well-meaning professionals who believe they know "what is best" for the elderly person. Ministry of presence, as elucidated earlier in the chapter, is absolutely vital. Humility, empathy, vulnerability—these qualities make the health or human service professional *safe* in her questions and in her presence; and these qualities in her interactions can, in and of themselves, be healing (Reimer-Kirkham et al., 2012). The understanding that another's journey is "holy ground" is important; for that ground that is sacred, the caring health care professional must "take off her shoes."[23] (This is, of course, intended in a metaphorical sense.)

In recognition that issues of forgiveness can pierce right through to the soul of some older adults, we recommend that professionals refer their aging clients to chaplains or clergy when these older adults appear particularly distressed spiritually. Clergy who are trained to deal with issues of forgiveness are often more adept at guiding their clients through the process of forgiveness. If older clients are deeply troubled by the need for forgiveness, but do not want to speak with clergy, nurses can refer them to professionals with advanced training in spiritual counseling (Milligan, 2011).

---

23. This metaphor is drawn from the biblical story of when Yahweh told Moses, at the burning bush, to take off his shoes, as "this is holy ground" (Exodus 3:4–6).

Case Example

Ron, 65 years old, is newly retired and living alone in his own home. You, as a community chaplain, were asked by Ron's brother to visit with him. You contacted him via phone and he agreed to meet with you.

As you enter Ron's home, you are struck by the number of trophies that are on shelves, as well as plaques and newspaper clippings on the walls. These mementoes attest to his accomplishments in sports, rock climbing, and sailing. You compliment him on his achievements and he sadly hangs his head and replies softly, "Yes, I used to be thrilled with what I did, but what do I have now? These trophies are my only companions and they can't talk . . . I am so alone."

Once you sit down, you ask Ron about his family. Who does he have in his birth family, and does he (or did he) have a wife or children? Ron admits that he had no time for relationships; between work and his physical exploits, there was no time for others. Tears spill down his cheeks as he comments, "Now no one has time for me. How could I have been so selfish?"

As you explore further any possible support systems, you gently inquire about what brings meaning into his life now. Also, did he have a belief system in the past that brought him comfort or direction in his life? Ron notes that he was raised in a religious home, but saw religion for the weak. "I thought I was so much stronger than those weaklings. Besides, my meaning came from conquering mountains, toughing it out in the elements (bad weather). Now, I have knee damage and cannot conquer nature. It seems enough to conquer the stairs in this place!"

Understanding that Ron's existential issues stem in part from not doing this introspective work in his earlier years, as well as from his new transition into retirement, you ask about his plans for the immediate future. You carefully weave into the conversation questions about what he wants to do to bring meaning into his life, and suggest activities such as volunteer work, connecting with siblings, and exploring beliefs that would bring him comfort. You suggest that he write down his ideas regarding what brings meaning into his life, spiritual beliefs that he might have held—however loosely in the past—that may bring him comfort now, and what he is learning through this new transition in his life. As you take your leave, you suggest that you meet together in a week to talk about his reflections.

Existential Work for Professionals

Why is it important for health and human service professionals to do their own existential work? Or in rephrasing the question, why would we suggest that professionals examine their beliefs about life, the world, the meaning of their existence, and so on?

From a professional perspective, having done one's own existential work prepares one to work with others experiencing the challenge of life transitions. A social worker, nurse, or chaplain will be alert to the existential issues of life, able to empathize with his patients, and be better equipped to ask questions of aging adults to help them process and come to terms with their lives.

Although important from a personal perspective, doing one's own existential work is also very necessary in working in human services. In the context of this text, professionals who do not do their own existential work may avoid working with older adults. They may feel that the issues of older adults "hit too close to home." In our experience, we have worked with colleagues in gerontology and palliative care who seem to enjoy their work, but at a certain time, move on to other specialties. This can be in part related to the desire to make a change, to acquire new knowledge and different skills. However, colleagues have also told us that they decided upon another focus in health care because working with aging and death and dying triggered issues in them.

To some degree, the calling of working with suffering others "forces" existential work. It taxes the nurse, the social worker, the chaplain, significantly. A recent study in Great Britain showed that 10% of the nurses surveyed missed more than six days due to illness in a three month period; and 20% admitted coming to work when they were too ill to perform the job.[24] One recent American study (Letvak, Ruhm, & McCoy, 2012) indicated that registered nurses suffered from depression at about twice the

---

24. The original study was commissioned by the British Department of Health, and surveyed National Health Services workers. For the study itself, see Van Stolk et al. (2009). For the response from the National Health Services, to deal with these issues, see Nash (2011).

regular rate of the population.[25] In both cases, the researchers stressed that these conditions affected the nurses themselves, the quality of care delivered, as well as their patients. It was recognized that the work itself led to physical and mental illness in nurses.

Strategies

Earlier on in this chapter Viktor Frankl (1986) was quoted as saying human beings exist in the somatic (body), the mental (psychological), and the spiritual. The lifelong development of personhood, it would follow, would focus on those three areas.

As all aspects of being human are interrelated, the following strategies touch upon the physical, the psychological, and the spiritual. As they relate to personhood (the spirit) it could be argued that they all are spiritual. Because we are all different, and express our spirituality in different ways, we suggest that the reader "pick and choose" that which resonates with his or her person.

Kalina (2007) counseled the following exercises: First, she recommended prayer. To pray (in whichever way one is accustomed) connects the health care professional with the Transcendent. It is one way to set down the burdens of the work and step away. It is another way to integrate the experiences of work and of life into one's soul.

Inspirational writings can be uplifting. The scriptures from one's faith can be a source of strength. So can popular books that appeal to the "faith, hope, and love" needs and sources of meaning in all of us.

Live graciously and in forgiveness. The qualities that we admire so greatly in those patients we work with—quiet strength, perseverance, ability to overcome adversity, forgiveness—were worked out in the trenches of life. The "muscles" that work for the aged—the muscles of the soul—have been developed over a lifetime and need to be exercised over the long haul to work effectively as one approaches the end of life.[26]

As health and human service practitioners, we are grateful for those who are grateful for our services. Gratitude is an exercise of the soul. Meister Eckhart said, "If the only prayer you said was 'thank you', that would be enough" (Quotes, 2015). Those who are grateful "embrace life" and find

---

25. Letvak, Ruhm, and McCoy (2012) conducted a study of 1,171 North Carolina hospital nurses. They found that 18% of nurses within this study suffered from depression and compared this with the American national rate of 9%. For more information on this study, see Letvak et al. (2012).

26. For a more complete discussion of these spiritual exercises, see Kalina (2007), pp. 62–69.

meaning in the "little things" (Moore et al., 2006, pp. 296–297). Fill your life with the things for which you are grateful; harness those things that bring you joy! For some, that means running outside on a crisp January morning; for others, it is sitting with a cup of coffee, reading a good book, on that same winter's day. In this way, meaning and joy are intentionally incorporated into each day.

Moore and colleagues (2006) suggested that individuals who have developed a philosophy that integrates adversity and challenge into the fabric of life do better in older adulthood. As with the other spiritual practices, this outlook involves work over the long term.

A health or human service professional can develop such a philosophy by drawing off of the experiences of the older adults she works with. Religious faith typically has such a philosophy built into it; so do many spiritual maxims. Susan, still working in her early senior years, was doing much existential work, born largely out of crisis: A dear friend had dropped dead at work. This woman was the same age as Susan and had died "for no apparent reason." Susan did not consider herself religious; but she was alert to what she felt life was teaching her. In her 60s, Susan had adopted the maxim "everything happens for a reason" and, in her grief and spiritual work, had this saying tattooed in large print down the underside of her forearm.[27] Although she did not know the reason of her precious friend's death, this proverb helped to anchor her.

For the experiences that an individual has particular difficulty with, it is recommended that he conduct his own quest. Finding meaning is truly a search, as Frankl's (2006) book title suggested. As has been mentioned earlier, working with people will tug at particular issues within each of us, based upon our experiences. When those tugs occur, it is wise for an individual to explore his reactions. For some, this is a natural exercise; for others, it is not.

Processing existential issues may be particularly difficult for the professional for whom meaning in life is in flux. For example, the nurse who was raised with a religious faith, but set that faith aside, may be particularly impacted by the spiritual/religious crisis of a patient. She may wonder how to view this event in the light of her current philosophical shift. Speaking with a counselor, a chaplain, or spiritual advisor may be helpful. While we recognize that spiritual development is a process that occurs over a lifetime, and also appreciate that individuals change in their understandings of the world as they experience challenges, it is essential that professionals

---

27. The authors of this book do not recommend a permanent action like getting a tattoo when one is in the throes of grief!

working in health and human services have a paradigm through which to process both the joys and sorrows of their personal and professional lives.

Doing one's own spiritual and existential work is all about the development of personhood over the lifespan. Attention to such matters will help professionals remain effective in their personal lives and professional practice over the long term.

SUMMARY

"To ride the truth of the soul can be a fearsome journey . . ." said Claire Nahmad (1994, p. 19). It can, indeed—for older adults and for those who work with them. But this journey is also awesome—for journeys fraught with challenge can also be very meaningful. In this chapter we looked at the concept of personhood and considered the existential issues of adults as they age. We addressed interventions within the family and the health care system that can help maintain and even further develop personhood in the latter years. And we encouraged health and human service professionals to do their own existential work. A few ethical issues, which will be dealt with more fully in Chapters 6 and 8, have been alluded to here. If we have "rattled the bars of the cage" (Fulghum) for you, the reader, just a bit, then we have succeeded.

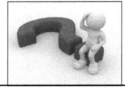

CRITICAL THINKING EXERCISES

- ▶ Review the case example again. If you were the community chaplain, what emotions would you experience as you look toward another visit with Ron? If, in the second meeting, he admits to not having done his "homework," how will you proceed in your spiritual care for him?

- ▶ What aspects of assessing for existential issues are most difficult for you?

- ▶ How do you address your own existential issues?

- ▶ What impact do you think aging will have upon your existential issues?

INTERESTING WEBSITES

▶ American Foundation for Suicide Prevention: www.afsp.org
▶ Attachment Parenting International: www.attachmentparenting.org
▶ Canadian Virtual Hospice: www.virtualhospice.ca

REFERENCES

Ainsworth, M. D. (1967). *Infancy in Uganda*. Baltimore: Johns Hopkins.

Ainsworth, M. D., & Bowlby, J. (1991). An ethological approach to personality development. *American Psychologist, 46*(4), 331–341. doi:10.1037/0003-066x.46.4.333

Allemand, M., Steiner, M., & Hill, P. (2013). Effects of a forgiveness intervention for older adults. *Journal of Counseling Psychology, 60*(2), 279–286.

Allport, G. W., & Ross, J. M. (1967). Personal religious orientation and prejudice. *Journal of Personality and Social Psychology, 5*(4), 432–443.

American Association of Suicidology. (2015). Risk factors for suicide. Retrieved January 5, 2015, from: http://www.suicidology.org/resources/facts-statistics

Anandarajah, G., & Hight, E. (2001). Spirituality and medical practice: Using the HOPE questions as a practical tool for spiritual assessment. *American Family Physician, 63*(1), 81–88.

Arnup, K. (2013). *Death, dying and Canadian families*. Ottawa, ON: Vanier Institute.

Attachment Parenting International. (1994–2014). Use nurturing touch. Retrieved March 24, 2015, from: http://www.attachmentparenting.org/principles/touch

Balboni, M. J., Sullivan, A., Amobi, A., Phelps, A. C., Gorman, D. P., Zollfrank, A., Peteet, J. R., Prigerson, H. G., VanderWeele, T. J., Balboni, T. A. (2013). Why is spiritual care infrequent at the end of life? Spiritual care perceptions among patients, nurses, and physicians and the role of training. *Journal of Clinical Oncology, 31*(4), 461–467. doi:10.1200/JCO.2012.44.6443

The Barna Group. (2009). New statistics on church attendance and avoidance. Retrieved February 10, 2015, from: www.barna.org/barna-update/article/18-congregations/45-new-statistics-on- church-attendance-and-avoidance

Benner Carson, V., & Koenig, H. G. (2004). *Spiritual caregiving: Healthcare as a ministry*. Philadelphia: Templeton Foundation Press.

Bibby, R. (2012). Religion and spirituality in Canada: Religion and spirituality remain pervasive: Latest national survey findings. Retrieved February 11, 2015, from: http://www.reginaldbibby.com/images/PCS_Release_Religion_Spirituality_Remain_Pervasive_in_Canada_Easter_2012.pdf

Blue, K. (1998). *Healing spiritual abuse*. Downer's Grove, IL: Intervarsity Press.

Bohlmeijer, E., Valenkamp, M., Westerhof, G., Smit, F., & Cuijpers, P. (2005). Creative reminiscence as an early intervention for depression: Results of a pilot project. *Aging & Mental Health, 9*(4), 302–304. doi:10.1080/13607860500089567

Bowlby, J. (1953). *Child care and the growth of love*. London: Penguin Books.

Bowlby, J. (1999). *Attachment and loss. Vol. II* (2nd ed.). New York: Basic Books.

Brainy Quotes. (2015). Retrieved January 31, 2015, from: www.brainyquote.com

Buber, M. (1958). *I and thou*. (Translated by Ronald Gregor Smith). New York: Charles Scribner's Sons.

Butler, R. N. (1963). The life review: An interpretation of reminiscence in the aged. *Psychiatry, 26,* 65–76.

Butler, R. N. (1969). Age-ism: Another form of bigotry. *The Gerontologist, 9*(4), 243–246.

Byock, I. (1997). *Dying well: Peace and possibilities at the end of life*. New York: Riverhead Books.

Caldwell, J. M., & Caldwell, D. (2010). Reading Luke for community formation against ageism. *Journal of Religion, Spirituality & Aging, 22*(3), 211–219. doi:10.1080/15528031003613359

Cappeliez, P., O'Rourke, N., & Chaudhury, H. (2005). Functions of reminiscence and mental health in later life. *Aging & Mental Health, 9*(4), 295–301. doi:10.1080/13607860500131427

Centers for Disease Control and Prevention (CDC) (2012). Suicide: Facts at a glance. Retrieved November 26, 2014, from: http://www.cdc.gov/violence prevention/pdf/suicide_datasheet-a.pdf

Chiang, K-J., Lu, R-B., Chu, H., Chang, Y-C., & Chou, K-R. (2008). Evaluation of the effect of a life review group program on self-esteem and life satisfaction in the elderly. *International Journal of Geriatric Psychiatry, 23*(1), 7–10. doi:0.1002/gps.1824

Chippendale, T., & Bear-Lehman, J. (2012). Effect of life review writing on depressive symptoms in older adults: A randomized control trial. *American Journal of Occupational Therapy, 66*(4), 438–446.

Cicirelli, V. G. (2001). Personal meanings of death in older adults and young adults in relation to their fears of death. *Death Studies, 25*(8), 663–683.

Coates, S. (1995). Spiritual components in spiritual care. *European Journal of Palliative Care, 2*(1), 37–39.

Coila, B. (2015). *The effect of human contact on newborn babies*. Retrieved February 10, 2015, from: www.livestrong.com/article/72120-effect-human-contact-newborn-babies/#ixzz2D9wp5WMD

Corner, L., & Bond, J. (2004). Being at risk of dementia: Fears and anxieties of older adults. *Journal of Aging Studies, 18*(2), 143–155. doi:10.1016/j.jaging.2004.01.007

Cram, R. H. (2003). *Bullying: A spiritual crisis*. St. Louis, Missouri: Chalice Press.

Crandall, L. G., White, D. L., Schuldheis, S., & Talerico, K. A. (2007). Initiating person-centred care practices in long-term care facilities. *Journal of Gerontological Nursing, 33*(11), 47–56.

Dark-Freudeman, A., West, R. L., & Viverito, K. M. (2006). Future selves and aging: Older adults' memory fears. *Educational Gerontology, 32*(2), 85–109. doi:10.1080/03601270500388125

Dennis, H., & Thomas, K. (2007). Ageism in the workplace. *Generations, 31*(1), 84–89.

Dobbs, D., Emmett, C. P., Hammarth, A., & Daaleman, T. P. (2012). Religiosity and death attitudes and engagement of advance care planning among chronically ill older adults. *Research on Aging, 34*(2), 113–130. doi:10.1177/0164027511423259

Downing, M. (2003). *Transitions in dying and bereavement: A psychosocial guide for hospice and palliative care.* Winnipeg: Health Professions Press.

Dufault, K., & Martocchio, B. C. (1985). Symposium on compassionate care and the dying experience. Hope: its spheres and dimensions. *Nursing Clinics of North America, 20*(2), 379–391.

Dunne, T. (2001). Spiritual care at the end of life. *Hastings Center Magazine, 31*(2), 22–26.

Dwyer, L-L., Nordenfelt, L., & Ternestedt, B-M. (2008). Three nursing home residents speak about meaning at the end of life. *Nursing Ethics, 15*(1), 97–109. doi:10.1177/0969733007083938

Egan, M., & Prud'homme Brisson, D. (2006). Outreach nurses' perceptions of the spiritual needs of their homebound older clients. *Journal of Religion, Disability & Health, 9*(4), 71–85. http://dx.doi.org/10.1300/J095v09n04_05

Elford, H., Wilson, F., McKee, K. J., Chung, M. C., Bolton, G., et al. (2005). Psychosocial benefits of solitary reminiscence writing: An exploratory study. *Aging & Mental Health, 9*(4), 305–314. doi:10.1080/13607860500131492

Enright, R. D. (1996). Counseling within the forgiveness triad: On forgiving, receiving forgiveness, and self-forgiveness. *Counseling & Values, 40,* 107ff.

Erikson, E. H. (1982). *The life cycle completed: A review.* New York: Norton.

Erikson, E. H., Erikson, J. M., & Kivnick, H. (1986). *Vital involvement in old age.* New York: Norton.

Frankl, V. E. (1986). *The doctor and the soul* (2nd ed.). New York: Vintage.

Frankl, V. E. (2006). *Man's search for meaning.* Boston: Beacon Press.

Free OnLine Dictionary. (2015). Retrieved January 31, 2015, from: www.thefreedictionary.com

Fry, P. S. (2000). Religious involvement, spirituality and personal meaning for life: Existential predictors of psychological wellbeing in community-residing and institutional care elders. *Aging & Mental Health, 4*(4), 375–387. doi:10.1080/713649965

Goffman, E. (1961). *Asylums: Essays on the social situation of mental patients and other inmates.* New York: Anchor.

Gress, L., & Bahr, R. (1984). *The aging person: A holistic perspective.* St. Louis, MO: Mosby.

Gunther, M. (2008). Deferred empathy: A construct with implications for the mental health of older adults. *Issues in Mental Health Nursing, 29*(9), 1029–1040. doi:10.1080/01612840802274974

Haight, B. K. (1988). The therapeutic role of a structured life review process in homebound elderly subjects. *Journal of Gerontology, 43*(2), 40–44.

Hall, P., McCarney, P., Hamilton, P. D., Robertson, C., & Yates-Fraser, J. (1996). Anne's garden: A journey of the human spirit. *Humane Health Care International, 12*(1), 24–26.

Hamilton, D. G. (1998). Believing in patients' beliefs: Physician attunement to the spiritual dimension as a positive factor in patient healing and health. *The American Journal of Hospice and Palliative Care, 15*(5), 276–279.

Hantman, S., & Cohen, O. (2010). Forgiveness in late life. *Journal of Gerontological Social Work, 53*(7), 613–630. doi:10.1080/01634372.2010.509751

Hawley, J. (1993). *Reawakening the spirit in work: The power of Dharmic management.* San Francisco: Barrett Koehler Publishers.

Hay, M. W. (1989). Principles in building spiritual assessment tools. *American Journal of Hospice & Palliative Care, 6*(5), 25–31. doi:10.1177/104990918900600514

Hayward, R. D., & Krause, N. (2013). Trajectories of change in dimensions of forgiveness among older adults and their association with religious commitment. *Mental Health, Religion & Culture, 16*(6), 643–659. doi:http://dx.doi.org/10.1080/13674676.2012.712955

Heliker, D., Chadwick, A., & O'Connell, T. (2001). The meaning of gardening and the effects on perceived well being of a gardening project on diverse populations of elders. *Activities, Adaptation & Aging, 24*(3), 35–56. http://dx.doi.org/10.1300/J016v24n03_03

Hemfelt, R., Minirth, F., & Meier, P. (1991). *We are driven: The compulsive behaviors America applauds.* Nashville: Thomas Nelson.

Herth, K. (1993). Hope in older adults in community and institutional settings. *Issues in Mental Health Nursing, 14*(2), 139–156.

Herth, K. A., & Cutcliffe, J. R. (2002). The concept of hope in nursing: Hope and gerontological nursing. *British Journal of Nursing, 11*(17), 1148–1156.

Heyse-Moore, L. H. (1996). On spiritual pain in the dying. *Mortality, 1*(3), 297–315. doi:10.1080/13576279609696250

Hinck, S. M. (2007). The meaning of time in the oldest-old age, *Holistic Nursing Practice, 21*(1), 35–41.

Hirst, S. P., Lane, A. M., & Reed, M. B. (2013). Personhood in nursing homes: Results of an ethnographic study. *Indian Journal of Gerontological Studies, 27*(1), 69–87.

Hood, R. W., Spilka, B., Hunsberger, B., & Gorusch, R. (2003). *The psychology of religion: An empirical approach* (3rd ed.). New York: Guilford Press.

Hughes, D., & Peake, T. (2002). Investigating the value of spiritual well-being and psychosocial development in mitigating senior adulthood depression. *Activities, Adaptation & Aging, 26*(3), 15–35.

Hunter, E. G. (2007–2008). Beyond death: Inheriting the past and giving to the future, transmitting the legacy of one's self. *OMEGA, 56*(4), 313–329. doi:10.2190/OM.56.4.a

Ingersoll-Dayton, B., Torges, C., & Krause, N. (2010). Unforgiveness, rumination, and depressive symptoms among older adults. *Aging & Mental Health, 14*(4), 439–449. doi:10.1080/13607860903483136

Jenko, M., Gonzalez, L., & Seymour, M. J. (2007). Life review with the terminally ill. *Journal of Hospice & Palliative Nursing, 9*(3), 159–167.

Kalina, K. (2007). *Midwife for souls: Spiritual care for the dying* (Rev. ed.). Boston: Pauline Books & Media.

Kind, V. (2010). *The caregiver's path to compassionate decision-making: Making choices for those who can't.* Texas: Greenleaf Book Group Press.

King, M. L., Jr. (1962). Towards freedom. Speech given at Dartmouth College, Hanover, NH. Retrieved February 10, 2015, from: www.dartmouth.edu/~towardsfreedom/transcript.html

Koenig, H. G. (2001). Spiritual assessment in medical practice. *American Family Physician, 63*(1), 30–31.

Korte, J., Bohlmeijer, E. T., Cappeliez, P., Smit, F., & Westerhof, G. J. (2012). Life review therapy for older adults with moderate depressive symptomatology: A pragmatic randomized control trial. *Psychological Medicine, 42*(6), 1163–1173. doi:10.1017/S0033291711002042

Korte, J., Cappeliez, P., Bohlmeijer, E. T., Westerhof, G. J. (2012). Meaning in life and mastery mediate the relationship of negative reminiscence with psychological distress among older adults with mild to moderate depressive symptoms. *European Journal of Ageing, 9*, 343–351. doi:10.1007/s10433-012-0239-3

Krause, N. (2004). Stressors in highly valued roles, meaning in life, and the physical health status of older adults. *Journal of Gerontology: Social Sciences, 59*(5), S287–S297. doi:10.1093/geronb/59.5.S287

Krause, N. (2007). Evaluating the stress-buffering function of meaning in life among older people. *Journal of Aging and Health, 19*(5), 792–812. doi:10.1177/0898264307304390

Krause, N. (2009). Meaning in life and mortality. *Journal of Gerontology: Social Sciences, 64B* (4), 517–527. doi:10.1093/geronb/gbp047

Kuhl, D. (2003). *What dying people want: Practical wisdom for the end of life.* Toronto, ON: Anchor Canada.

la Cour, P. (2008). Existential and religious issues when admitted to hospital in a secular society: Patterns of change. *Mental Health, Religion and Culture, 11*(8), 769–782. doi:10.1080/13674670802024107

Lawler, K., Younger, J., Piferi, R., Jobe, R., Edmondson, K., & Jones, W. H. (2005). The unique effects of forgiveness on health: An exploration of pathways. *Journal of Behavioral Medicine, 28*(2), 157–167. doi:10.1007/s10865-005-3665-2

Letvak S., Ruhm, C. J., & McCoy, T. (2012). Depression in hospital-employed nurses. *Clinical Nurse Specialist, 26*(3), 177–182. doi:10.1097/NUR0b013e3182503ef0

Lewis, M. M. (2001). Spirituality, counseling, and elderly: An introduction to the spiritual life review. *Journal of Adult Development, 8*(4), 231–240.

Ley, D. (1992). Spiritual care in hospice. In G. R. Cox and R. J. Fundis (Eds.), *Spiritual, ethical and pastoral aspects of death and bereavement* (pp. 207–215). Amityville, NY: Baywood Publishing Company.

MacKinlay, E., & Trevitt, C. (2010). Living in aged care: Using spiritual reminiscence to enhance meaning in life for those with dementia. *International Journal of Mental Health Nursing, 19*(6), 394–401. doi:10.1111/j.1447-0349.2010.00684.x

MacMillan, K., Peden, J., Hopkinson, J., & Hycha, D. (2000). *A caregiver's guide: A handbook about end of life care*. Edmonton: The Palliative Care Association of Alberta.

May, G. G. (1982). *Care of mind, care of spirit: A psychiatrist explores spiritual direction*. San Francisco, CA: Harper.

McKernan, M. (2005). Exploring the spiritual dimension of social work. *Critical Social Work, 6*(2). Retrieved February 10, 2015, from: http://www1.uwindsor.ca/criticalsocialwork/exploring-the-spiritual-dimension-of-social-work

McSherry, C. B. (2011). The inner life at the end of life. *Journal of Hospice & Palliative Nursing, 13*(2), 112–120. doi:10.1097/NJH.0b013e318207af49

Merriam-Webster Online Thesaurus. (2015). Retrieved January 31, 2015, from: http://www.merriam-webster.com/dictionary/thesaurus

Milardo Floriani, C. M. (1999). The spiritual side of pain. *American Journal of Nursing, 99*(5), 24PP–24RR.

Milligan, S. (2011). Addressing the spiritual care needs of people near the end of life. *Nursing Standard, 26*(4), 47–56.

Moore, S. L. (1997). A phenomenological study of meaning in life in suicidal older adults. *Archives of Psychiatric Nursing, 11*(1), 29–36.

Moore, S. L., Metcalf, B., & Schow, E. (2006). The quest for meaning in aging. *Geriatric Nursing, 27*(5), 293–299.

Mount, B. (1993). Beyond psychosocial and physical needs. *The American Journal of Hospice and Palliative Care, 10*(1), 28–37. doi:10.1177/104990919301000109

Munsey, B. (1980). *Moral development, moral education, and Kohlberg: Basic issues in philosophy, psychology, religion, and education*. Birmingham, AL: Religious Education Press.

Nahmad, C. (1994). *Garden spells*. London: Pavillion Books.

Nash, S. (2011). Health and wellbeing part 1: Helping ourselves and others. *Nursing Times, 107* (22), 19–20.

Newport, F. (2011). More than 9 in 10 Americans continue to believe in God. Retrieved February 4, 2015, from: www.gallup.com/poll/147887/americans-continue-believe-god.aspx

Nietzsche, F. (1911). *Twilight of the idols*. (Translated by A. M. Ludovici). New York: Macmillan.

Pittroff, G. E. (2013). The humbled expert: An exploration of spiritual care expertise. *Journal of Christian Nursing, 30*(3), 164–169.

Poor, B., & Poirrier, G. P. (2001). *End of life nursing care.* Sudbury, MA: Jones and Bartlett.

Power, J. (2006). Religious and spiritual care. *Nursing Older People, 18* (7), 24–27.

Public Health Agency of Canada (PHAC). (2010). The Chief Public Officer's report on the state of public health in Canada in 2010. Retrieved November 25, 2014, from: http://www.phac-aspc.gc.ca/cphorsphc-respcacsp/2010/fr-rc/cphorsphc-respcacsp-06-eng.php

Purcell, B. (2008). *Spiritual terrorism: Spiritual abuse from the womb to the tomb.* Bloomington, IN: AuthorHouse.

Reimer-Kirkham, S., Sharma, S., Pesut, B., Sawatsky, R., Meyerhoff, H., Cochrane, M. (2012). Sacred spaces in public places: Religious and spiritual plurality in health care. *Nursing Inquiry, 19*(3), 202–212. doi:10.1111/j.1440-1800.2011.00571.x

Reker, G. T. (1997). Personal meaning, optimism, and choice: Existential predictors of depression in community and institutional elderly. *The Gerontologist, 37*(6), 709–716. doi:10.1093/geront/37.6.709

Religious Tolerance. (1999–2007). How many North Americans attend religious services (and how many lie about going)? Retrieved February 04, 2015, from: www.religioustolerance.org/rel_rate.htm

Reyna, C., Goodwin, E. J., & Ferrari, J. R. (2007). Older adult stereotypes among care providers in residential care facilities. *Journal of Gerontological Nursing, 33*(2), 50–55.

Ryan, P. Y. (2005). Approaching death: A phenomenologic study of five older adults with advanced cancer. *Oncology Nursing Forum, 32*(6), 1101–1108. doi:10.1188/05.ONF.1101-1108

Satterly, L. (2001). Guilt, shame and religious and spiritual pain. *Holistic Nurse Practice, 15*(2), 30–39.

Speck, P. (1998). Spiritual issues in palliative care. In D. Doyle, G. W. Hanks and N. MacDonald (Eds.), *Oxford textbook of palliative medicine* (2nd ed.; pp. 805–814). Oxford, UK: Oxford University Press.

Stoneking, C. B. (2003). Modernity: The social construction of aging. In S. Hauerwas, C.B.

Stoneking, K.G. Meador, and D. Cloutier (Eds.), *Growing old in Christ* (pp. 63–89). Grand Rapids, MI: Eerdmans.

Sulmasy, D. (2006). Spiritual issues in the care of dying patients: "It's okay between me and God." *Journal of the American Medical Association, 296*(11), 1385–1392.

Thomas, C. L., & Cohen, H. L. (2006). Understanding spiritual meaning making with older adults. *Journal of Theory Construction & Testing, 10*(2), 65–70.

Thompson O'Maille, T., & Kasayka, R. E. (2005). Touching the spirit at the end of life. *Alzheimer's Care Quarterly, 6*(1), 62–70.

Timmer, E., Westerhof, G. J., & Dittmann-Kohli, F. (2005). "When looking back on my past I regret . . .": Retrospective regret in the second half of life. *Death Studies, 29*(7), 625–644. doi:10.1080/07481180591004660

Toussaint, L. L., Williams, D. R., Musick, M. A., & Everson-Rose, S. A. (2008). The association of forgiveness and 12-month prevalence of major depressive episode: Gender differences in a probability sample of U.S. adults. *Mental Health, Religion & Culture, 11*(5), 485–500. doi:10.1080/13674670701564989

Tse, M. M. (2010). Therapeutic effects of an indoor gardening programme for older people living in nursing homes. *Journal of Clinical Nursing, 19*(7-8), 949–958. doi:10.1111/j.1365-2702.2009.02803.x

Turesky, D. G., & Schultz, J. M. (2010). Spirituality among older adults: An exploration of the developmental context, impact on mental and physical health, and integration into counseling. *Journal of Religion, Spirituality & Aging, 22*(3), 162–179. doi:10.1080/15528030903437406

VandeCreek, L., & Burton, L. (2001). Professional chaplaincy: Its role and importance in healthcare. *The Journal of Pastoral Care, 55*(1), 81–97.

Van Stolk, C., Hassan, E., Austin, C., Celia, C., Disley, E., Hunt, P., Marjanovic, S., et al. (2009). *The NHS workforce health and wellbeing review.* London: Department of Health.

Walsh, F. (1999). *Spiritual resources in family therapy* (Ed.). New York: The Guilford Press.

Walsh, F. (2009). Religion, spirituality and the family: Multi-faith perspectives. In F. Walsh (Ed.), *Spiritual resources in family therapy* (2nd ed.; pp. 3–30). New York: The Guilford Press.

Weingarten, K. (1999). Stretching to meet what's given: Opportunities for a spiritual practice. In F. Walsh (Ed.), *Spiritual resources in family therapy* (pp. 240–255). New York: The Guilford Press.

Westerhof, G. J., Bohlmeijer, E., & Webster, J. D. (2010). Reminiscence and mental health: a review of recent progress in theory, research and interventions. *Aging and Society, 30*(4), 697–721, doi:http://dx.doi.org/10.1017/S0144686X09990328

World Health Organization (2014). *First WHO report on suicide prevention.* Retrieved on January 5, 2015, from: http://www.who.int/mediacentre/news/releases/2014/suicide-prevention-report/en/

Worthington, E. L. (1989). Religious faith across the lifespan: Implications for counseling and research. *Counseling Psychologist, 17*(4), 555–612. doi:10.1177/0011000089174001

Wright, L. M. (2005). *Spirituality, suffering and illness: Ideas for healing.* Philadelphia: F. A. Davis.

CHAPTER 6

DEATH: THE FINAL TRANSITION

*The boundaries which divide Life from Death are at
best shadowy and vague. Who shall say where the
one ends, and where the other begins.*
(Edgar Allan Poe)

*There is no Death;
What seems so is transition.*
(Anonymous, quoted in Ley & van Bommel, 1994, p. 42)

Death is the final transition that older adults face. This transition is imbued with mystery; what an individual's dying process will look like and what will happen afterward are not known for certain. These mysteries result in the shadows and vagueness described by American writer Poe. For some aging individuals, death is a welcomed transition out of this world into the next. Others fear death greatly and move into this transition with considerable trepidation. Coming face-to-face with death not only entails the physical act of dying, but also involves a psychological and spiritual response. And facing one's mortality can result in existential issues, as discussed in Chapter 5. From many spiritual perspectives—and what is increasingly being understood within the discipline of palliative care—is that physical death is not "the end," but rather a transition.

Within this chapter, we examine myths and issues that surround the dying and death of aging adults, both for the aging individuals themselves, as well as for their family members. As we look at these issues, we weave into these discussions what the work of health and human service professionals involves in assisting dying older adults, as well as their family members. Finally, we raise ethical issues in relation to dying, older individuals. We suggest that Chapters 5 and 6 be read in tandem, because many of the concepts appear in both. As well, examples from Chapter 5 will be referred to in Chapter 6, further examining these examples using concepts from the latter chapter. Of significant difference, Chapter 6 will focus upon the *vulnerability* of the dying older adult, with care and interventions tailored specifically to uphold dignity and personhood in this circumstance.

Before we delve into the content of the chapter, a foundational concept needs to be explained. In dealing with the dying of any individual across the lifespan, the terms *palliative care* or *hospice* come up. Canadian Virtual Hospice Team (2011) defined palliative care as:

> *a type of health care for patients and families facing*
> *life-threatening illness. (It) helps patients to*
> *achieve the best possible quality of life right up until the end of life.*
> *Palliative care is also called end-of-life, or comfort care.*

Further, palliative care focuses on the concerns of the patient: physical symptoms and the emotional and spiritual concerns of the patient and family. Its goal is to maintain and uphold dignity; it seeks to honor the religious and cultural practices of the patients; and after the patient passes, the family receives bereavement support (Canadian Virtual Hospice Team, 2011).

This definition of *palliative care* can contain the concept of *hospice* within it; hospice care being understood to focus on end-of-life, with a time frame attached to it. A number of sources differentiate between the two concepts, stating that palliative care focuses on the reduction of physical symptoms (such as pain, nausea, or constipation), which can occur at any time during a serious illness, while hospice care encompasses this and the psychosocial and spiritual supports, as well as reflecting that these are provided at the very end of life (for example, Buchanan, Choi, Wang, & Ju, 2004). In fact, in the US, the term "palliative" is associated with symptom reduction at any stage in a serious (not necessarily terminal) illness (National Cancer Institute, 2010) and an individual may receive palliative care much earlier in their illness (Jackson, 2015). As this chapter focuses on death and dying, and as (in Canada) the terms *hospice, palliative care,* and *end-of-life care* tend to be used interchangeably in common usage (as the definition from Canadian Virtual Hospice suggests), so they will be utilized here.

The definition from Canadian Virtual Hospice describes the breadth of hospice palliative care; however, it does not capture its heart. Here, Dorothy Ley provides us with that dimension:

> *Palliative care is about living and the meaning of life.*
> *It's about loss and grief and joy. It's about caring and sharing.*
> *It's about tears and laughter . . . They are very powerful words*
> *when acted upon . . . Palliative care is about life, not death.*
> *(Ley & van Bommel, 1994, p. 30)*

Myths About Dying in Advancing Years

There are myths that surround death and dying in older individuals. These myths are taken up in everyday conversation about the final transition in life and impact how individuals view and respond to death in the aged. In the following discussion, we attempt to debunk these myths, as unwittingly, health and human service professionals can adopt some of these ideas.

Dying and Death Are Not as Difficult for Older Adults as They Are for Younger Individuals

Death and dying are difficult for many people, irrespective of age. It is true that some older adults want to die, perhaps due to significant illness or pain, as well as having lost close friends and family members. Others, however, do not. They may not feel ready, still enjoying life. Others may fear the unknown; the mysteries surrounding dying, as well as what will happen after death, may still trouble and even haunt some older adults, despite having had many years to wrestle with such concerns (Reed, 2015). Family members and health care professionals may inadvertently assume that the dying process is easier for their older patients (Sidell, Samson Katz, & Komaromy, 2000) and thus fail to provide the level of attention to psychological and spiritual issues that they might for younger patients.

A chaplain had a number of delightful interactions with a terminally ill gentleman who was admitted to a palliative care ward within a hospital. He was well into his 90s and was now bedridden. "I just don't understand it," he said in reference to being confined to bed. "Just a year ago I was golfing." The chaplain responded with a comment about his age and that he had done so well for so long. "Yes, I know that," he replied, "but I just don't understand it!" Upon reflection, it became clear to the chaplain that his "lack of understanding" was really an existential statement about still feeling young inside and, hence, the surprise at being physically limited. This realization shifted the focus of the conversations from that which was more corporeal (issues of the body) to that which was more spiritual (issues of the heart).

In Chapter 5, I (MBR) referred to the grandmother of my spouse, Brian. Grandma Reed said on numerous occasions to my husband, "On the inside, I'm not old; I'm still the same me I've always been." A lovely statement of personhood! A very active woman, she had once enjoyed swimming in the Georgian Bay. Visiting at "the cottage" (she was now in her 90s and a resident in a nursing home), she said to my husband on a sweltering August day, "What I wouldn't give to feel the coolness of the bay!" Brian took her hand and walked her down to the water; she took her shoes off and being supported by her grandson, dipped her hands and feet in, enjoying the sensation of cold water on her warm skin. Unexpectedly, to my husband as well as his siblings on the shore, she plunged in for a brief swim! She spent the next couple of hours in borrowed clothes in the cottage, as her own clothes were being dried; but this experience of swimming was, she said, totally worth it!

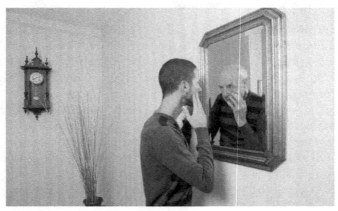

tommaso lizzul/Shutterstock, Inc.

In both of these examples, there were no significant existential issues and no fear in getting very old and facing into death; there was simply incredulity in both of these very elderly people; they could not quite believe they were at the end of their lives. For older adults who have lived life fully, in their spirits they may still be young ("young at heart"); and so being very old, with its limitations, may seem like a surprise or even an offense.

Chapter 5 provided a number of examples of older adults with existential issues surrounding age and dying. These issues can be profound. Older adults can and do find peace in dealing with these concerns, and they seem to become uniquely sensitive to spiritual matters as they age (Meraviglia, Sutter, & Gaskamp, 2008; Reed, 2014). One man said that his palliative experience caused him "to come alive spiritually." That growth came as a result of his spiritual pain in dying, and his willingness to reach out for and receive help. He died peacefully.

But not all older adults leave this life serenely. In Shakespeare's play, *Henry VI*, Joan of Arc famously says, "Fight till the last gasp" (Searchquotes, 2015). Though the context of this quote is different than twenty-first century North America, many people do just that. It would seem that we are "wired" for life, and a person does not simply turn off the "switch for living" as she would turn off a light. That same strength of spirit that kept this woman going through difficulties in life can keep the dying older adult alive—sometimes longer than she herself would wish! Even when an individual has done her existential work, the goodbyes have been said, and practical affairs are in order, it can still take some time for the passage to happen. This can be very distressing to family members. But discussion with them generally reveals that their loved one has been a strong, independent person who has tended to live life on his or her own terms. "Each person dies in his or her own way" (Halifax, 2009, p. 65).

Older Adults Experience Less Pain

Perhaps because aging individuals do not often complain to health or human service professionals about pain, or because some conditions preclude the voicing of pain to others (e.g., aphasia related to strokes or dementia), it is sometimes assumed that older adults experience less pain in dying than their younger counterparts (Gropelli & Sharer, 2013). This is not true; older adults can experience just as much pain as younger individuals in the dying process. Believing that pain is just a part of aging can result in health care professionals responding less vigorously to complaints (Gammons & Caswell, 2014). Also, many elderly people hold the same opinion, and so may not voice their discomfort (Gammons & Caswell, 2014); they also may be concerned about worrying their adult children, or that voicing persistent pain may precipitate a change in living arrangements (from home to a long-term care facility, for example), thereby resulting in a loss of independence.

Gropelli and Sharer (2013) examined the attitudes of 16 nurses (registered nurses and licensed practical nurses) working in long-term care facilities in the United States. Within their interviews, nurses stated that pain control had significantly improved in their facilities, but noted that there still needed to be more improvement in this area. They made reference to the attitudes of other nurses (in other parts of their facility) who had antiquated beliefs about pain control (such as, older adults complain histrionically about pain, that pain control can lead to addiction), and also admitted to not having up-to-date in-services on pain control. They also mentioned that institutional patterns, such as only calling physicians for medication when pain was severe or a lack of individualized care plans, impacted older residents negatively (Gropelli & Sharer, 2013).

Despite the believed improvement in pain control, however, chronic pain remains an issue in long-term care facilities. For instance, it is estimated that 38% in Canada (Statistics Canada, 2010) and 75–85% in the US (National Institute of Health Medline Plus, 2011) of older adults living in long-term care facilities suffer chronic pain.

Although data from Statistics Canada (2010) and the NIH Medline Plus (2011) were not specifically palliative in nature, many elderly people die in nursing homes. Currently it is estimated that about 10% of older Canadians die in long-term care facilities (Cairns & Ahmad, 2011). In America in the first decade of the twenty-first century, it is estimated that about 20% of older adults died in long-term care facilities. As we are living longer, and as the length of hospital stays continue to decrease, it is estimated that the percentage will double by 2020 (Muramatsu, Hoyem, Yin, & Campbell, 2008).

There are unique challenges when a person is unable to express her pain accurately, due to dementia or other physiological conditions. There are a number of assessment tools that professionals can use to determine pain levels, such as the Numeric Rating Scale (NRS), the Verbal Descriptor Scale (VDS),[1] the SOCRATES pain questionnaire, the Faces Pain Scale-Revised (FPS-R), Pain Assessment in Advanced Dementia (PAINAD) and

---

1. The Iowa Pain Thermometer is a more recent adaptation of the VDS and is considered to be an effective scale for rating pain in the young and old cognitively impaired population. See Herr, Spratt, Garand, & Li (2007).

the Pain Assessment Checklist for Senior Adults with Limited Ability to Communicate (PACSLAC).[2]

Ersek and Polomano (2011) recommended the following in assessing pain in older adults, including those who are dying. First, older adults *deserve* effective pain assessment and control. Sometimes, the most difficult person to convince of this fact is the dying person himself! (One dying man in a palliative setting continually refused pain medications. He used the "tough guy" approach, but as his cancer pain increased, he became increasingly agitated in his mood and behaviors. As staff got to know him, it became apparent that he felt he did not deserve good pain management. Dealing with issues of shame psychosocially and spiritually aided him in receiving the analgesics he so obviously needed. The soul work also may have lessened some of his physical pain.)

Second, counseled Ersek and Polomano (2011), what the patient *says* about her pain should take precedence over other indicators. Pain thresholds are different from person to person; pain is subjective. Individuals who have experienced chronic pain may be more sensitive to it—in their living and in their dying. Pain assessment tools, including observation for physiological and behavioral indicators of pain, must only replace the patient's verbal report if the dying individual is not able to communicate herself.

A number of the pain assessment tools mentioned previously recommend the family's knowledge of their dying adult as a resource for assessing pain. We would like to stress that here. Health care providers can be limited in pain assessment, particularly if the older adult is cognitively impaired or unable to communicate, due to lack of experience with and historical knowledge of that individual. For instance, hospital stays can be short, and nurses may not care for a patient more than once or twice. The family who has been caregiving for their loved one has the inside track.

In one example of this guideline, a delightful very elderly woman was in a residential hospice. In her late 90s, she presented with humor and spunk. Her dementia did not seem really pronounced on first glance; she sat in her chair with her newspaper daily. (Over time the extent of the dementia became clearer; she did not really read and forgot whether she had seen the paper that day.) To questions of pain she would respond, "Oh, no!" She came from a very professional family; her father had been a doctor, her husband had been a doctor, and an adult daughter and grandson were

---

2. For information on all of these tools except for the SOCRATES pain questionnaire, see www.geriatricpain.org. For more information on the SOCRATES pain questionnaire, see Hughes (2012).

doctors also. It was her daughter who initially tipped the nurses off that her mom would routinely say, "no" to questions of pain. This loving daughter encouraged staff to look deeper than the verbal response. She knew her better than anyone![3]

The Death of Older Adults Should Not Be Too Hard on Adult Family Members

It is commonly assumed that the deaths of aging relatives, while sad, should not be too upsetting for adult family. After all, it is reasoned, death is to be expected in older adults and they have lived their lives. It is not unusual for adult children to be asked the age of a parent when it is known that the parent is dying or has passed away. If the grieving adult children admit that the parent was over 80 years of age, the response is often something like, "Well, she had a long life," or "At least his suffering is over." While these comments are well intended, they often speak more about the discomfort of those who offer the comments, than the actual impact of the death of a parent upon the adult child(ren).

Adult children can sometimes express surprise in their own responses to a parent's (impending) death. They may express disbelief. One man was speaking about the imminent death of his elderly father. He expressed disbelief that his father's life was ending. "I'm a science kind of guy, and it should be possible for people to live well into their hundreds," he said. When the health care provider sought to touch upon the emotional aspects of his impending loss, he rebuffed her: "It's just wrong that he should die; there should be still lots of years left." He was not comfortable in dealing with the existential issues of death and his emotional response. Rather, he chose to speak about the impending death "scientifically" as a way to vent his distress.

And sometimes adult children are surprised (and ashamed) of the depth of their emotions in response to an elderly parent's death. "I should be handling this better," is sometimes expressed with tears. This may reflect an acceptance of the societal myth that the death of an older adult—specifically a parent—should not be too hard on adult family members. To this, McDaniel and Clark stated, "No human being can know how he or she will feel when a parent dies" (2009, p. 45).

---

3. Of course, caution is in order here. Sometimes family members, in their anxiety, are not accurate in their assessment of their loved one's pain levels. However, they can give health care providers clues about what to look for.

Health and human service professionals are not immune to buying into this myth. They may assume that family members will be able to accept the passing more easily; after all, their loved one "was old!" I (MBR) remember being called in on a sunny Saturday afternoon to provide support for the family of a woman who was well into her 90s and had just passed in a residential hospice. My own thoughts, as I shifted from gardener (I was pruning shrubs) to chaplain, was "Oh, this shouldn't be too difficult," as the nurse who paged me had let me know that the deceased woman was very elderly. I arrived unprepared for the level of grief I found in the room. An adult granddaughter was distraught; her grandma had raised her and was closer to her than anyone else in her life. And an older sister (who was nearing 100 years of age) cried, as her wheelchair was pushed into the room, "Why wasn't it me?! I'm older. Now there is no one left but me!" It was truly humbling for me—at that time I was a relatively new palliative care chaplain. I believe that I brought the requisite clinical skills to the situation, but my ability to provide the ministry of presence was not there. I was caught off guard, unprepared to tread on this very sacred ground with my shoes off!

When the relationship is close

Even if the death of an aging parent is expected, it still can result in a significant grief reaction in family members. One factor in grief is the depth of the relationship; the closer the connection, the greater the grief (Rando, 1984). The assumption that family is prepared for the death of an older loved one, simply because their loved one is older, is fallacious. Preparation is vital and support is invaluable.

In one instance, a very elderly man came into the hospital for palliative care. His daughter, who had worked as an aide in a long-term care facility for decades, could not accept that her father was dying. (This was a surprise to a number of staff members, who assumed that her professional experience would provide some preparation for the challenges of her personal life; but witnessing others' deaths did not prepare her to come to grips with her own father's imminent passing). As the trust relationship was established and deepened, she revealed that she did not believe in an afterlife and could not bear to "lose" her dad. Cremation was the plan, so it was suggested to her that she purchase a locket, in which she could keep a few of her father's cremains. Wearing this locket on a chain would keep her dad "close to her heart." This seemed to resonate with this adult daughter and she did just that. In that act she could carry some of her father with her in her daily life and derive comfort from his presence.

When the relationship is conflicted

As will be discussed in Chapter 7, traumatic or conflicted issues of the past may be dredged up through the process of caring for the dying parent; this, too, makes the death of a parent difficult. Being present to the dying parent is painful, not simply because of the imminent death; it is also painful because of past wounds/experiences that the contact brings up.

Here, the adult children experience anticipatory grief as well as conflicted grief. They know the death is coming, and they experience the anticipated loss. The grief is conflicted, because while this individual was a parent that they were connected with (and have likely loved), the complicating factors (abuse in the past, neglect or indifference, unresolved conflicts, or other serious issues) make the situation even more painful. Adult children often feel the need to speak of past experiences to health and human service professionals and need to be heard. Even if they have had counseling to deal with the past, they are now experiencing those issues in another way. This parent who once abused or neglected them is now vulnerable, and they are, perhaps, in a position of "power" for the first time in their lives (the adult children are now the ones possessing the health and youth). There is a notable shift in the dynamics of the relationship. (However, it should be noted that although dying older adults are vulnerable, some still wield considerable power over their children on their deathbed.)

It is essential that health and human service professionals provide a safe place for these adult children to work through their grief *as it is,* rather than what the nurse, doctor, social worker, or chaplain feels it should be. Old experiences are reprocessed in the new reality (the impending death of the parent). Here it is very helpful to have an interprofessional approach, with a referral to a social worker or chaplain, to provide that place for the grief work (regarding both anticipatory and conflicted grief) to happen. It is often a time when some significant internal growth can happen in the adult children.

Case Example

Jean and Sandra were adult daughters of Bob, who had been admitted to a hospital palliative care unit with end stage renal failure. In their formative years Sandra and Jean had been terrified of their alcoholic father. Understandably, some of this fear remained. Of their own accord, they confronted their dying father of his abuse in the past. This confrontation occurred on a weekend, and they tearfully informed the chaplain and social worker on the following Monday. They were struggling to sort through the tangled web of emotions they were feeling. The social worker and chaplain helped them to do this, through listening and validating the emotions of these women. While the confrontation was frightening, it turned out to be empowering. Although Sandra and Jean felt that the apology for the past abuse was "weak," they saw their father through new eyes. He was no longer the terrifying figure who abused them; he was now vulnerable and, in some ways, pitiful. While feeling proud of themselves, the women wondered whether it had been morally wrong to confront the dying man; could they have been "pushing him over the edge"? The social worker and chaplain helped them work through the tangled strands of what they needed, and what confrontation afforded and cost Bob: the opportunity to receive forgiveness, but with the discomfort of the discussion. As professionals, the chaplain and social worker understood that they could not tell these women who had been victimized what they should feel or how to proceed from here. They knew that their role was to help them sift through the experience of confrontation and bring some understanding to their conflicted emotions; Jean and Sandra had to make their own choices, as they bore the consequences of them.

Existentially speaking

Not only do adult children grieve the loss of an aging parent and recognize that their life histories, up to this point in time, have been ensconced within their parents' lives, but the death of one, particularly both parents, signals that they themselves are entering a later phase of their own lives. Adult children may talk about the stark realization that they will die next, barring some unfortunate twist of fate that younger family members die before them. The growing recognition that they are aging and that death is not as far away as once thought can be unsettling for some individuals. Existential questions such as "Have I done what I've wanted to do with my life?" may be triggered (Milligan, 2011). And a very real sense of aloneness may be experienced; these adult children may exclaim, "I'm an orphan now!" (McDaniel & Clark, 2009).

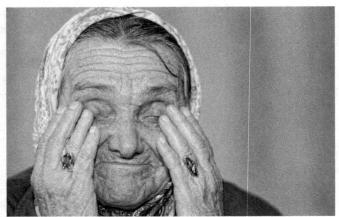

Whatever individuals' lives have entailed, their past history and a significant part of who they are has been intertwined with the lives of their parents. As so aptly stated by Maya Angelou, "I've learned that regardless of your relationship with your parents, you'll miss them when they're gone from your life" (Good Reads, 2015). We recognize that not all readers will agree with this statement; nevertheless, it is poignant. Parents have played a significant role in their children's lives; for acquaintances or professionals to assume that the loss is not significant because the parent was older, is doing a disservice to grieving adult children or family members.

In order for health and human service professionals to appropriately and effectively assist older adults and their family members through the final transition of life, it is important that they are apprised of the issues experienced in dying. Dying is challenging for the aged adult as well as for their adult children (and grandchildren), and age does not prevent pain in the dying process. Dying is also a formidable process for those who work with them. "Live to the point of tears," said Albert Camus (Thinkexist. com, 2015); in working with the dying, all involved experience life to this degree—to the point of tears.

Issues Related to Dying for Older Adults

There are physical issues related to dying, as well as spiritual ones. Many of the issues related to dying are the same as the existential issues discussed in Chapter 5. However, the existential issues are often magnified in dying, as there is finality in the experience, as well as a limited time frame in which to deal with them. The need to deal with the existential issues of dying is central to personhood; one's sense of mortality may have been avoided over the course of the lifespan, but when dying, an individual has little choice. Palgi and Abramovitch (1984) stated, "Death awareness is a natural sequel to self-awareness—an intrinsic attribute of humankind" (p. 385).

Next within this chapter, we will look at *the* major physical (and psychological) concern that older adults have in dying: pain (Creedon & O'Regan, 2010). We also will look at the existential issues in the light of impending death: loss of control, aloneness, meaning in life and in death, and relationship with self and others. Additionally, we explore a common term in palliative care: a *good death*. Is this possible? What is a good death? We will also look at the impact of dementia upon the dying process.

Pain

Earlier in the chapter we discussed the prevalence of pain in the elderly. We also looked at their reticence to speak of it and sometimes health care providers' reluctance to treat it assertively (Hughes, 2012). It is now possible with palliative medications to very effectively deal with pain.

As was mentioned in Chapter 5, some believe that pain can *always* be managed. Byock (1997), for example, believed this is possible and looks toward the day when this will be a reality.[4] Dealing with pain effectively is a distinguishing strength of hospice and palliative care. But pain in end-of-life care can be complex; families caring for loved ones at home, staff on acute care units within hospitals, and staff in long-term care often do not feel equipped to handle it.

When a terminally ill older adult experiences pain, she likely already has a number of co-existing medical conditions; she may also have allergies and sensitivities to certain standard pain medications (such as codeine). The number of medications she is taking can be dizzying (to her and her health care providers!). Compounding the difficulties, these pharmaceuticals may be interacting with each other. Herbal remedies, unknown to her family doctor, may also be a part of her health repertoire, as well as over-the-counter medications, and these may be interacting with the prescribed

---

4. The World Health Organization has developed cancer pain guidelines for treating those with cancer. McHugh and colleagues estimated that 10–20% of advanced cancer patients do not get adequate pain control within the parameters of these guidelines (or suffer from intolerable symptoms from the medications prescribed). These researchers called for more research and an expansion of treatment options. See McHugh, Miller-Saultz, Wuhrman, and Kosharskyy (2012).

medications. Other factors, such as being bedridden, may be contributing to her pain. As well, she may have a number of complex psychosocial and spiritual burdens that contribute to her overall malaise.

So in a palliative setting, professional caregivers are educated and experienced in dealing with the whole person. A medication review will take place; some medications may be removed from her list; others, specific to palliative care, may be added. A patient's goals of care will be delineated. Pain control is generally a part of a patient's goals. In a palliative situation, health professionals will not worry about opioid addiction as they would in other situations (Gropelli & Sharer, 2013). This type of specialized medical and nursing care will be provided around the clock. Evidence reveals that pain management is better for those receiving palliative care than those who do not (Miller, Mor, Wu, Gonzalo, & Lapane, 2002; Regan, Tapley, & Jolley, 2014).

In the palliative care construct, psychosocial and spiritual supports will also be put into place, using social work, chaplains, and volunteers. Family members will be supported too (Nunn, 2014). In this type of setting, pain is generally managed very well. Quality of life is maintained and even enhanced. Patients and family members work together and grow in the process.

However, does this mean that pain is nonexistent? For a variety of reasons, involving the patient, the setting, the circumstances of the pain, and the expertise of the staff in the home or health care setting, truly, it does not (Hughes, 2012; Regan et al., 2014). A terminally ill man may come into a palliative setting with pain issues that take some time to sort through. Or a medication may come to the end of its effectiveness. Additionally, new pain may develop as cancer spreads. It is erroneous to assume that because there *are* effective pain medications available that a person will *never* experience pain. This is stated bluntly here because sometimes patients and their families come into a palliative care setting with this idea firmly entrenched; then, if pain is experienced, they feel let down and sometimes become angry at the health care providers.

And not everyone receives the benefits of palliative care. Within the United States and Canada, the nature of and the benefits of palliative care, either through home care services, hospice care within a long-term care facility, or within residential hospices, are being increasingly understood.[5]

---

5. Understanding, however, is only one step in the process of change. For example, while 87% of American long-term care facilities hold contracts with hospice services, only 30% of these facilities have a resident receiving hospice services at any given time (Hospice Action Network, 2013).

It would be ideal if everyone *who wanted to* experience this care could. However, health care realities at this time do not make this possible; sometimes, there are not open beds within a local hospice facility and so older adults cannot be transferred.[6] Unfortunately, then, effective pain control does not always occur.

It also happens sometimes that a person will pass away quickly from a catastrophic event, such as a pulmonary embolism, unrelated to his terminal condition.[7] Medication can help to ease the suffering if an embolus occurs. However, the event may happen so quickly that nursing staff are not able to get that medication to the individual to ameliorate the suffering. In this case, the individual may pass in distress, and this is very distressing to family members! Some of the challenges of this will be discussed further on in this chapter.

Occasionally, a terminally ill person will ask to "be put out of (my) misery." Or, a family member will say, "If this were our dog, we'd have had her put down!" These expressions of distress can involve physical pain and often existential pain, as well. From a palliative care perspective, the physical pain is generally resolved through adjusting medications and/or dosages. However, the cries are more than physical; they are existential, revealing a sense of suffering without meaning (Frankl, 2006). From psychosocial and spiritual perspectives, social workers, chaplains, and nurses come alongside these suffering individuals and their family members (Creedon & O'Regan, 2010) to provide support and assist with meaning (Nunn, 2014). Many important things, such as relationship restoration and the blessing of family members, happen in a person's final weeks or days. And the healing impact of relationship restoration or blessings from the dying person to family members cannot be emphasized enough; such end-of-life work is enormously helpful for family members in their grieving after the older adult has passed away.

One woman came into a palliative care setting "just done." She had had enough, she stated, and hoped that the end came sooner, rather than

---

6. For example, in Canada, it is estimated that only between 16–30% of dying Canadians have access to hospice palliative care, and access to it is highly dependent upon the region in which one is living (Canadian Hospice Palliative Care Association Fact Sheet, 2012).

7. In palliative care, the focus is on quality of life, rather than on prolonging life. So a dying person who is bedridden may develop a blood clot from continuously lying down; this is not directly related to the condition that is making him terminally ill. In a palliative setting, a patient often does not want medications such as blood thinners, as his focus is not on the prolonging of life, but rather on the quality of the remaining days. Due to blood stasis in the deep veins, a clot may develop and travel to his lungs (a pulmonary embolism) and death may result sooner than anticipated.

later. Through the care of the interprofessional staff, and the support of her family, she gained a new lease on life. Her days were meaningful and her interactions rich. "I hope God gives me many more days!" she stated as I (MBR) was offered cake at a little party in her room. The value of this time for her and for her family cannot be overstated: Bonds were deepened, the things that needed to be said were, she prepared herself emotionally and spiritually for her own passing, and the family became better prepared to handle her death after demise.

To complete this section on pain, there is in some of the literature a distinction between "pain" and "suffering" (Halifax, 2009). An individual can be in *pain*, but not be *suffering*. Physical pain is distinguished from the existential messages about the pain (the suffering) that overtake us—as Halifax said, the "story" surrounding the pain. She quoted the Buddha:

> *When touched by . . . pain, the ordinary, uninstructed person sorrows, . . . becomes distraught. So he feels two pains, physical and mental, just as if he was shot with an arrow, and, right afterward, was shot with another one, so that he felt the pain of two arrows. (Halifax, 2009, p, 72)*

Halifax's point is poignant. She was not minimizing physical pain, but rather encouraging those experiencing it not to interpret it as we so often do in North America—as something that is an aberration! Dr. Paul Brand, a Christian surgeon who worked for decades in India on the hands and feet of those ravaged by leprosy, echoed the same concerns about western society. Brand (Yancey & Brand, 1997) encouraged us that we need to master pain, before it masters us. How an individual views her physical pain is a key factor in how she deals with it and experiences life.

Need to Have Control in the Dying Process

For many dying individuals, including older adults, maintaining meaningful control of their lives, in their dying, is vital. Decision-making is foundational in personhood (Hirst, Lane, & Reed, 2013), and hence is essential in an older adult's experience of the dying process.

Dying involves many losses of control. The loss of control a dying individual faces includes: over his body, disease and pain, emotional boundaries, and life itself (Strohbuecker, Eisenmann, Galushko, Montag, & Voltz, 2011). For many, loss of control over bodily functions is deeply distressing. When needing incontinence products, they may exclaim, "I started life this way, and now I guess I'll be finishing it this way too!" This is not only an expression of concern regarding the need to address incontinence, but is an existential expression of sorrow. Other existential statements concerning loss of other forms of control—and perhaps, diminishment of the person one once knew—could be: "I didn't used to look this way, you know," and "It seems like I cry so easily right now!" (Ozanne, Graneheim, & Strang, 2013).

Besides the loss of control that terminally ill people face because of disease and/or effects of medication, Goffman (1961) and others spoke of the loss of control (and hence personhood) in institutionalized settings, such as a hospital. An example comes to mind. When I (AML) was a fairly new graduate nurse, I worked on a medical/oncology unit. I cared for a man dying of stomach cancer. The man was in hospital receiving a particular form of nutrition through intravenous tubing (called TPN or total parenteral nutrition). This fluid was very thick, sugary, and sticky (if some landed on the floor). This man was very particular about needing his square pad placed near his pillow, with his spit basin placed in a specific position, as well as his square box of tissues arranged just right. Being young and not knowledgeable about his need for control in his dying process, I was sloppy about how I arranged his basin and tissues, as well as in spilling TPN fluid when changing the intravenous bag. He would become very annoyed as a small amount would land on the floor. By the end of four 12-hour shifts, I was frustrated and frazzled by his attempts to control his environment. Being much older now, and also being aware of the importance for human beings to have some semblance of control in their lives, particularly in the dying process, I truly regret not being more attentive to his need for some mastery over his environment. I also recognize, however, that my inability to give him more control was also related to the environment—a busy hospital unit. Even if I had been more knowledgeable and aware of the significance of facilitating control on his part, the busyness of the unit would have precluded my attempts, at least to some degree, to allow him more control. As is being highlighted in this chapter, palliative care seeks to restore that sense of personhood, of dignity, and of control by providing the environment within which individuals can make meaningful decisions surrounding their own bodies, their care, and their lives (Nunn, 2014).

Ozanne and colleagues (2013) spoke of the need for a dying person to have emotional flexibility—letting go of control and taking it back—

in order to negotiate the path of decline to death. This resonates with us. The elderly adult, in the interest of total control, who will not allow others within her space, tends not to benefit from the very activities that could enhance her personhood: visits from significant others, the massage of a nurse, a phone call from a childhood friend. If she retains no control (the other extreme), her room may be overrun with visitors, or she may not make her wishes known. Healthy control is the balance, and, in terminal illness, this balance is not easily achieved.

The threads of loss of control are many and are often interwoven. For instance, the dynamic between the individual and his medications and the wishes of the family and the dying older adult with respect to those medications, can be complicated. To illustrate, a family may strongly desire their loved one to be more awake, hence discouraging the older gentleman from taking medications that could alleviate pain (but might also lead to drowsiness). Sometimes the dying older adult wishes to be more alert, but his family struggles emotionally with his physical pain.

Besides the effects of the particular medications upon the patient, the power structure within the family may be revealed and challenged. A healthy sense of personhood in the dying adult is so vital. If he has capacity, his wishes, in consultation with medical staff (and in accordance with the law), are followed. However, sometimes the elderly dying individual does not have a sufficient sense of self to insist upon what he desires; this is generally a part of a lifelong pattern of giving in to the wishes of others. Hence, whatever control he had in life is further jeopardized in his dying process.

Aloneness

The older adult who is dying may feel very alone. This may involve a lack of visitors to her nursing home room or to her social isolation from being confined to her home. But there is different "aloneness" that some people who are dying feel keenly: This is an existential aloneness (Ozanne et al., 2013). Caregivers can only journey so far with their loved ones and their patients. In conversation with these individuals, they sometimes remind this chaplain (MBR) that while they appreciate the company, they "cross over" on their own. How true this is.

Sourkes (1982) used the term "the deepening shade" to describe the impact of a terminal illness upon the psyche, and she spoke of the aloneness that dying people feel. As already discussed, they fear a loss of control; they also fear the loss of identity and the loss of relationships (the separation from loved ones at death). Briefly stated, the loss of identity involves losing the person as she once was. This can involve physical changes, due to disease and medication. One woman said of her elderly mother, before cancer literally ate her face away, "I wished you had known her as she was; she was beautiful!" No doubt that she had been lovely before the cancer struck; however, in this dying woman's gracious response to her disease, her willingness to accept new people into her life and her resilience, I (MBR) found her person to be very beautiful!

Loss of identity can also entail the cessation of activities (such as work or defining hobbies) that an individual once performed. The very elderly have had more time to deal with those losses, so this loss may not be as pronounced. For men, however, their sense of personhood is often attached to what they have *done,* thus in their dying they look back longingly at the past with their instrumental role in this world. And they feel alone in their current reality. With a greater proportion of women now in the workforce than during the 1960s and 1970s, we suggest that this loss of identity may become more pronounced for aging North American women in the coming decades.

In the deepening shade, an older adult may fear the loss of relationship—she may fear losing her loved ones—certainly in the short term and perhaps in the long haul. For those who do not believe in an afterlife, the impending loss of relationship may propel them to do some rethinking and research on this topic. One gentleman, who had been raised within a major faith tradition but set it aside during his lifetime, picked up threads of it again in his dying. Of prime importance to him was being able to see his loved ones again in the afterlife. For him, the exact parameters of the afterlife were not defined; it was enough to know (for him) that there *is* one (he appreciated some stories about deathbed phenomena/near death experiences), and he wanted to prepare himself for that. Always a man of great integrity, he said, "You don't think it's duplicitous of me to now, in my dying, come back to faith, do you?" And, of course, it was not duplicitous; as part of his integrity and his spiritual growth, he reconnected to that which had previously been meaningful to him.

Existential aloneness and its "solution" was expressed so well by family therapist Kathy Weingarten (1999), who herself has faced into death more than once. In the following quotation, she spoke of the need for connection, and then the reality that at some point in her dying, she will not have it. She wondered how she will fare.

For me, connection remains the answer. I value connection,
although I know that I will not always have it. Stretching to
face the inevitability of my death, not just once but recurringly,
forced a relationship to aloneness. Tending to this relationship
is part of my spiritual practice. (p. 249)

The dying older adult may actually have an advantage over his younger terminally counterpart in that he has had years to tend to this aloneness through introspection, prayer, and solitude. But not all adults have worked with their existential aloneness. Wilma, discussed in Chapter 5, could only bear her aloneness in the reassuring presence of others. In her dying, she needed the physical and psychological presence of others to bring her security.

Integration of Life Experiences

The need for integration of life experiences has been discussed at length in Chapter 5. In dying, the need is greater for many, and the time frame in which to complete the work is more compact. Older dying adults may do this work through asking adult children to write down for them their family history. Others will compose their own obituary, having their children act as scribes. Some will plan their own funerals, calling in people to ask of them special requests. Tara, a teacher for many years, asked a number of individuals to represent her at her funeral service. One old family friend was asked to speak of Tara when she was a girl and discuss her life into her growing up years. Another was asked to speak of Tara's work professionally; yet another of Tara in her later years. In this way, she integrated life experiences within her soul by reflecting back on her life, "commissioning" others to tell her story, and setting the scene for her life history to be viewed at her funeral. The eulogies and the video tribute honored this well-deserving woman.

There is, today, a tendency to forego a formal service to remember one's life. This may be, in part, a reflection of the secularization of North America (particularly Canada); it also may reflect our discomfort with death (Rando, 1984). We would like to suggest that the ritual of having some kind of formal remembrance is very important. The ritual need not be religious. And it gives the dying elderly person a chance to reflect upon her life by being involved in the planning; it also provides those who grieve the opportunity to *celebrate* her. The work of integration is hers, but it also belongs to her loved ones.

Sometimes family members say of a dying relative, "Jim does not want a formal service." On the surface, this would seem noble to honor the loved one's request. However, not having a formal remembrance can impact the grieving process for family members, as will be discussed later in the chapter. Perhaps it also reveals an inability of the dying older adult to come to *integrity* (as discussed in Chapter 5), being trapped in *despair* (Erikson, 1982; Thomas & Cohen, 2006). A frank discussion with the dying older adult and his family members can often result in a compromise, balancing the dying person's desire and the grieving family's needs. Sometimes, the reason behind not wanting a service or ritual can open up a valuable opportunity to speak of unresolved aspects of a dying person's life and can lead to some further integration.

For instance, in one case an elderly gentleman in a hospice said that he did not want a service after his passing. "I don't think that anything good will be said of me!" In this situation, there had been profound family issues; there was some restitution and reconnection in the latter part of his life, but he feared that he would be remembered for "the bad years." His family felt the need to have some kind of formal remembrance. This issue was, at the request of the family, addressed by the chaplain; the dying man spoke of his fears but also his willingness to speak with his children about their desire. The two adult children approached their father with their hope: to have a small private family gathering in the hospice's chapel, led by the chaplain that this gentleman had come to trust. Some details were discussed, and this older adult added his suggestions. A quiet candle lighting service was held for his immediate family (about 10 present); several of his favorite poems and prayers were read. His two adult children gave tributes, acknowledging the struggle but also the victories of this man and his family. And, at his insistence, the family went out for a nice supper at a favorite restaurant afterward, at his expense. The service and the dinner served to bring some measure of closure and hope in this man's passing.

Meaning in Life and Death

Chapter 5 spoke about the need for meaning in life, in every stage, and the challenges for older adults as transitions lead to significant changes in their lives. These changes can lead to great wrestling with how to attain meaning and purpose (Erikson, Erikson, & Kivnick, 1986; Walsh, 2009).

The terminally ill older adult may approach this transition with a sense of immediacy, needing to make each moment count (Hantman & Cohen, 2010). This is seen often in legacy work, in celebrating, in a big way, last experiences (such as having the house decorated from top to bottom to celebrate Christmas, one last time). Within palliative settings, terminally ill persons may have their birthdays celebrated early. Anticipated weddings within the family may be expedited, so that Grandma can be there. This reveals the urgent need to find meaning in what time is left in life.

These older adults sometimes seek to attach meaning to their deaths. One significant way is organ donation. Depending upon the diagnosis, and the age of the older adult, her eyes and perhaps other organs may be harvested to bring *life* to others. Sometimes older individuals desire to donate their bodies to science that others may learn from them.[8] Monetary donations from the terminally ill person while still alive and then again in the will are other ways that people seek to bring meaning to their passings. It cannot be overstated here that in the case of donation of organs or funds, strict ethical practices and procedures must be adhered to. The dying older adult is very vulnerable, and he can be exploited by others. Health care in the western world has firm codes of conduct for health care workers and the institutions themselves in this area.

For some older adults, final days and death are deemed to be meaningless; the experience is one of despair, rather than integrity (Erikson, 1982; Thomas & Cohen, 2006). Hence, a dying older adult in this position may emotionally and spiritually withdraw (Georgesen & Dungan, 1996), not wishing to connect with others, self, and/or God. This is a profound form of existential distress. Presence, if the patient is willing, can be a gentle intervention; in this, nothing is asked of the dying older adult, but spiritual care may be felt by the empathic, humble caregiver, whether that individual is a family member or professional.[9]

---

8. It is vital that individuals and their families are informed in their donating. From time to time individuals think that donating their body to science may lead to the cure for a disease, when, in fact, the donated body is used for students learning to do dissections. Social workers in hospitals and palliative settings can walk individuals and families through the process, ensuring this understanding and consent.

9. One chaplain sat with a blind, dying woman. There was no dialogue, and the two were not touching. The dying older adult said, "I can't see you, but I can feel you." She was comforted by the chaplain's quiet, caring presence.

This condition can be temporary, with the palliative interprofessional approach ameliorating suffering, bringing about opportunity for further quality of life and opportunities for integrity (Erikson, 1982; Thomas & Cohen, 2006). Georgesen and Dungan (1996) told of a dying gentleman who had withdrawn in such an experience of existential despair. Medication for his depression, the work of a nurse clinician, spiritual counseling, and the rites of his faith all contributed to his return to his family and his God. One last goal remained; this was a trip to see a family member out of state. Although the trip was not completed (he could only make it partway due to physical deterioration), the family member they had planned to see was able to meet them partway. As a family they returned home, within several hours, the patient passed, having completed his final desire.

Forgiveness at the End of Life

The meaning and need for forgiveness has been discussed in Chapter 5. The struggles of forgiving, and the benefits thereof, were spelled out. Forgiveness is often a theme in religion. The Dalai Lama said, "All major religious traditions carry basically the same message that is love, compassion and forgiveness; the important thing is they should be part of our daily lives" (Brainy Quotes, 2015). In addition, forgiveness is at times larger than a few individuals, encompassing sociological and political concerns, as illustrated by the lives and work of people like Mahatma Gandhi and Nelson Mandela. South African Bishop Desmond Tutu, speaking politically as well as theologically, said, "Without forgiveness, there is no future" (Brainy Quotes, 2015). And forgiveness is a deeply personal issue. A hospital psychiatrist, in seeking to encourage an estranged elderly parent into reuniting with his adult children, was verbally ousted out of the room with "Don't you *dare* talk to me about forgiveness!"

The discussion here in Chapter 6 about forgiveness will focus, gently, on the topic of the meaning of forgiveness for vulnerable people—those elderly adults who are dying. The need to forgive and be forgiven seems almost to be universal; it is inextricably tied to love. Thomas Fuller said, "He that cannot forgive others breaks the bridge over which he must pass himself; for every man has need to be forgiven" (Brainy Quotes, 2015). Dying people, especially the elderly who have experienced so much of life, seem to know this instinctively. They also know, having been through the difficulties of life, that forgiveness is not always easily achieved.

General principles on forgiveness

As health and human service professionals, we must be very gentle in our approach to those in our care, those in need of forgiveness from God, others, or self. From this foundation of care, we offer the following suggestions.

Forgiveness is a key component to meaning and purpose, as personal relationships are intrinsic to a meaningful life (Allemand, Steiner, & Hill, 2013; Hantman & Cohen, 2010). As discussed in Chapter 5, a key component of spiritual distress is disconnection from self, others, and God (Heyse-Moore, 1996). These disconnections lead to profound pain; forgiveness, extended and received, brings completion to relationship (Allemand et al., 2013; Byock, 1997). The health care provider can feel confident in this understanding. Sometimes patients with the greatest bravado are actually masking great pain, the suffering coming through disconnection. Within Chapter 5 we suggested that health and human service professionals be open to speaking about such issues. In the context of a dying older adult sharing life experiences that have involved ruptured relationships, or if the dying individual demonstrates spiritual distress, it is appropriate for the professional caregiver, with a ministry of presence and valuing the patient, to gently raise the issue and to do so with a quiet confidence.

Providing the opportunity for the patient to speak, it is vital that the professional listens much more than she speaks. This can be difficult, as she may feel that she needs to give answers. However, this listening validates personhood (Hirst et al., 2013); it also allows the professional to discern deeper meaning, the themes of the patient's life, which she can draw out as pertinent. Unconditional love both affirms personhood by demonstrating to the suffering individual that he is known for who he is and that he is loved (Satterly, 2001). Being accepted by others allows an individual to believe that he is accepted by God.

This sense of being accepted and loved by others, translating (eventually) to a sense of being loved by self, others, and/or God (wherever the need lies), takes time. Initially, conversations surrounding deeper issues may not occur. It takes great courage for the older adult to expose her soul. By dignifying the dying older individual with sensitive care, the professional may demonstrate that unconditional love. Over time, as trust develops, the older adult may open up. Interesting, nurses sometimes report that individuals with complex issues of disconnection often begin to open up to their caregivers during the night, in the dark, as a nurse is tending to them.

In this way, perhaps, the dying older adult feels less exposed; the darkness of the night provides him with some protection, allowing him to raise painful issues. Ultimately, the goal is that the dying individual can experience unconditional love that strengthens him to forgive others, to forgive himself, and to perhaps receive forgiveness from God, if this is his need.[10]

It is in this safety of acceptance that dying individuals can pursue the reconnections that they feel they need. Upon their request, nurses may help facilitate this through connecting the dying older adult with family members or by sending a referral to the social worker or chaplain.

The dying individual often knows what he needs. I (MBR) was called in after hours to be with an elderly individual in great spiritual distress. I asked him what he needed. "I need to reckon with the Savior," he replied. We sat together and I prayed with him. I was deeply moved by the pouring forth of his soul to reconnect with his God—the literal calling out in his weak voice, occurring upon the "amen" of my prayer. He sought and received the forgiveness he needed. This experience, for both of us, was holy ground.

Cautions

The stories of the lives of dying older adults are deeply layered and truly filled with mystery. Health and human service professionals enter into their stories in the last chapter (sometimes on the last page of the final chapter). We do not understand all the whys and hows of their lives, and we cannot begin to know exactly what they need. (Ryan [2005], as well as Field and Cassel [1997], reported on how often health care providers make assumptions about what patients need, without really understanding.) So as caregivers, we must enter their stories with care, with respect, and with humility.

---

10. The ability to give and receive unconditional love is rooted in our experience as children; conditional love and acceptance from family members (parents) and from God (through unforgiving religious teaching) negatively impacts our ability to give and receive unconditional love and acceptance ourselves (Satterly, 2001), and the ability to be simply ourselves in relationship is not established in our formative years (Ainsworth & Bowlby, 1991; Bowlby, 1999). According to our experience, major personality and family issues are generally not resolved in the weeks before a person's death. However, significant steps can be taken that can bring peace to the dying individual and her family. And if this individual never is able to complete all of that work, at least she has *received* that type of love in her dying. This is akin to the work of Mother Teresa of Calcutta, who gave the dying unconditional love and care as an antidote to individuals' suffering, knowing that there would never be any tangible payoff.

Myrla Seibold (2001) wrote a beautiful article about forgiveness from a Christian perspective. She cautioned against the imposition of a quick-forgiveness approach toward those who have experienced deep wounding, stating that well-meaning people can re-victimize those who have known deep hurt. She encouraged narrative work—the telling of people's stories—and stated clearly that recounting one's experiences in life is not evidence of unforgiveness. And, akin to Satterly (2001), she spoke of forgiveness ultimately flowing out of love—love that is replenished in the life of the hurt individual by *safe* others. From that position of safety, the violated individual can do the forgiveness work he or she needs to do.

Although not written for dying older adults, the principles of Seibold's article apply. The role of the professional caregiver, in the life of a dying individual, is to be a source of that unconditional love to assist in providing the environment that the older adult needs. The caregiver must resist being invested in a result, or else she risks meeting her needs, rather than the patient's need.

Restoration of relationship?

There is much confusion regarding what forgiveness means; many assume that it involves the restoration of relationship, no matter what has occurred in the past. However, a number of authors who addressed the need for forgiveness clarify that forgiveness does not necessarily mean the restoration of relationship. Smedes (1997) emphasized that a person can forgive without there being a restoration of relationship; the restoration of relationship takes two people and sometimes one of the parties is not interested. In the case of terminally ill older adults, there can be a great sense of urgency to repair broken relationships, but their families are not always interested. Here, Smedes' principle can be helpful. From a palliative perspective, the older adult can do his forgiveness work in preparation for death (asking for or extending forgiveness), and perhaps leave a letter for the adult child to receive later.

Enright (1996) cautioned that it may not always be safe to restore relationship. In situations where there has been significant violation, the offended individual may not feel emotionally safe to re-engage. The urgency of a parent's imminent passing and the common misunderstanding that forgiveness means restoration of relationship—imposed by others—can cause great psychological and emotional distress. An individual's wishes and boundaries must be respected by health care professionals. I (AML) recall a situation of an elderly father in hospital. In earlier days, he had been abusive toward his children. His sensitive daughters could not visit. But they did what they could. They baked cookies, brought clothes and cigarettes, and left them at the nursing station in the hospital, to be given to their father. This was, in my mind, noble.

This caution regarding the restoration of relationship also applies to family members of the dying older adult. Adult children who have not been in relationship for years can be "thrown together" in a parent's dying. This causes enormous stress on all. A dying person may say, "I just want my children to let the past go and to get along." A very human desire! Family members will often set aside differences for the sake of the situation at hand. But this does not mean that relationship can or should continue after the parent's death, especially if the relationship has involved violation.

The emphases of Enright (1996) and Smedes (1997) are that the requesting and extending of forgiveness is a deeply personal action; one can do her own soul work apart from the readiness of the other within the relationship. Forgiveness can, but not necessarily does, mean the restoration of relationship.

The "Good Death"

There is much in the literature of death about what constitutes a "good death" (Ryan, 2005). This goal is expressed in a number of ways: the "peaceful death" (Callahan, 1993), the "appropriate death" (Weisman, 1988), the "happy death" (Corless, 1994), and "dying well" (Byock, 1997). The literature reveals a discrepancy between what health care providers consider to be a good death and what patients perceive (Watts, 2012). Health care providers have tended to view pain and symptom management as key in deciding whether a death is good. Patients have described a good death as "sudden death" or "dying in one's sleep" (Arnup, 2013; Ryan, 2005), as well as having family support and anticipatory planning (Lawton, Towsey, & Carroll, 2013).[11] One commonality between health care providers and patients is that a "good death" is one in which pain is controlled (Hughes, 2012).

This discrepancy of opinion is not surprising. The dying and their family members often query: "What would be better? A death that takes time or something quick and easy?" This question is generally existential, as it takes courage for the dying older adult and family members to face into

---

11. Though this is a hope of many people, it generally does not happen. A recent Canadian study reported that only 10% of Canadians die suddenly. See Arnup (2013).

death. (The value of the palliative experience will be discussed in the grief section, as well as the ethical issues section later in this chapter.)

The literature increasingly reflects the need for those dying to be met in *their* places of need (Ryan, 2005). And based upon studies of patients on dialysis, with HIV or in nursing homes, Singer, Martin, and Kelner (1999) identified five key domains for end-of-life care, from *patients'* perspectives: pain and symptom management, the avoidance of inappropriate prolongation of life, patients achieving a sense of control, relieving the burden of care on the loved ones, and the bolstering and deepening of relationships with loved ones. This, in a nutshell, is the thrust of hospice palliative care. And, more than just the focus of palliative work, the provision of this type of care is an ethical obligation (Singer et al., 1999).

What is striking within a clinical context is that the dying and their families can feel much pressure to experience a good death. Could this reflect the North American compulsion to "succeed"? I (MBR) have been present at many passings. The dying express concerns that they will not display sufficient courage. Family members, in a typical grief response and perhaps societal pressure, query whether they have done a "good enough job" in supporting their loved one. Again, this pressure—almost moral in nature—to succeed is present even in death! An older woman had struggled tremendously with faith and with fear in her dying; she agonized through the entire process. At her funeral, the celebrant stated numerous times that "she died well." In this context, the focus was that she died in faith. Whether she did was not the issue; the fact that the minister felt the need to stress this repeatedly to members of the congregation revealed the pressure that is applied to people to die a certain way. Placing this type of weight upon a dying individual and her family members is not helpful.

Roshi Joan Halifax (2009) takes a very practical approach to dying. She told of an individual who died with great struggle, and Halifax wrestled with whether this was a good death. Here is her conclusion:

The concept of a good death can put unbearable pressure upon the dying and their caregivers . . . Our expectations of how someone should die can give rise to subtle or direct coerciveness. And no one wants to be judged for how well she dies! (Halifax, 2009, p. 65)

Part of bereavement work with grieving individuals is to help them work through this pressure of having performed adequately during their loved one's illness and dying. One woman came into the palliative setting in the last stages of a chronic condition. She was expected to live for a number of weeks. In the course of events, she passed within a couple of hours after her arrival with what appeared to be a pulmonary embolism. Her dying was very quick and she was anxious. Her daughter, who had wanted to make sure that everything was "perfect" for her mom, was devastated. As I came into the room moments after her mother's passing, the adult daughter collapsed into my arms. "Why did it have to happen this way?" was her cry. No doubt, there is much mystery and we live in "the richness of not knowing" (Halifax, 2009, p. 65). I responded to her that we often come into this world crying, and sometimes we leave that way too. Being birthed into this life is a transition that comes with stress; being birthed into the next life sometimes involves stress also.

From our perspective, the primary factor in determining whether a death is good is the presence of love. If the dying individual and his family *know* that they are loved, and diligent efforts are made to cover off on the other factors (described by Singer et al., 1999), the death has been good. "The salvation of man is in love and through love" (Frankl, 2006, p. 37).

Issues for Family Members

Even though family members of an aging adult are not personally dying, they typically experience significant grief and grapple with a number of issues related to the impending death of the older adult, whether this person is a spouse, parent, or other relative. The experience of personally standing by someone who is loved and is dying can impact a person to his core—to the depths of his spirit. It impacts his identity; it changes his world forever. For the family, this process is about detaching from their loved one as they currently experience her, just as the dying individual is letting go of them. It is also about developing a new relationship to the deceased.

Anticipating the Death of an Elderly Spouse

The death of a spouse is one of the most profound losses of a person's life (Hamilton, 2005). As people are living longer, many older adults will experience the death of a partner of many years. Having lived so long, and experienced so many things, older adults often have coping mechanisms that help them deal with loss; however, the sheer number and magnitude of the losses can compromise their ability to handle the impending loss (Gibson, 2009). The soon-to-be surviving spouse may refer to the day the terminal diagnosis came as when life, as he had known it, was changed forever (Hamilton, 2005). The bonds that have been formed and strengthened throughout the years are many; the thought of separation can be unbearable. How the older adult left behind copes—in the time of anticipating this loss and after the spouse's death—may be dependent upon a person's personality and how he has coped with challenges in the past.

Decision-Making Regarding End-of-Life Care

It is not uncommon for family members to hold opposing views on end-of-life decisions for the dying individual. One family member may be adamant that treatment must be continued regardless of the diagnosis, prognosis, or response to treatment; another family member may argue just as vehemently that care should be just supportive with no extenuating measures. And ironically, the aging, dying older adult may be lying comatose on the hospital bed between these two family members who are engaged in the verbal tussle.

Family members' decision-making may be complicated when an older adult has not made her wishes known or prepared a living will (Arnup, 2013; Clabots, 2012). The older, dying adult may assume that she can let the family know "when time comes," but then suffers a stroke or becomes comatose, and it becomes too late for wishes to be spoken out loud. While in some developed countries, individuals and/or family members designate the level of care (e.g., no invasive treatment) they wish the aging and/or dying adult to receive when entering long-term care or palliative care facilities, this may not occur within hospitals. Then, when a major event occurs, such as a massive cardiac event or a stroke, families may be paralyzed in their decision-making on behalf of their hospitalized elder.

Decision-making regarding end-of-life care can be straightforward for some families and less smooth for others. When older adults have prepared a living will and have designated a family member to make decisions on their behalf, the process may be clearer. Although family members may not necessarily agree with the stated wishes, they at least know that their spouse, parent, or relative made the decision when of sound mind. This may relieve family members of great angst and guilt at a time of vulnerability and turmoil: when their family member is dying.

Health and human service professionals need to broach the conversation of end-of-life care decisions with their aging and ailing patients.

However, studies have revealed that nurses and physicians may be reluctant to talk to aging adults about end-of-life wishes (Boyle, Miller, & Forbes-Thompson, 2005; Kahana, Dan, Kahana, & Kercher, 2004). As the focus of care within acute care hospitals is often to sustain life, such conversations may be seen as giving up hope (Clabots, 2012). Also, health and human service professionals may be uncomfortable with end-of-life discussions, as these may raise their own existential issues. Therefore, professionals need to consider their own beliefs, values, and fears about dying and death, as well as meaning and purpose in life (Clabots, 2012).

Supporting Older Adults in the Dying Process

Not only will some family members require support in their grieving and concerns about a dying older adult, but they may also *require support to support the dying, aged individual.* The need for support may be related to other reasons besides a tumultuous relationship with the dying parent (as has been discussed already within this book). For example, a family member of a dying elderly person may have significant mental illness and may be experiencing an exacerbation of her symptoms due to the stress of grieving. Or, an adult child with an intellectual disability may not know how to express his grief regarding the impending death of his parent, or, on some level, may not understand what death entails. A spouse with dementia who is visiting her dying husband will need much support in her process.[12]

Dealing with Caregiving Exhaustion

Standing *with* an aging family member who is dying is exhausting in every way: physically, mentally, and spiritually. Just the anticipation of the dying of a family member results in profound weariness; however, other factors exacerbate this fatigue. For example, an adult daughter may have spent months being up frequently during the night to assist her terminally ill mother and hence is sleep-deprived. When Mom is hospitalized, she may

---

12. There is some literature on helping those with dementia cope with the (impending) deaths of loved ones. For example, Miller Lewis and Trzinski (2006) stated that those with dementia have the same grief needs as others, and so need help in their grieving. With impaired cognition, they may forget that their spouse has passed, and so may experience acute reactions repeatedly. For this situation, Miller Lewis and Trzinski (2006) recommended *spaced retrieval* and *group buddies* as approaches to helping the cognitively impaired with their grieving. In these approaches, the bereaved person with dementia retains cognition that there has been a death, and, over time, that the person who died was her spouse. In this way, the bereaved does not experience the loss repeatedly in an acute fashion, every time the passing of their spouse is mentioned.

spend nights sitting in the hospital chair, straining her back to hold her mother's hand. The walks that were a part of her routine may be given up; her practice of yoga set aside. In the understandable preoccupation of caring for the needs of her mother, she may have neglected to eat and drink in a healthy manner, losing or gaining weight. Without adequate sleep, nutrition, and hydration, she finds herself to be prone to colds (due to stress on the immune system), headaches, and backaches, and the "well" of her spirit may be dry.

Health and human service professionals often encourage self-care for caregivers. "Oh, don't worry about me. I'll take care of myself after this is all over" is a common reply from family members. However, when the caregiving goes on for longer than expected, caregivers can find themselves exhausted and ill. They themselves can suffer with depression.

Bioethicist Viki Kind (2010) discussed the notion of care-grieving. The stresses of caregiving, combined with anticipatory grieving—for either the death that will occur or the loss of the older adult one once knew—as well as perhaps the loss of the job or social relationships that one limited or gave up to provide care, can leave family members exhausted, burned out, and depressed. Walker and Pomeroy (1996) sought to distinguish between clinical depression and anticipatory grieving in their research regarding the caregivers of those with dementia. Whether the caregiver is depressed or engaged in anticipatory grieving,[13] the sense of being overcome by circumstances bigger than self is very real; one's own personhood can feel threatened. Kind (2010) stated: "Care-grieving can become so overwhelming that it creates in us a desperation and a need to survive. It's not that we wish our loved one was gone, we just wish our pain was gone" (p. 106).

There are many factors in the dying process that are outside of the caregivers' control. This sense of being out of control (and exhausted) is associated with the "burden" of caregiving (Walter & Pomeroy, 1996). Having said that, elderly people who have provided care for their dying spouses derive great comfort, during the bereavement process, from having done so (Chan & Chan, 2011; Hamilton, 2005).

---

13. It is interesting that the construct of pre-death grief is now suggested for caregivers of those with dementia, rather than anticipatory grief. This is because caregivers are not only grieving in anticipation of the impending death of their loved ones, they are already grieving the loss of their family members' cognition and personality (see Lindauer & Harvath, 2014).

Grieving the Death of the Older Adult

Grieving is intensely demanding work. Even when the death is expected, due to the age and illness of a spouse or parent, the amount of grief can overwhelm some family members. "Death creates chaos. It creates a total upheaval in the entire family structure," stated Kagawa-Singer (1998, p. 1752). The following is a brief discussion of the types of grief as they impact the passing of an older adult. Because this text is geared toward the transitions of older adults, and the impacts upon family members, the discussion about some of the forms of grief will be limited to those that impact and have relevance to the grieving family.[14]

Some of the types of grief and their application

Anticipatory grief has been touched upon a number of times in this text. The term was coined by Lindemann in 1944, in his seminal work on acute grief (see Lindemann, 1944). He wrote of wives of soldiers at war (World War II) who so anticipated the deaths of their husbands overseas that if they returned, the wives had already successfully detached emotionally from them (Siegel & Weinstein, 1983). Since then the term has been used extensively in the field of grief to describe a form of grieving that begins before a person actually dies. Family members and the dying adult experience this as they begin to come to grips with the reality that death is coming. Often, the loss comes in stages: a loss of health due to disease; a loss of body image due to the impact of treatment; a loss of capacity; and eventually, the actual loss of the loved one.

Johansson and Grimby (2012) suggested that the time of anticipatory grief in caregivers can be, for some, more intense than the grief that follows after their loved one's passing. This means that in the dying process, the dying older adult and the loved ones suffer a number of losses, as is typical of grief, but the process is elongated: a series of "small deaths" (Zerwekh, 2006). The existential question raised by many dying people, as well as their loved ones, was asked earlier: "What would be better: a death that takes time or something quick and easy?" Ryan (2005) cited that patients sometimes desire the latter. The existential concerns discussed in Chapters 5 and 6 figure in heavily here. "I'm not sure that I'm up to this," an elderly gentleman said, about his dying process. He had experienced a number of "small deaths" and was not sure he had the resources to face the big one.

---

14. For a detailed discussion of the various forms of grief, see Rando (1984).

Within practice, it is generally assumed that knowledge ahead of time that a loved one is going to die leads to better grief resolution. However, from a grief research perspective, the evidence is not conclusive. According to Parkes (1975), a family having time to prepare for a passing leads to better grief outcomes; Golsworthy and Coyle (1999), in their study examining older adults who had lost a spouse, concurred, as did Shah and colleagues (2013). Maddison and Walker (1976) and Gerber, Rusalem, Hannon, Banin, and Arkin (1975) did not find that knowing of the death ahead of time aids in the bereavement process.

Some of the conflicting evidence appears to be tied to the lack of clarity in defining anticipatory grief (D'Antonio, 2014). Siegel and Weinstein (1983) spoke of the need to have the empirical foundations of the concept of anticipatory grief firmly established; they noted that the concept is too ambiguous to be clearly tested. D'Antonio (2014) has divided the concept of anticipatory grief into two: anticipatory grief and anticipatory mourning. Anticipatory grief refers to the grief in anticipation of the losses that have not yet occurred. Anticipatory mourning is anticipatory grief, plus the efforts of the individual to cope; past losses are reviewed in order to elicit coping mechanisms from the past. From her research, D'Antonio concluded that anticipatory grief may be more intense than the grief experienced after a loss; however, anticipatory mourning and the mourning activities post death are equally intense. The discussion of how to define anticipatory grief and all that comes with it continues (D'Antonio, 2014).

It is our experience that preparation for a death *is* helpful, *if* the family has received support through the process. Adult children have stated that the palliative experience, with the support provided, both before and after their parent's death, was far superior to their experience of the death of another parent that was sudden and unexpected; in one situation the family (with five adult children) commented on how helpful this experience was for their teenage children, to learn about death and to develop coping skills, as well. But here, too, the concept of anticipatory grief is not specifically isolated; our generalization is made with another factor involved, and that is palliative care. A lengthy illness and then passing of a loved one, without the supports of hospice and palliative care, may simply wear a family down, without leading to better grief resolution. The literature demonstrates that the hospice palliative experience, which includes support in anticipatory grief, provides the dying individual and the family a better experience (D'Antonio, 2014; Shah et al., 2013; Teno et al., 2011; von Gunten, 2012).

Normal grief is the process of emotional detachment that occurs after a death. It is an intense process, involving physical symptoms (chest pain

and tightness, tightness in the throat, sleep disturbances, appetite disturbances, dry mouth, sensitivity to noise), emotional symptoms (fear, crying,
emotional numbness, anger, guilt, depression), psychological symptoms
(trouble with concentration and decision-making) and spiritual symptoms
(existential angst) (Rando, 1984). It is helpful for the reader to note that
these symptoms are "normal." Meaningful attachment to people (as spoken of in Chapter 5) leads to a strenuous time when that relationship, as it
was experienced, is altered through death. That being said, physical symptoms in the bereaved, such as chest pain and tightness, need to be checked
out medically to rule out serious health problems. And the depression of
grief can lead to suicide; nurses and other health care professionals need
to be aware of this fact and prepared, in their work with grieving people,
to assess for suicide risk. In order to move through this "normal" phase
of detaching, individuals need to be able to attach meaning to the death.
Meaninglessness in death is associated with anger and an indefinite grieving period (Chan & Chan, 2011).

When an elderly person has lost her spouse of many years, the process of grief will be especially arduous; also, the length of the bereavement
period may be especially long (Golsworthy & Coyle, 1999). Older grieving
adults have higher morbidity rates (Elwert & Christakis, 2008); they experience a higher level of mental health issues after the death of a partner
(Ott, Lueger, Kelber, & Prigerson, 2007). Men, in particular, are even more
susceptible to the impact of losing a spouse (Bennett, 2005). Their adaptive
capacities in their later years may be stretched beyond their limit with the
number of challenges they are facing (Gibson, 2009). Given the length of
many marriages of the elderly (50-plus years), the shared identity and life
histories, many older adults never really emotionally detach. Here, we like
the term of J. William Worden, that of *emotionally relocating* the loved one
who has passed (Worden, 2009). The loved one does not cease to exist in
the life of the one who remains on earth; in this way, the personhood of the
deceased is not nullified.

As such, one of the *tasks of grieving* (Worden, 2009)[15] is to emotionally relocate the deceased person; this is so some form of relationship with
the deceased remains. The carrying out of this task is evidenced in many

---

15. There are a number of grief models: Elisabeth Kubler-Ross' (1969) Five Stages of Grief
is probably the most famous. We like Worden's model—the *Tasks of Grieving* because it
seems less passive. Those in grief apply themselves to tasks, rather than moving passively
through stages. It should be noted, though, that grief is far too complex a process to distill
down to a set of stages or tasks; this is being increasingly recognized in the literature (see
Hamilton, 2005, and Copp, 1998).

ways. For some, their loved one resides in a cemetery. The surviving spouse may go, on special occasions, to "speak" with her deceased husband. An adult daughter, earlier in this chapter, kept some cremains of her father in a locket that she wore close to her heart. Literally and figuratively, her dad stayed in (or upon) her heart.

Another woman, herself now in a palliative setting, kissed her husband's photograph and said, "He's always with me." The nature of the relationship changed (he was no longer physically present), but she still felt his influence and his presence in her life. She also expressed that tender connection through looking at, and periodically kissing, his picture.

Michael and colleagues (2003) conducted a literature review examining the impact of religion and spirituality in aiding widows to cope with the loss of their husbands. They found research demonstrating that faith and spirituality help older women cope with the deaths of their husbands, in part, because they were able to form a new relationship with the deceased loved one, in essence, to emotionally relocate the departed; the loved one may be always in his or her heart ("I always feel her with me") or in heaven ("we'll be together again"). They found that having spiritual/religious beliefs assists the older adult in the grief process, because older individuals are able to make some meaning of the passing and are also able to place this loved one in the next life. Religious involvement is associated with the support of a faith community, as well (Michael, Crowther, Schmid, & Allen, 2003).

Conflicted grief occurs when the relationship with the deceased has been ambivalent. It is characterized by the exaggeration of one aspect of normal grief, with the suppression of other aspects. Rando (1984) spoke of guilt and anger being two common elements in conflicted grief. For example, in situations where there has been a very dependent relationship, grief can be very difficult. An adult son may feel much anger toward his elderly mother, the anger coming from his own dependence upon her, and her leaving him in death, after "all he's done for her!" He may not feel able to express this, and so outwardly emphasizes to others only the positive things (their shared love). But internally, there is guilt over his internal relief that the relationship is done, fear of what the future holds (he has not reached his developmental milestones and only knows a life of dependence upon her), as well as sadness for the loss of his mother. In essence, the conflicted grief results in a tangled mass of emotions that the son is unable to understand.

For the health and human service professional, an acknowledgment that both the positive feelings (love, affection) and the "negative" ones (anger, hurt) are present and normal, in this context, is vital. It is important that the bereaved adult child grieve the loss of that which was good and that which was not. (It is common for these adult children to grieve the loss of the type of parent they never had.) Many hospice programs in the community have bereavement follow-up; in situations where the grief is conflicted, these services are even more important. Researchers have found, however, that even within hospice settings, the majority of people do not access these bereavement services (Cherlin et al., 2007; Holland, Futterman, Thompson, Moran, & Gallagher-Thompson, 2013).

We would be remiss if we did not spend some time discussing grief in situations of ambiguous loss. The term *ambiguous loss* (Boss, 1999) was explained in Chapter 3. For those experiencing ambiguous loss, where their loved one is still physically present, but emotionally or psychologically absent (with dementia or brain injury) their grief can be confusing. The loved ones—spouses, adult children, caregivers—feel the loss keenly, but may not recognize that it is grief they are experiencing, because the loved one is still physically present (Gibson, 2009). As well, there are not the rituals in our society to mark this type of loss (such as a funeral), and others may not recognize it and provide support (Kind, 2010).

Gibson (2009) noted that when older adults are experiencing this ambiguous loss caused by dementia in their partner, they are also experiencing a number of other challenges: the passings of friends, difficulties with their own health, and the deaths of siblings. Hence, the resources for coping are limited. On top of this, the social network that used to provide help, such as neighbors and relatives, is often no longer there (Gibson, 2009) because of the length of the illness (as discussed in Chapter 2).

The strain on the older adult without dementia, as well as on adult family members, is enormous. Feelings of anger and guilt will often be present, as they wish that "this were all over." The need for adequate provision of appropriate long-term care placements cannot be overemphasized. By the time families reach a palliative setting (if they do), they often need reassurance that their expressions of frustration have come from exhaustion, not lack of love. They also need to be reassured of the personhood of their loved one.

It is no wonder that when a loved one does pass, there are a myriad of feelings: relief that one no longer needs to give care, guilt that one has felt this way, as well as sadness for the passing of one he loved. A gentleman was admitted into hospice with end stage Alzheimer's disease. His two sons showed staff members many pictures on their computer of the man he used to be. The gentleman in the bed—no longer eating or drinking, eyes open but not making contact—was not the person they had known. They had a great need to tell story after story of who he was and what he did when he was well: "So that you will know that he wasn't always like this!" They needed to be reassured that their feelings of loss as well as relief were normal and *okay*.

For all people, including the elderly and their adult children, meaning is a significant issue in life and in death. The loss of a partner and the loss of a parent represent the loss of meaning. And so, the bereaved must be able to accommodate the massive loss of her spouse into her life, to "make sense" of it (Holland et al., 2013). There are many deaths that are difficult to make sense of. The elderly parent who loses an adult child and the very old woman murdered for change in her purse are two examples. Here, the grief is difficult, and coming to acceptance is impeded by the fact that the nature of these deaths goes against everything we believe should happen. Chan and Chan (2011) used the term *timely* in relation to a death that is more easily made sense of and accepted. They suggested that the death that is *untimely*—where it is unexpected, hastened by medical error, or where there are people older than the deceased still alive—makes acceptance more difficult. They added that just because a person is aged does not necessarily mean that the death is timely.

How does one make sense of death, and hence be able to move beyond a loss? For the elderly, research is showing more and more that some sort of relationship with the deceased continues (Golsworthy & Coyle, 1999; Ho, Chan, Ma, & Field, 2013). This sense of relationship can be sustaining. Health professionals can help bereaved individuals tap into coping mechanisms from the past; that which brought meaning in the past can be utilized to bring meaning into the present and for the future (Chan & Chan, 2011). As mentioned, religious faith and spirituality that relocate the deceased can aid bereaved people (Golsworthy & Coyle, 1999). Sometimes, forms of meaning can be made through transcendence. "My loved one died of cancer, but perhaps research on her body can lead to the cure for someone else." Chan and Chan (2011) spoke of the importance of volunteer work, which brings an "other-centeredness" to the bereaved person, and which may help a spouse in accepting the death of her husband.

Funeral Services

As was mentioned earlier in the chapter, many people are opting out of having funeral/memorial services for a departed loved one.[16] Obituaries

---

16. Technically, a funeral is a service where the deceased is present in body—in the casket. A memorial service may include an urn, but there is no body. More and more, people are entitling their services, in whatever format they are held, as "Celebrations of Life."

regularly mention phrases such as "according to John's wishes, there will be no funeral service." This, on first glance, appears respectful of the person who has died. But the question must be asked, who is the service for? Gire (2002) noted that a funeral service is a *rite of passage* for both the dying person and the living. First, terminally ill people utilize the funeral service as an opportunity to impart "one last message" or to celebrate the life they have lived, in anticipation of the life they are now entering. Many put extensive effort into planning their service, and discussing their plans and purposes with family members and friends.

However, primarily, the service (in whichever form it takes) is for the living. Researchers have noted a number of purposes of the memorial (Gire, 2002; Kastenbaum, 2004). First, the funeral provides a context in which everyone formally recognizes that the death has really happened. Second, the function of the funeral is to realign relationships among the living. The bereaved wife is now a widow, in need of care and support in a way that she previously has not needed; the community comes together to provide that care for her in her new context, in the service itself and afterward. Third, it provides the rituals within which the bereaved can "send off" the deceased person into his new life. These rituals can continue after the funeral; for example, prayers for the "repose of the soul" may continue for a period of time after a passing. And finally, funeral services may provide a place for the bereaved to deal with their guilt and grief. One astute minister, in the funeral for a congregant who passed unexpectedly, stated, "I meant to get together with this gentleman. I did not, and feel guilty. You may feel guilty too. In our presence here, we are 'getting together' with him and honoring him. We need to forgive ourselves for where we feel we have been lacking in relationship to him." In this way, he gave the mourners permission to admit to themselves their guilt, to forgive themselves, to honor the deceased, and to grieve in a healthy manner. Funerals can provide the context for individuals to act out their grief—through mourning—in a place of support (Gire, 2002). In all these things, the service helps mourners to "make sense" of the connection between life and death (Holloway, Adamson, Argyrou, Draper, & Mariau, 2013, p. 35), bridging the transitional place "between dead and alive and the sacred and the human, (and bringing) together the past, present, and future of the deceased and their 'surviving' loved ones" (Davis, 2008, p. 421).

As has been expressed a number of times in this text, the western world is uncomfortable with death and expressions of grief. I (MBR) have officiated at many funerals (in whatever form they have taken). Grown men, weeping over their loved ones, have sometimes expressed, "I shouldn't be crying like this!" In one service, the sons-in-law of the deceased elderly woman—burly, strong men—wore sunglasses to cover their swollen eyes and wept copiously. They loved her! While their weeping may not be common in North America, in many societies, overt weeping (and even wailing) is both typical and helpful (to release grief).

Sometimes memorial services/celebrations of life occur a lengthy time after the passing. In one circumstance, the elderly man had passed three years earlier. His nieces said, "We need to have this service; we can't just can move on!" Whether they occur immediately after a death, or sometime later, a woman whose mother-in-law had just passed, said it best: "This day cannot be just like any other; we have to remember and celebrate her!"

As has been mentioned, the form of the ritual is not nearly as important as the *meaning* that the chosen ritual holds to the person who has passed and to his or her loved ones. Gatherings can take many forms; but the gathering needs to fulfill the needs of the mourning community to recognize the loss, to realign the relationships among the bereaved, and to provide a place to deal with grief needs, such as mourning.

Tending to Issues Related to Will, Estate, Finances

Ideally, work related to establishing wills and keeping financial matters current should be ongoing and, therefore, minimize the responsibilities of a grieving spouse or adult children after the death of an older individual. However, even when the aging adult has tended to matters of finances, the will, and the estate, there still is work involved for the executor of the estate. Adult children may fight over issues in the will or dividing up of the estate. Fighting about these matters may begin even before the aging adult has died.

In situations that are complex, and where difficulties are expected, some elderly people are opting to have an independent third party (such as a representative from a bank) look after matters of the estate. This can be costly but may ameliorate difficulties among adult children. As legal issues are beyond the scope of this text, we encourage readers to access texts addressing legal matters in relation to older adults.

Ethical Issues

Ethical issues, where there are competing values in difficult decision-making, render the process of resolution strenuous. Those who deal with these issues—in whatever field—wrestle significantly with dilemmas.

This is not a text on ethics, so the discussion will be limited. But briefly, in the area of biomedical ethics, there are four foundational concepts[17] to guide decision-making: autonomy, beneficence, nonmaleficence, and distributive justice.[18] These foundational principles form the base for ethical decision-making. While the meaning of each of the concepts appears to be straightforward, there are situations in life where the relationship between foundational principles is strained. It is in these circumstances, where there is conflict between these guiding values, where the ethical dilemmas arise. For example, an older man may have suffered with kidney disease for many years. For the last ten years, he has had to have dialysis three times a week. Recently, he received a cancer diagnosis. He does not want to receive treatment for the cancer, and he feels like he is just "done" with dialysis. His desire to refuse forms of medical treatment that will prolong his life (chemotherapy and dialysis) come into conflict with his family and their values; they believe he has the obligation to receive the treatment that is available. His assertion of autonomy and their understanding of beneficence (doing what is good) come into conflict.

In such situations, decision-making models such as the Latimer Ethical Decision-Making Model and the Kuhl Ethical Grid can be helpful (see Downing & Wainwright, 2006; and Kuhl & Wilensky, 1999). As discussed in Chapter 5, a fully developed person learns from a young age and in ever-deepening ways throughout his life, that he matters, and so do others! The needs of the individual are balanced with the needs of others (Kissane & Kelly, 2000).

The following two issues, as they arise in end-of-life, are ethical issues because the foundational values of autonomy, beneficence, nonmaleficence, and distributive justice—or the *interpretation* of these values—come into conflict. So much could be said about suicide and euthanasia from legal and religious perspectives; entire books have been written on the

---

17. The foundational concepts of ethical decision-making are also values and principles. So the terms will be used interchangeably, where appropriate.
18. Autonomy refers to an individual having the right to his or her own values and beliefs and, when possible, decision-making. Hence, regarding older adults, living wills are vital. Second, there is beneficence; this mean to do good. Third, nonmaleficence refers to "doing no harm." This is central to all health care! And finally, there is distributive justice, which means that there is to be fairness among people. This four-principle model, with the discussion of scope of each in relationship to the others, was first postulated by Beauchamp and Childress in text form in 1985. Since then, their text *Principles of Biomedical Ethics* has become a classic in biomedical ethics; there have been a number of editions of this text, with some significant revisions. The reference list provides information for the most recent edition (2012).

subjects. This text is not a legal text, nor is it a religious one, however. So the following topics will be covered primarily from a grief and loss as well as palliative care perspective.

Suicide

It has been discussed in other chapters within this text that suicide in older adults is a major issue. But it is not something we are comfortable speaking about. So I (MBR) was surprised, when guest lecturing about grief in a university class, when a delightful older adult broached the subject in front of his many, and much younger, classmates.

This gentleman shared openly that his wife had died and that when he felt that he was "done," he would spare his family and society the burden of caring for him and simply end his life. "What do you think about that?" he questioned me in front of the large class. I acknowledged the loss of his wife and the difficulties that elderly people have with grief and finding (new) meaning. As the issue of suicide is emotionally charged and value-laden, I paused before responding.

Gathering my thoughts, I explained to the class that each individual has a right to her own life (autonomy), but that there are always more people involved than simply an individual (family and friends). From a grief perspective, death always leaves guilt (some of it justified; some of it not). However, suicide leaves a mountain of guilt and regret that is not easily reckoned with or resolved. Bereaved family members struggle to make sense of the death and often feel that they are at least in part responsible for it. ("If only I had taken her out for breakfast that day..." "I never should have moved across the country to take this job!") The grief that follows a suicide is very complex; it is traumatic (Rando, 1984; Swarte, van der Lee, van der Bom, van den Bout, & Heintz, 2003).

In the western world we are strongly oriented toward the youth and the individual. While this affords certain advantages in terms of self-actualization, the lifelong development of personhood, through all of its transitions, may actually be hampered, because we attempt to cope with transitions on our own. And when we reach our final years, we may feel that we have little to contribute to, or receive from, our families. It could be said that suicide in the elderly is a symptom of this isolation and disconnect with others.

One health care professional declared to me (MBR) that if he received a terminal diagnosis, he would end his life immediately. "No one should have to go through that," he said. But when a valued member of his family passed away from suicide, he struggled tremendously. At this point, the perspective changed, as he was one who was left behind; what was once "logical" to him was no longer so.

Physician-Assisted Suicide and Euthanasia

There is much in the news regarding physician-assisted suicide and euthanasia today. Physician-assisted suicide is when a doctor intentionally provides, at patient request, the drugs needed for that patient to kill herself; euthanasia is the doctor's intentional killing of a patient by drugs, as a response to the patient's intentional and competent (with capacity) request (Frileux, Lelievre, Munoz Sastre, Mullet, & Sorum, 2003; Materstvedt et al., 2003).[19] Both of these actions are legalized in certain regions in the western world. The reasons why a patient may request such a procedure are complex; often, they reveal the physical, psychological, and spiritual suffering (such as pain, feelings of aloneness, spiritual distress) that palliative care seeks to address (Ley & van Bommel, 1994; Materstvedt et al., 2003). In general, physician-assisted suicide is viewed more kindly than euthanasia, because of the patient's intention of dying (by asking the physician, sometimes repeatedly, for the medications to terminate her own life) and her action to carry out the desire on her own (Frileux et al., 2003).

Within western regions that permit physician-assisted suicide and euthanasia, there is great concern about what constitutes *consent*. In the Netherlands, for example, euthanasia can be carried out without a patient's current consent, because he had mentioned previously to his physician that he feared suffering (Materstvedt et al., 2003); sometimes *there is no patient consent* at all, hence the terms nonvoluntary and involuntary euthanasia[20] (Hendin, Rutenfrans, & Zylicz, 1997). Hendin (1998) spoke of a physician who carried out the euthanasia of a nun, who was suffering terribly, but whose religious convictions did not condone her asking for it; hence, her

---

19. Euthanasia must not be confused with palliative sedation. In palliative sedation, the patient is within days or hours of death, the symptoms being uncontrolled without some sedation (mild or heavier). In this circumstance, the guidelines for the procedure are clear, consultation among palliative physicians must occur, and the intent is to control symptoms, not to end life (Materstvedt et al., 2003).

20. Nonvoluntary euthanasia refers to euthanasia where the patient is not able to consent. Involuntary euthanasia is euthanasia against the patient's will. (See Materstvedt et al., 2003.)

convictions were violated.[21] Some bioethicists worry that a non-voluntary euthanasia may become justified for individuals with severe dementia (Sharp, 2012).

Dorothy Ley (Ley & van Bommel, 1994) separated euthanasia from the popular phrase: "dying with dignity":

---

*The current fashion to equate dying with dignity
with euthanasia reflects the mistaken belief that death
whose moment is chosen is somehow more dignified
than one not chosen (p. 67).*

Ley (Ley & van Bommel, 1994) alluded to a Western ideal that equates dignity with health, looking good, and control over all bodily functions. She suggested that we revisit this concept and understand that dignity is not something that can be taken away by bodily changes. For instance, the loss of continence is often more distressing for family members than it is for the patient herself (Kissane & Kelly, 2000). Dignity resides in the quality of care, and in the attitudes of those giving and receiving care (Arnup, 2013). Fenigsen (2012) said, "We are told that to be assisted by medical technology entails loss of dignity, as if the dignity of honest, caring, courageous people, our parents and spouses, could somehow be drained out of them through medical devices" (p. 73).

Ley (Ley & van Bommel, 1994) continued to caution that the "right to die" easily gets converted into a "duty to die" (p. 67). This conviction was echoed by a number of researchers into the Dutch medical system, which practices euthanasia (see Fenigsen, 2012; Materstvedt et al., 2003). Ley (Ley & van Bommel, 1994) also mentioned that vulnerable populations are most at risk for this pressure: the elderly, the poor, the handicapped.

Regarding older adults, Kissane and Kelly (2000) stated that "the practice of euthanasia and physician-assisted suicide is clearly related to age" (p. 330), and they caution against using the ethical principle *autonomy* as

---

21. The literature reveals that within the Netherlands, the boundaries of what is considered acceptable in euthanasia continue to widen; doctors who oppose the practice receive professional pressure and ostracism; and when instances of euthanasia are carried out that are outside of the boundaries of the law, they are not prosecuted (Boer, 2014; Fenigsen, 2012; Hendin, 1998; Hendin, Rutenfrans, & Zylicz, 1997; Kissane & Kelly, 2000; Materstvedt et al., 2003).

the predominant standard for making decisions regarding end of life, as this autonomous choice may be unachievable in the context of advanced age or severe illness. And it is worth noting that one never acts in isolation; autonomous actions always impact others. (The interdependence of individuals in the experience of transition [Hutchison, 2008] was discussed in Chapter 1.) A study carried out by Segers (1988) observed that vulnerable peoples (particularly the elderly) are less likely to agree with euthanasia, as they fear the procedure may be carried out on them against their will.[22]

Loss of dignity is something that involves the negating of personhood. A thrust of this text has been to affirm the personhood of older adults, in all of their transitions. And effective palliative care both maintains and even develops personhood at the end of life. Research shows that when issues such as total pain are dealt with, patients who had been thinking about euthanasia no longer wish to die in that way (Materstvedt et al., 2003; Segers, 1988; Teno et al., 2011; von Gunten, 2012).

From a grief perspective, as has been touched upon, grieving is made much more difficult for the bereaved when a death does not make sense (Holland et al., 2013) and is not seen to be timely (Chan & Chan, 2011). Confusion over consent, premature ending of life, the violation of convictions (whether the patient's or her family members) all lead to pronounced and prolonged grief. When family members are called upon to help plan the death (physician-assisted suicide or euthanasia), they often experience a conflict of values—wanting to honor their loved one's wishes, but struggling because to honor their loved one's wishes may lead to violating their values (Starks et al., 2007). Starks and colleagues (2007) spoke of the family of a "Mrs. Bowen," who were involved in hastening her death, at her request. Two and a half years after Mrs. Bowen's death, a daughter said this:

> *The impact of this is so huge . . . I've become socially*
> *isolated, exhausted . . . It's been three years since I've*
> *had a life . . . I'm not sleeping well . . . Sometimes I'll*
> *wake up around 4 (a.m.) thinking, "Did I kill her?" (p. 117).*

---

22. Dr. J. Segers (1988), in a Dutch study, found that 66% of older adults living independently, and 95% of older adults living in care facilities opposed government support of euthanasia, and they expressed fear of involuntary euthanasia.

Chapters 5 and 6 in this text have illustrated the personal growth and relational work that can occur in the context of end of life, particularly when there is effective palliative care. When the medical expertise and the social and spiritual supports are in place, dying older adults may experience profound meaning in their last days, and families are aided greatly in their journeys of grief, as well as their own development of personhood. Suicide, physician-assisted suicide, and euthanasia precludes dying individuals and their families the opportunity for profound growth and meaning, and those left behind face very complex journeys of grief. Good palliative care is the response to end-of-life issues. Chapter 8 will include a brief section on the need for palliative care to be available to everyone who needs it.

Concluding this discussion, Dutch ethicist Theo Boer supported physician-assisted suicide and euthanasia for years. For nine years he sat on a regional euthanasia review committee, working with committee members to evaluate individual cases to ensure that they complied with Dutch law. Boer, in a 2014 letter originally sent to Britain's *Daily Mail* (and then published internationally), indicated that "I was wrong: euthanasia has a slippery slope." (See Doughty, 2014). In the Netherlands, what qualifies within the law for the option of euthanasia has precipitously widened. In this country, the suffering that would permit this response has broadened from intractable physical suffering to those who are aged, lonely, bereaved, experiencing psychiatric illness or dementia. The numbers of cases of physician-assisted suicides and incidents of euthanasia have increased dramatically. Using the term "slippery slope" Boer concludes:

> *I used to be a supporter of legislation (for euthanasia).*
> *But now with 12 years of experience, I take a different*
> *view . . . Once the genie is out of the bottle, it is not*
> *likely to ever go back in again. (Boer, 2014, n.p.)*

SUMMARY

Within this chapter, we have examined some myths that surround the dying and death of aging adults. We also addressed issues related to dying in older adults, both for the aging individuals themselves, as well as for their family members; health care interventions were woven into the discussion.

And finally we looked at ethical issues surrounding death and dying. To quote Jesse, a dying individual who participated in a study conducted by Patricia Ryan (2005), "Dying is no easy thing; there's a lot to it" (p. 1106).

CRITICAL THINKING EXERCISES

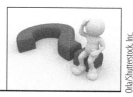

▶ Review the case example. If you had been the social worker or chaplain working with Jean and Sandra, would you have handled the situation differently? What thoughts and emotions did this case evoke in you?

▶ What has been your experience with death up to this point in time?

▶ What concerns do you have in assisting a dying older adult, as well as his family members?

▶ How do you mentally and spiritually process death?

INTERESTING WEBSITES

▶ Canadian Virtual Hospice: www.virtualhospice.ca

▶ National Hospice and Palliative Care Organization: www.nhpco.org

▶ Hospice Action Network: www.hospiceactionnetwork.org

REFERENCES

Ainsworth, M. D. S., & Bowlby, J. (1991). An ethological approach to personality development. *American Psychologist, 46*, 331–341.

Allemand, M., Steiner, M., & Hill, P. (2013). Effects of a forgiveness intervention for older adults. *Journal of Counseling Psychology, 60*(2), 279–286.

Arnup, K. (2013). *Death, dying and Canadian families*. Ottawa, ON: Vanier Institute.

Beauchamp, T. L, & Childress, J. F. (2012). *Principles of biomedical ethics* (7th ed.). New York: Oxford University Press.

Bennett, K. M. (2005). 'Was life worth living?' Older widowers and their explicit discourses of the decision to live. *Mortality, 10*(2), 144–154. doi:10.1080/13576270500102906

Boer, T. (2014, July 17). I was wrong: Euthanasia has a slippery slope. *The Calgary Herald.*

Boss, P. (1999). *Ambiguous loss: Learning to live with unresolved grief.* Cambridge, MA: Harvard University Press.

Bowlby, J. (1999). Attachment. *Attachment and loss, Vol. I* (2nd ed.). New York: Basic Books.

Boyle, D. K., Miller, P. A., & Forbes-Thompson, S. A. (2005). Communication and end-of-life care in the intensive care unit: Patient, family, and clinician outcomes. *Critical Care Nursing Quarterly, 28*(4), 302–316.

Brainy Quotes. (2015). Retrieved February 1, 2015, from: www.brainyquote.com

Buchanan, R. J., Choi, M., Wang, S., & Ju, H. (2004). End-of-life care in nursing homes: Residents in hospice as compared to end-stage residents. *Journal of Palliative Medicine,* (April), *7*(2), 221–232.

Byock, I. (1997). *Dying well: Peace and possibilities at the end of life.* New York: Riverhead Books.

Cairns, B., & Ahmad, M. (2011). Choosing where to die: Allowing for choices: dying at home, in a hospice or in palliative care. *CBC News,* May 17. Retrieved February 12, 2015, from: http://www.cbc.ca/news/health/choosing-where-to-die-1.1002383

Callahan, D. (1993). Pursuing a peaceful death. *Hastings Center Report, 23*(4), 33–38.

Canadian Hospice Palliative Care Association. (2012). Fact sheet: Hospice palliative care in Canada. Canadian Hospice Palliative Care Association. Retrieved January 31, 2015, from: http://www.chpca.net/media/7622/fact_sheet_hpc_in_canada_may_2012_final.pdf

Canadian Virtual Hospice Team. (2011). What is palliative care? Canadian Virtual Hospice. Retrieved February 12, 2015, from: www.virtualhospice.ca/en_US/Main+Site+Navigation/Home/Topics/Topics/What+Is+Palliative+Care_/What+Is+Palliative+Care_.aspx

Chan, W. C. H., & Chan, C. L. W. (2011). Acceptance of spousal death: The factor of time in bereaved older adults' search for meaning. *Death Studies, 35,* 147–162. doi:10.1080/07481187.2010.535387

Cherlin, E. L., Barry, C. L., Prigerson, H. G., Schulman-Green, D., Johnson-Hurzeler, R., et al. (2007). Bereavement services for family caregivers: How often used, why, and why not. *Journal of Palliative Medicine, 10*(1), 148–158. doi:10.1089/jpm.2006.0108

Clabots, S. (2012). Strategies to help initiate and maintain end-of-life discussion with patients and family members. *MEDSURG Nursing, 21*(4), 197–203.

Copp, G. (1998). A review of current theories of death and dying. *Journal of Advanced Nursing, 28*(2), 382–390. doi:10.1046/j.1365-2648.1998.00794.x

Corless, I. B. (1994). Dying well: Symptom control within hospice care. *Annual Review of Nursing Research, 12,* 125–146.

Creedon, R., & O'Regan, P. (2010). Palliative care, pain control and nurse prescribing. *Nurse Prescribing, 8*(6), 257–264.

D'Antonio, J. (2014). Caregiver grief and anticipatory mourning. *Journal of Hospice and Palliative Nursing, 16*(2), 99–104. doi:10.1097/NJH.0000000000000027

Davis, C. S. (2008). A funeral liturgy: Death rituals as symbolic communication. *Trauma and Loss, 13*, 406–421. doi:10.1080/15325020802171391

Doughty, S. (2014, July 9). Don't make our mistake: As assisted suicide bill goes to Lords, Dutch watchdog who once backed euthanasia warns UK of 'slippery slope' to mass deaths. *The Daily Mail*. Retrieved February 1, 2015, from: http://www.dailymail.co.uk/news/article-2686711/Dont-make-mistake-As-assisted-suicide-bill-goes-Lords-Dutch-regulator-backed-euthanasia-warns-Britain-leads-mass-killing.html#ixzz3QWxKjmjm

Downing, G. M., & Wainwright, W. (2006). *Medical care of the dying*. Victoria, BC: Victoria Hospice Society.

Elwert, F., & Christakis, N. A. (2008). The effect of widowhood on mortality by the causes of death of both spouses. *American Journal of Public Health, 98*(11), 2092–2098. doi:10.2105/AJPH.2007.114348

Enright, R. D. (1996). Counseling within the forgiveness triad: On forgiving, receiving forgiveness, and self-forgiveness. *Counseling & Values, 40*, 107ff.

Erikson, E. H. (1982). *The life cycle completed: A review*. New York: Norton.

Erikson, E. H., Erikson, J. M., & Kivnick, H. (1986). *Vital involvement in old age*. New York: Norton.

Ersek, M., & Polomano, R. A. (2011). Nursing management of pain. In S. L. Lewis, S. R. Dirksen, M. M. Heitkemper, L. Bucher, & I. M. Camera (Eds.), *Medical-surgical nursing: Assessment and management of clinical problems* (8th ed.; pp. 127–152). Philadelphia: Elsevier.

Fenigsen, R. (2012). Other people's lives: Reflections on medicine, ethics and euthanasia. *Issues in Law and Medicine, 28*(1), 73–87.

Field, M. J., & Cassel, C. K. (Eds.) (1997). *Approaching death: Improving care at the end of life*. Washington, DC: National Press Academy.

Frankl, V. E. (2006). *Man's search for meaning*. Boston: Beacon Press.

Frileux, S., Lelievre, C., Munoz Sastre, M. T., Mullet, M., & Sorum, P. C. (2003). When is physician-assisted suicide or euthanasia acceptable? *Journal of Medical Ethics, 29*(6), 330–336. doi:10.1136/jme.29.6.330

Gammons, V., & Caswell, G. (2014). Older people and barriers to self-reporting of chronic pain. *British Journal of Nursing, 23*(5), 274–278.

Georgesen, J., & Dungan, J. M. (1996). Managing spiritual distress in patients with advanced cancer pain. *Cancer Nursing, 19*(5), 376–383.

Geriatricpain.org. (2012). Geriatric pain. Retrieved February 1, 2015, from: www.geriatricpain.org

Gerber, I., Rusalem, R., Hannon, N., Banin, D., & Arkin, A. (1975). Anticipatory grief and aged widows and widowers. *Journal of Gerontology, 30*(2), 225–229. doi:10.1093/geronj/30.2.225

Gibson, J. (2009). Living with loss. *Mental Health Practice, 12*(5), 22–24.

Gire, J. T. (2002). How death imitates life: Cultural influences on conceptions of death and dying. In W. J. Lonner, D. L. Dinnel, S. A. Hayes, & D. N. Sattler (Eds.), *Online readings in psychology and culture* (Unit 14, Chapter 2). Bellingham, WA: Center for Cross-Cultural Research, Western Washington University. Accessible at: www.wwu.edu/culture/gire.htm

Goffman, E. (1961). *Asylums: Essays on the social situation of mental patients and other inmates.* New York: Anchor.

Golsworthy, R., & Coyle, A. (1999). Spiritual beliefs and the search for meaning among older adults following partner loss. *Mortality, 4*(1), 21–37.

Good Reads. (2015). Retrieved February 1, 2015, from: www.goodreads.com

Gropelli, T., & Sharer, J. (2013). Nurses' perceptions of pain management in older adults. *MedSurg Nursing, 22*(6), 375–382.

Halifax, J. (2009). *Being with dying: Cultivating compassion and fearlessness in the presence of death.* Boston: Shambhala Publications.

Hamilton, N. (2005). Grief and bereavement: Anticipating the loss of a spouse. *Nursing and Residential Care, 7*(4), 167–169.

Hantman, S., & Cohen, O. (2010). Forgiveness in late life. *Journal of Gerontological Social Work, 53*(7), 613–630. doi:10.1080/01634372.2010.509751

Hendin, H. (1998). *Seduced by death: Doctors, patients, and the Dutch cure.* New York: Norton.

Hendin, H., Rutenfrans, C., & Zylicz, Z. (1997). Lessons from the Dutch. *Journal of the American Medical Association, 277*(21), n.p. Retrieved February 4, 2015, from: www.life.org.nz/euthanasia/abouteuthanasia/history-euthanasia10/Default.htm

Herr, K., Spratt, K., Garand, L., & Li, L. (2007). Evaluation of the Iowa Pain Thermometer and other selected pain intensity scales in younger and older adult cohorts using controlled clinical pain: A preliminary study. *Pain Medicine, 8*(7), 585–600. doi:10.1111/j.1526-4637.2007.00316.x

Heyse-Moore, L. H. (1996). On spiritual pain in the dying. *Mortality, 1*(3), 297–315.

Hirst, S. P., Lane, A. M., & Reed, M. B. (2013). Personhood in nursing homes: Results of an ethnographic study. *Indian Journal of Gerontological Studies, 27*(1), 69–87.

Ho, S. M., Chan, I. S., Ma, E. P., & Field, N. P. (2013). Continuing bonds, attachment style, and adjustment in the conjugal bereavement among Hong Kong Chinese. *Death Studies, 37*(3), 248–268. doi:10.1080/07481187.2011.634086

Holland, J. M., Futterman, A., Thompson, L. W., Moran, C., & Gallagher-Thompson, D. (2013). Difficulties accepting the loss of a spouse: A precursor for intensified grieving among widowed older adults. *Death Studies, 37*(2), 126–144. doi:10/1080/07481187.2011.617489

Holloway, M., Adamson, S., Argyrou, V., Draper, P., & Mariau, D., (2013). "Funerals aren't nice but it couldn't have been nicer." The makings of a good funeral. *Mortality, 18*(1), 30–53. http://dx.doi.org/10.1080/13576275.2012.755505

Hospice Action Network. (2013). Hospice in the nursing home. Hospice Action Network, Series 1, Number 4. Retrieved February 4, 2015, from: http://hospiceactionnetwork.org/linked_documents/get_informed/issues/nursing_home/NH_Fact_Sheet.pdf

Hughes, L. D. (2012). Assessment and management of pain in older patients receiving palliative care. *Nursing Older People, 24*(6), 23–29.

Hutchison, E. (2008). *Dimensions of human behavior: The changing life course.* Thousand Oaks, CA: Sage.

Jackson, V. (Speaker). (2015). Navigating discussions of prognosis: Balancing honesty with hope. *Schwartz Center Webinar Series,* (January 13, 2015). Information available at: www.theschwartzcenter.org/media/Navigating-Discussions-of-Prognosis-HANDOUT.pdf

Johansson, A. K., & Grimby, A. (2012). Anticipatory grief among close relatives of patients in hospice and palliative wards. *American Journal of Hospice Palliative Medicine, 29*(2), 134–138.

Kagawa-Singer, M. (1998). The cultural context of death rituals and mourning practices. *Oncology Nursing Forum, 25*(10), 1752–1756.

Kahana, B., Dan, A., Kahana, E., & Kercher, K. (2004). The personal and social context of planning for end-of-life care. *Journal of the American Geriatrics Society, 52*(7), 1163–1167. doi:10.1111/j.1532-5415.2004.52316.x

Kastenbaum, R. (2004). Why funerals? Generations, 28(2), 5–10.

Kind, V. (2010). *The caregiver's path to compassionate decision-making: Making choices for those who can't.* Austin, TX: Greenleaf Book Group Press.

Kissane, D. W., & Kelly, B. J. (2000). Demoralisation, depression and desire for death: Problems with the Dutch guidelines for euthanasia of the mentally ill. *Australian and New Zealand Journal of Psychiatry, 34*(2), 325–333.

Kubler-Ross, E. (1969). *On death and dying.* London: Tavistock Publications.

Kuhl, D. R., & Wilensky, P. (1999). Decision making at the end of life: A model using an ethical grid and principles of group process. *Journal of Palliative Medicine, 2*(1), 75–86.

Lawton, S., Towsey, L., & Carroll, D. (2013). What is a 'good death' in the care home setting? *Nursing & Residential Care, 15*(7), 494–497.

Ley, D., & van Bommel, H. (1994). *The heart of hospice.* Toronto: NC Press Limited.

Lindauer, A., & Harvath, T. A. (2014). Pre-death grief in the context of dementia caregiving: A concept analysis. *Journal of Advanced Nursing, 70*(10), 2196–2207. doi:10.1111/jan.12411

Lindemann, E. (1944). Symptomatology and management of acute grief. *American Journal of Psychiatry, 101,* 141–148.

Maddison, D., & Walker, W. L. (1967). Factors affecting the outcome of conjugal bereavement. *British Journal of Psychiatry, 113,* 1057–1067.

Martinson, I. M. (1998). Funeral rituals in Taiwan and Korea. *Oncology Nursing Forum, 25*(10), 1756–1760.

Materstvedt, L. J., Clark, D., Ellershaw, J., Forde, R., Boeck Gravgaard, A. M., Muller-Busch, H. C., Porta i Sales, J., & Rapin, C. H. (2003). Euthanasia and physician-assisted suicide: A view from an EAPC ethics task force. *Palliative Medicine, 17*(2), 97–101. doi:10.1191/0269616303pm673oa

McDaniel, J. G., & Clark, P. G. (2009). The new adult orphan: Issues and considerations for health care professionals. *Journal of Gerontological Nursing, 35*(12), 44–49.

McHugh, M. E., Miller-Saultz, D., Wuhrman, E., & Kosharskyy, B. (2012). Interventional pain management in the palliative patient. *International Journal of Palliative Nursing, 18*(9), 426–433.

Meraviglia, M., Sutter, R., & Gaskamp, C. D. (2008). Providing spiritual care to terminally ill older adults. *Journal of Gerontological Nursing, 34*(7), 8–14.

Michael, S. T., Crowther, M. R., Schmid, B., & Allen, R. S. (2003). Widowhood and spirituality: Coping responses to bereavement. *Journal of Women & Aging, 15*(2/3), 145–165.

Miller Lewis, M., & Trzinski, A. L. (2006). Counseling older adults with dementia who are dealing with death: Innovative interventions for practitioners. *Death Studies, 30*(8), 777–787. doi:10.1080/07481180600853199

Miller, S. C., Mor, V., Wu, N., Gonzalo, P., & Lapane, K. (2002). "Does receipt of hospice care in nursing homes improve the management of pain at the end of life?" *Journal of the American Geriatrics* Society, *50*(3), 507–515.

Milligan, S. (2011). Addressing the spiritual care needs of people near the end of life. *Nursing Standard, 26*(4), 47–56.

Muramatsu, N., Hoyem, R., Yin, H., & Campbell, R. (2008). Place of death among older Americans. *Medical Care, 46*(8), 829–838.

National Cancer Institute. (2010). Palliative care in cancer. Retrieved January 27, 2015, from: http://www.cancer.gov/cancertopics/factsheet/Support/palliative-care

National Institute of Health Medline Plus. (2011). Seniors and chronic pain. Retrieved November 13, 2014, from: www.nlm.nih.gov/medlineplus/magazine/issues/fall11/articles/fall11pg15.html

Nunn, C. (2014). It's not just about pain: Symptom management in palliative care. *Nurse Prescribing, 12*(7), 338–344.

Ott, C. H., Lueger, R. J., Kelber, S. T., & Prigerson, H. G. (2007). Spousal bereavement in older adults: Common, resilient, and chronic grief with defining characteristics. *Journal of Nervous & Mental Disease, 195*(4), 332–341. doi:10.1097/01.nmd.0000243890.93992.1e

Ozanne, A., Graneheim, U. H., & Strang, S. (2013). Finding meaning despite anxiety over life and death in amyotrophic lateral sclerosis patients. *Journal of Clinical Nursing, 22,* 2141–2149. doi:10.1111/jocn.12071

Palgi, P., & Abramovitch, H. (1984). Death: A cross-cultural perspective. *Annual Review of Anthropology, 13,* 385–417.

Parkes, C. M. (1975). Determinants of outcome following bereavement. *Omega, 6*, 303–323.

Rando, T. A. (1984). *Grief, dying and death: Clinical interventions for caregivers.* Champaign, IL: Research Press.

Reed, M. B. (2014). Me and my shadow: Interprofessional training in and modeling of spiritual care in the palliative setting, *Indian Journal of Gerontology,* (November), *28*(4), 501–518.

Reed, M. B. (2015). Caring for older adults at the end of life. In S. P. Hirst, A. M. Lane, & C. Miller (Eds.) *Miller's Nursing for Wellness in Older Adults* (pp. 588-602). Philadelphia, PA: Lippincott.

Regan, A., Tapley, M., & Jolley, D. (2014). Improving end of life care for people with dementia. *Nursing Standard, 28*(48), 37–43.

Ryan, P. Y. (2005). Approaching death: A phenomenologic study of five older adults with advanced cancer. *Oncology Nursing Forum, 32*(6), 1101–1108. doi:10.1188/05.ONF.1101-1108

Satterly, L. (2001). Guilt, shame and religious and spiritual pain. *Holistic Nursing Practice, 15*(2), 30–39.

Searchquotes. (2015). Retrieved February 24, 2015, from: www.searchquotes.com

Segers, J. H. (1988). Persons on the subject of euthanasia. *Issues in Law & Medicine, 3*, 407–424.

Seibold, M. (2001). When the wounding runs deep: Encouragement for those on the road to forgiveness. In M. R. McMinn & T. R. Phillips (Eds.), *Care for the Soul* (pp. 294–308). Downer's Grove, IL: InterVarsity.

Shah, S. M., Carey, I. M., Harris, T., DeWilde, S., Victor, C. R., & Cook, D. G. (2013). The effect of unexpected bereavement on mortality in older couples. *American Journal of Public Health,* e1–e6.

Sharp, R. (2012). The dangers of euthanasia and dementia. How Kantian thinking might be used to support non-voluntary euthanasia in cases of extreme dementia. *Bioethics, 26*(5), 231–235.

Sidell, M., Samson Katz, J., & Komaromy, C. (2000). The case for palliative care in residential and nursing homes. In D. Dickenson, M. Johnson, and J. Samson Katz (Eds.), *Death, dying and bereavement* (2nd ed.) (pp. 107–121). London: Sage.

Siegel, K., & Weinstein, L. (1983). Anticipatory grief revisited. *Journal of Psychosocial Oncology, 1*(2), 61–73. doi:10.1300/J077v01n02_04

Singer, P. A., Martin, D. K., & Kelner, M. (1999). Quality end-of-life care: Patients' perspectives. *Journal of the American Medical Association, 281*(2), 163–168.

Smedes, L. B. (1997). *The art of forgiving: When you need to forgive and don't know how.* New York: Ballantine Books.

Sourkes, B. M. (1982). The deepening shade: Psychological aspects of life-threatening illness. Pittsburgh: University of Pittsburgh Press.

Starks, H., Back, A. L., Pearlman, R. A., Koenig, B. A., Hsu, C., Gordon, J. R., & Bharucha, A. J. (2007). Family member involvement in hastened death. *Death Studies, 31*(2), 105–130. doi:10.1080/07481180601100483

Statistics Canada. (2010). *Healthy people, healthy places—82-229-X.* Author. Retrieved November 13, 2014, from: http://www.statcan.gc.ca/pub/82-229-x/2009001/inf-eng.htm

Strohbuecker, B., Eisenmann, Y., Galushko, M., Montag, T., & Voltz R. (2011). Palliative care needs of chronically ill nursing home residents in Germany: Focusing on living, not dying. *International Journal of Palliative Nursing, 17*(1), 27–34.

Swarte, N. B., van der Lee, M. L., van der Bom, J. G., van den Bout, J., Heintz, A. P. M. (2003). Effects of euthanasia on the bereaved family and friends: A cross sectional study. *British Medical Journal, 327* (7408), 189–192.

Teno, J. M., Gozalo, P. L., Lee, I. C., Kuo, S., Spence, C., Connor, S., & Casarett, D. J. (2011). Does hospice improve quality of care for persons dying of dementia? *Journal of the American Geriatrics Society, 59*(8), 1531–1536. doi:10.1111/j.1532-5415.2011.03505.x

Thinkexist.com. (2015). Retrieved February 1, 2015, from: www.thinkexist.com

Thomas, C. L., & Cohen, H. L. (2006). Understanding spiritual meaning making with older adults. *Journal of Theory Construction & Testing, 10*(2), 65–70.

von Gunten, C. F. (2012). Evolution and effectiveness of palliative care. *American Journal of Geriatric Psychiatry, 20*(4), 291–297. doi:10.1097/JGP.0b013e3182436219

Walker, R. J., & Pomeroy, E. C. (1996). Depression or grief? The experience of caregivers of people with dementia. *Health Social Work, 21*(4), 247–254.

Walsh, F. (2009). Religion, spirituality and the family: Multi-faith perspectives. In F. Walsh (Ed.) *Spiritual resources in family therapy* (2nd ed.; pp. 3–30). New York: The Guilford Press.

Watts, T. (2012). End-of-life care pathways as tools to promote and support a good death: A critical commentary. *European Journal of Cancer Care, 21,* 20–30.

Weingarten, K. (1999). Stretching to meet what's given: Opportunities for a spiritual practice. In F. Walsh (Ed.), *Spiritual resources in family therapy* (pp. 240–255). New York: The Guilford Press.

Weisman, A. D. (1988). Appropriate death and the hospice program. *Hospice Journal, 4,* 65–77.

Worden, J. W. (2009). *Grief counseling and grief theory: A handbook for the mental health practitioner* (4th ed.). New York: Springer Publishing.

Yancey, P., & Brand, P. (1997). *The gift of pain.* Grand Rapids, MI: Zondervan.

Zerwekh, J. V. (2006). Nursing care at the end of life. Philadelphia: FA Davis Company.

CHAPTER 7

THE FAMILY

Happy or unhappy, families are all mysterious.
We have only to imagine how differently we would
be described—and will be, after our deaths—
by each of the family members who
believe they know us.
Gloria Steinem (American feminist and writer)

Reflective Questions

- ▶ What are several potential challenges that families may face when assisting an older adult through a transition?

- ▶ What are three guiding principles that may help you as a professional in facilitating older adults and their family members in navigating a transition?

- ▶ How do societal definitions of *family* impact your understanding of family and how you practice as a professional working with older adults?

Regardless of whether we agree with the quote from Gloria Steinem, she raises some important aspects about families. Families are indeed mysterious, and defining their composition is not as easy as it may seem. They are made up of much more than a number of physical bodies; they entail characteristics that are not so visible, such as beliefs, patterns, alliances, and norms (Wright & Leahey, 2013). What regulates families, in terms of patterns, norms, roles, and beliefs can be a source of great comfort and

251

stability, and can be, paradoxically, endlessly frustrating and befuddling. How members of a family relate to each other, understand and describe each other can change over time and can vary from context to context. And, after the death of a family member, our understandings, descriptions, and relationships to the departed family member can change markedly.

Despite the challenge of understanding families and the work involved in unraveling family patterns and relationships, it is vital that older adults be considered within the context of their family. While an individual is always best understood within the context of the family (Wright & Leahey, 2013), this is particularly so for older adults, especially when older adults are experiencing transitions. For a number of older adults, as they reach more advanced ages of 80 years and above, the physical and cognitive problems that become more prevalent at that time in life have made them more vulnerable and in greater need of support. They are less able to compensate for their disabilities and hence may need to rely upon others. Even if family members have been estranged, at this time of life, some adult children become involved. This means that it is imperative for health and human service professionals to assess and intervene, not just with the older adult who is experiencing transitions, but also with the family. It is not simply the older adult who may be feeling traumatized, but family members as well.

Within this chapter, we begin with attempting to define *family*. We briefly mention the idea of developmental tasks for aging families, then proceed to address some challenges health and human service professionals might encounter when working with families in facilitating transitions of their older adults. We offer some specific ideas as to how to address the difficulties professionals may face. Next, a case example is presented that reflects some of the challenges professionals experience when working with families. Finally, we cover some guiding principles that can assist health and human service professionals in working with older adult families experiencing transitions and, where applicable, apply the case example through this discussion.

Definition of the Family

Decades ago, it was generally accepted that the family was composed of individuals who were biologically related. Typically, a family was made up of a father, mother, and a number of children. Some families might also have an aging grandparent living within the home. Roles were clearly defined with men as "breadwinners" and women as "homemakers." Today, roles have become more relaxed; women predominantly work outside the home, there are increased rates of divorce resulting in single parent families, there is greater awareness and visibility of gay and lesbian families (The Vanier Institute of the Family, n.d.), and correspondingly, the definition of family has stretched beyond the borders of biologically related individuals.

So what is the definition of a family? Certainly, the legal definition varies from country to country and has changed over time. For instance, in 2005, the Statistics Canada definition of family was:

[A] now-married couple, a common-law couple or a lone-parent with a child or youth who is under the age of 25 . . . Now-married couples and common-law couples may or may not have such children and youth living with them. (Statistics Canada, 2012)

In the 2011 Canadian Census, the definition of family became broader. This Census definition stated:

A census family is composed of a married or common-law couple, with or without children, or of a lone parent living with at least one child in the same dwelling. Couples can be of the opposite sex or of the same sex. (Statistics Canada, 2012)

Thus, the Census definition of family has expanded to include gay and lesbian couples. Further, step-families and foster children were counted for the first time in the 2011 Census (Statistics Canada, 2012). Thus, the legal definition is expanding to include the multiple forms of families present in Canada and other developed nations.

Developmental Tasks of an Aging Family

Wright and Leahey (2013) provided a lens through which to understand family processes: the family life cycle (originally discussed by Carter and McGoldrick, 1989). Within the family life cycle, families progress through various stages. As part of moving through the various stages in the growth and development of the family, Wright and Leahey (2013) discussed the idea of the completion of tasks for families at various developmental stages. For instance, one stage is entitled "Marriage: The Joining of Families" (p. 100). In this stage, two individuals marry and thus form their own family unit. The tasks at this developmental stage involve the establishment of an identity as a couple, as well as making choices about having children (Wright & Leahey, 2013). These tasks, then, are part of the fabric and work of that stage of life, the stage of the formation of the couple relationship.

The last stage of development in the family life cycle is "Families in Later Life" (Wright & Leahey, 2013, p. 108). This stage may begin with the commencement of retirement and extends until the death of both spouses. However, as noted by Wright and Leahey (2013), it is hard to know when this stage now begins. The suggested tasks for this phase (we quote verbatim) include:

▶ Maintaining own or couple functioning and interest in the face of physiological decline: exploration of new familial and social role options.

▶ Making room in the system for the wisdom and experience of seniors.

▶ Dealing with loss of spouse, siblings, and other peers and preparation for death. (Wright & Leahey, 2013, pp. 109–110, quoted verbatim)

As will be evident from the forthcoming discussion in this chapter, the ability for older adults and their family members to address the tasks of aging families may be compromised by transitions caused by illness (e.g., dementia, depression), relocation (e.g., to a long-term care facility) or extremely troubling existential issues.

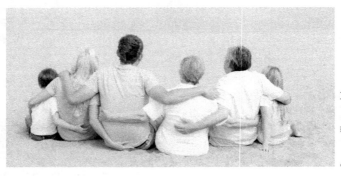

Challenges in Working With the Family

There are a number of challenges inherent in working with families of older adults who are undergoing transitions. The challenges may be related to family composition, past family experiences, and the challenges in transitions such as the placement process.

Defining the Family: Who Really Is the Family?

Although there are legal definitions, as well as definitions used for statistical purposes within countries, there is little agreement among scholars or the public regarding what constitutes a family (Edwards & Graham, 2009). Broadly speaking, families can be conceptualized and categorized according to structure, psychosocial aspects, and transactional processes. The structural understandings of family emphasize biological and adoption ties, as well as the extended family. Psychosocial definitions focus on whether particular family tasks are performed. Thus, psychosocial definitions assume that there is at least one adult who is responsible for the nurturance and socialization of children. Finally, the third category focuses upon transactional processes. This understanding of family highlights families as sharing rituals, identity, loyalty, and belonging. Within this understanding, there is great variance in conceptions of the "family" (Edwards & Graham, 2009). One such example of a definition that privileges transactional processes is that of family therapists Lorraine Wright and Maureen Leahey. They suggested that the family is "who they say they are" (Wright & Leahey, 2013, p. 55).

While we appreciate this definition, we also recognize that when dealing with transitions in older adults, health care and legal processes may demand greater tightness in the definition. For instance, health care professionals will generally seek input from biological family members, rather than from a neighbor or a friend. Even if a friend or neighbor has more contact and a closer relationship with an older adult, professionals will generally seek to involve family members in decision-making, rather than a neighbor, in order to avoid legal issues if family members contest the decisions. As such, sometimes professionals in the community, as well as those in hospital or in long-term care facilities, need to spend significant time navigating through "who is who" in the older adult's family, their connection, and who makes decisions. Older adults, as well as family members, need to be counseled regarding the importance of personal directives or (American) durable power of attorney for health (for health

care decisions often involving end-of-life care), guardianship (for decisions regarding treatment and issues such as placement), and enduring
power of attorney or trusteeship in Canada or durable power of attorney
in the US (for financial decisions).

What if Family Members Are Not Involved?

Occasionally, within our clinical work with older adults, we have come
across older adults where there seems to be no family involvement. In these
situations, there may be family members, such as adult children, but for
various reasons they have chosen not to be involved. Or, the older adults
may be single (never married or divorced) with no children and no other
family members, such as nieces, nephews, or cousins, have presented to
the professionals involved. These situations pose difficulties, in whatever
the setting in which the older adult is currently situated. For instance, a
nurse or occupational therapist who visits an older adult in the home may
be concerned about the safety of the older adult. If the therapist enters the
home of an older woman and finds little food in the refrigerator and cup-
boards, many stairs and scatter rugs, papers and objects scattered across
the floor (fall risk), he may ask if family members are concerned about
safety. If the elderly woman tells him that she has no family, he might
become even more concerned that there are no family members to provide
ongoing support and monitoring. He may wonder if he needs to refer his
older patient for a psychiatric consultation; and he may struggle, knowing
that if this woman is deemed unsafe and mentally unable to care for herself
at home, she might be removed to live in another setting.

This same older woman may be brought to hospital and placed on
a geriatric or a mental health unit; there she will be assessed for mental
competency (capacity),[1] and her ability to care for herself within her own
home (independently). All staff—psychiatry, nursing, social work, occupational therapy, and recreational therapy—will conduct assessments to
ascertain the soundness of this woman's cognition, her ability to plan a
meal, buy the groceries, and cook for herself. They will determine if she is
able to take care of personal hygiene, dress, and complete other functions
related to independent living (Lane, 2007). If they decide that their older
patient is unable to care for herself independently, they may need to look
at placement. However, there is a problem. If this woman truly has no

---

1. When assessing for cognitive functioning, in medical settings, the term is *capacity*
(i.e., an individual has or does not have capacity). In legal terms, cognitive functioning is
termed *mental competence* (or incompetence).

family members, the social worker may need to contact the Office of the Public Guardian in order to have a guardianship order put in place (Office of the Public Guardian, 2015). However, if there are family members, but they are unwilling or reluctant to become involved, the situation becomes stickier. The Office of the Public Guardian may be reluctant to secure the guardianship order if there are family members who are deemed fit to assume guardianship of this older woman. This means that this woman may spend longer on the hospital unit than she would like, as the professionals on the unit address issues with the Office of the Public Guardian.

What if the Older Adult Has Different Views of What Should Happen in the Transition?

It is not uncommon that an older adult disagrees with family members regarding what should happen in his care. He may think that despite his health problems, he can manage well enough in his home or apartment. He may remain within his home, but when a health crisis hits, he will often be brought to hospital by family members or ambulance. Once in hospital, health care professionals will work to stabilize his health and then may wonder if he is fit to return home. They may begin some mental status assessments, as well as physiotherapist and occupational therapist assessments, to determine his abilities to function alone within his home. When consulting family members, professionals may find that adult children are worried about the safety of their father and that they would like to see him move to an assisted living facility or be placed in a long-term care facility. When talking with the older patient, he may be adamant about his desire to remain in his home and his ability to manage.

The work of health and human service professionals involves careful and sensitive assessment of this older man's abilities to manage independently. The assessment of the occupational therapist, in terms of this man's ability to plan meals, shop for groceries, cook food, manage money, and call 911 in a crisis, becomes front and central in the decision-making of the health care team (Lane, 2007). While they cannot force a move to an assisted living or long-term care facility (unless the man is deemed to not have capacity, at which point a family member becomes the legal guardian and decides that her father needs placement) the health care team can make recommendations.[2]

---

2. We encourage professionals to access The Office of the Public Guardian in their province or state for information specific to their geographical region.

When making recommendations, it is very important that the older patient, not just family members, is present to hear the deliberations of the interprofessional team. If the health care team believes that their older patient still has capacity to make decisions and is still able to cope independently, they can help the older man and family with suggestions regarding additional supports in the home to enhance his safety and living. These suggestions can include mechanical devices such as a raised toilet seat, a railing by the toilet, and a bath stool for the shower. They can also suggest a homemaker for cleaning and a personal aide to assist with showering (depending upon the coverage of the province or state, or the personal finances of this man or family members). If the health care team agrees with family members that the older man lacks capacity or is not able to function independently within the home, the general axiom of placement (as discussed in Chapter 4) is to suggest the *least restrictive environment* for the patient (Lane, 2007). Hence, in this situation, the team might recommend an assisted living facility with additional supports if they determine that this man is still cognitively intact, but just needing additional reinforcements.

What if There Are No Family Members Available, and Both Members of the Couple Are Experiencing Cognitive Impairment?

It is not that uncommon to have both members in a couple experiencing some degree of dementia, particularly if they are both well into their 80s (Alzheimer's Association, 2014). It is, however, uncommon to have both members of a couple experiencing dementia in their early to mid 70s, where there are no children and no nearby relatives to be involved. In such a situation, health care professionals may need to take additional steps.

I (AML) remember one situation where both the husband and wife suffered from a dementia. Their caring doctor recognized that each member of this couple was experiencing significant memory loss. Out of concern regarding their living situation, she visited their home to find that the house was a mess, the couple had many dogs and cats, and the couple ate poorly, preferring to feed their animals their supply of vitamins and food. This physician contacted our unit psychiatrist to arrange a day where the couple could be admitted to our unit. She herself personally arranged for the husband and wife to be brought to the hospital and admitted to our unit. By making all the arrangements, she circumvented the normal multi-stepped process of being admitted to hospital. Once in hospital, the professionals in the health care team began their assessments, according to their disciplinary focus. This couple was situated together in the hospital room, prior to the practice of men and women sharing hospital rooms. The couple pushed their beds together to make a double bed, rather than two single beds. They could be seen walking the unit together, hand in hand, with the husband carrying his briefcase. They were obviously very attached to each other, both physically and emotionally. Every now and then, the husband might say to me, "Excuse me, we've had a very nice stay in this hotel, but can we pay our bill and leave now?"

This couple was eventually placed in an assisted living facility that had a locked unit for those with dementia. They were able to share a room together on this unit. They also had a paid companion who took them out on day trips. I remember one day running on a lovely pathway along the side of a large body of water within the city. There were benches strategically placed at various points on the path, so that individuals could enjoy the scenery, including the lovely blue water, the deciduous and coniferous trees and grass. The couple sat on the bench, gazing at the blue water in the distance, enjoying the gentle, soft wind blowing in their faces, looking truly contented. Knowing that they would not recognize me, I stopped anyways to chat about the weather and the lovely view. The couple happily agreed about the beauty and the weather. As I took my leave from them and commenced jogging again, I felt extremely glad that they appeared happy and at peace, and that they remained together. This situation was one in which the husband and wife, while having no children, had a caring physician who took additional steps, probably outside her scope of responsibility. The couple also had significant monetary resources that could ensure their placement in a nice facility, as well as pay for extras, such as a companion to take them out on day trips. Unfortunately, not all situations where there are few or no family members resolve so well.

In situations where both members of the couple are experiencing cognitive impairment, and there appears to be no available family members to directly intervene, a member of a mental health team, a family doctor, or a psychiatrist may need to get involved. The couple may have to be brought to hospital under the provincial mental health act (or state act, depending upon the country) to be assessed. If at all possible, it is important to keep the couple together, both in hospital and in placement in the upcoming facility. This fosters the "couple functioning" (Wright & Leahey, 2013, p. 109), despite the cognitive impairment. While it is true that sometimes one member of the spousal couple wants to be placed on a different unit in the long-term care facility than the spouse, usually spouses that have

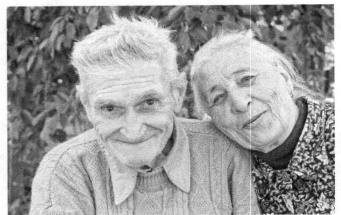

Dundanim/Shutterstock, Inc.

been together for decades prefer to remain together. This may necessitate a longer wait within hospital. During the wait in hospital, the unit social worker can continue the search for some family members, be they nephews or nieces or cousins.

When Grandchildren Are Caregiving

It is not unusual today to hear of grandparents raising grandchildren due to parents being unable to give care. The parents may have severe mental illness, be incarcerated, frequently be in other parts of the world, have HIV/AIDS, or have passed away from AIDS. It is far less common to hear of grandchildren providing care for their grandparents. However, there is a growing cohort of grandchildren between the ages of 18 to 30 who are providing significant care for aging grandparents, about which we know little[3] (Blanton, 2013; Fruhauf & Orel, 2008; Ihara, Horio, & Tompkins, 2012; Levine et al., 2005). Within the literature, questions are raised about the impact of providing care to grandparents at this developmentally crucial time. During these years, individuals go to college or university to study, work on a career, marry, and have children.

Generally, there is little research on this cohort of individuals. Some research examines grandchildren's role when they are not primary care-

---

3.   While there is also a small body of research on adolescents as caregivers for grandparents, these individuals are caregiving within their family structure and home. Therefore, they are not the primary caregivers, but rather, assist parents in caregiving (Hamill, 2012). As such, this section will not address adolescents who assist in care.

givers; they may be assisting parents, but do not carry the bulk of the load. They may provide instrumental care such as shopping, transportation, and housework (Levine et al., 2005), but are less likely to provide more personal care. The research suggests that when grandchildren are not the primary caregivers, the negative impact is relatively small. Interestingly, the extent and impact of caregiving upon grandchildren appears to be influenced by the prior relationship with the grandparents, as well as intergenerational family dynamics. For instance, Blanton (2013) found that the care provided by grandchildren was determined by the previous relationship; for instance, where relationships with grandparents were more difficult, the care was more peripheral. However, when relationships were close over the years, grandchildren were more extensively involved and were more likely to speak about the positives of caregiving. That being said, grandchildren mentioned that they felt caught between parents and the grandparents, or between parents and other family members. And, if there was intergenerational tension, grandchildren caregivers reported feeling burden, stress, and conflict (Blanton, 2013).

An interesting subset within this category is the group of English-speaking young adults who become essentially responsible for their relatively recently immigrated extended families. In such situations, these grandchildren may provide vital service to their non-English speaking grandparents in their dying. While the adult children are present, language barriers make the necessary conversations between health care staff and the patient very difficult; hospitals and hospices may frequently access these English-speaking grandchildren for assistance in communication. The role these grandchildren fulfill is more than simply translation, however. It can also be bridging two traditions: North American mores (in which they are immersed) and the traditions of their grandparents/parents. These grandchildren may find themselves caught between cultural norms and unwittingly in a double bind. Not uncommon in palliative care settings with recently immigrated Asian families is the reluctance to speak to the terminally ill family member about her impending death. Family may state to the terminally ill individual that she is coming to a very nice hospital to get better. While this is a cultural practice, it does not fit in with the North American practice of being open with a dying person about her looming death. Palliative care staff can feel a conflict in not being able to speak of the dying person's impending death; grandchildren, accustomed to North American norms, may also feel conflicted about keeping this information about their grandparent's health a secret.

In one situation, a grandfather's impending death was not revealed to the patient himself or to members outside of the immediate family. In the elderly gentleman's dying, the family used computer technology to connect relatives in Asia to what was happening in the hospital room, so that they would understand that their relative was truly dying. The adult grandchildren felt truly conflicted and may well have violated their parents' wishes; but they felt they had to let extended family know of the situation before Grandfather passed.

Health and human service professionals assessing and intervening with families where grandchildren are caregivers need to assess how much care grandchildren are providing for the older adult and the impact of caregiving upon their lives in terms of their ability to work, date, and lead normal lives, as well as upon their emotional/mental health. Professionals need to ask grandchildren caregivers what kinds of support they need in providing care: Are there formal supports that can be accessed to relieve them of some of their duties? Are there supports, such as counseling or support groups that might provide a venue for venting the stress of caregiving, for receiving emotional support, as well as helpful caregiving information? Further, are there family members that could be involved to lessen the load? Grandchildren caregivers should be reassured that committed caregivers *do* access formalized supports and share the work load (Piercy, 2007). This may be particularly significant for those from other cultures (Benner Carson & Koenig, 2004); in these situations, accessing professional help can sometimes be seen as a disgrace or a failure. Professionals should also commend them for their resilience and acknowledge that their role gives a sense of purpose and meaning to their lives (Piercy, 2007). With the growing numbers of grandparents who are raising young grandchildren, there may be many more grandchildren as primary or secondary caregivers of older adults in the future (Levine et al., 2005).

The Dynamic Exerted by Family Members Not Present

Unbeknownst to health and human service professionals, family members who do not present to the interprofessional team may be exerting a powerful influence upon family members. These family members may be distant geographically or may simply choose not to present themselves to the team on the unit or in the long-term care facility. In such situations, these absent family members may be influencing the decision-making of the present family members around decisions such as trusteeship, placement, and health care. These unseen alliances are one reason why it is important for health and human service professionals to complete a genogram (picture of a family tree) (Wright & Leahey, 2013) to understand who is a part of the family system. Also, it is important to meet with the family members together in a scheduled family meeting. The professional can question the family members present about siblings or other members of the family who are not in attendance but are part of the caregiving and decision-making on behalf of the older adult.

Also, the genogram provides the opportunity for the professional to assess who is in the family, but no longer physically present due to death. Sometimes, a family member may not be present bodily, because he or she is deceased, but the individual is still a powerful presence in the family (McGoldrick, 1991). When completing the genogram, the nurse or professional can ask about the deceased member. When did the individual die? What were the circumstances? How is the family member remembered? If the family member were present today, what would he or she suggest happen with the older adult? The health or human service professional is not only attempting to examine the influence of unseen family members, but also to assess the responses of family members to these questions. Are family members uncomfortable? Do family members appear to be hiding a family secret about the unseen individual? Sometimes those who are not present, particularly due to death, can exert powerful influences in the decisions that are made and how family members relate to each other and talk about the past (McGoldrick, 1991).

Unpleasant memories of the deceased family member, or a negative experience in the death of that individual, can strongly influence the emotions and choices of adult children in the end-of-life decisions for the second parent.[4] The answers to the questions asked and the emotions displayed, as well as how family members react to each other's responses, give the health care team valuable information about what the family, not simply the patient, will need.

Who Really Is the Patient?

Sometimes in working with families, we realize that the "identified patient" is not really the problem. Or perhaps better stated, the identified patient

---

4. Responses to the questions asked by the professional also can elicit positive information. Favorable memories of a deceased parent and meaningful experiences in that parent's death can, for example, reveal to professionals the "tools in the toolbox" for the end-of-life decisions for the second parent. "We've been through this before" gives professionals the reassurance that a family has some preparation for what lies ahead.

is behaving in certain ways that are considered problematic, due in part because of unhealthy family patterns. This is sometimes the case when adolescents present as the family problem. When a therapist works with a family where an adolescent is causing significant problems, sometimes the problem is not simply that of the adolescent, but in actuality, the adolescent is responding to family patterns. Part of the work of the therapist involves deconstructing the reasons behind the adolescent's behavior and connecting it to the family pattern that is troubling, and then working to disrupt this family pattern.

Interestingly, a similar dynamic may sometimes occur in families with older adults. Sometimes older adults are admitted to hospital units for problems related to addictions. The adult children may be sincere in their wish for their parent to be free of addiction; the statement "We just want our mom (or dad) back!" is completely heartfelt. However, the adult children may not realize to what extent particular family patterns depend upon the older adult being addicted to a substance, and therefore not fully functional as an adult/parent. In a drunken state, the older man may capitulate to his adult children's requests for money. While the adult children truly *want* a fully functional father, they also *need* his money. When through professional treatment the older man becomes sober, he may start to develop a sense of self that feels more confident and able to make decisions. When his children ask for more money, he may now say "no," recognizing that the request is unreasonable and that he does not have to give in to gain acceptance. (He now recognizes that his own self-respect and self-acceptance mean much more than the approval of his children.) The children, not anticipating that their financial source would dry up as a result of treatment, may stop visiting their father. The father will then need support to not give in to his children or return to his drinking patterns, out of frustration over the rupture in this relationship. Although the children were genuine in their desire to have a sober father, their continued use of his monies depended upon him being mentally compromised through drinking.

The above scenario is not infrequent in relation to addictions in a family or other family patterns that develop around an illness. In these situations, the older adult may be the identified patient, but in actuality, there may be several individuals who are in need of professional assistance.

Health and human service professionals may also see this type of situation occur with spouses of older adults. Although an older woman is admitted to hospital due to her inability to cope with multiple sclerosis and refusal to manage the activities of daily living (when health care professionals believe, based upon their assessments, that she is capable of completing these tasks), her husband may be unwittingly contributing to these issues. For instance, if the husband is busy and does not offer time or emotional support to his wife unless she is symptomatic, she may become focused upon her pain and disability in order to gain her husband's support and attention. In these circumstances, neither individual is "bad"; however, the wife cannot secure the emotional and physical support she wants when she is self-sufficient, and the husband may be oblivious to the emotional yearnings of his wife. By being overly engaged in his own pursuits when his wife is reasonably stable and by only providing nurturance when his wife is ill, he inadvertently gives the message that sickness is necessary to bring attention and support. In a situation like this, the professional works to disrupt this pattern so that the couple provides nurturance to each other, in both ill and stable health.

The work of health and human service professionals involves recognizing the patterns that are occurring among family members and gently identifying the patterns. In regard to the first example with the alcohol-dependent father and the adult children, the professional can reinforce to the father the importance of not jeopardizing his sobriety due to his children's withdrawal. The strength of this older man is reinforced and hospital staff can question the man about what his ability to stop drinking says about himself; the goal of this question is to help this man begin to develop a sense of self that includes personal strength and resilience. Staff can inquire of this man about other times in his life when he demonstrated strength and resilience. If the individual responds with descriptions of physical feats, such as mountain climbing, running, or sports, professionals can use metaphors in their work with him to reinforce his strength: "Mr. Smith, you are a champion!" Knowing that individuals who struggle with addictions can return to substances when returning home or when under stress, professionals ensure that this man has supports for sobriety when he returns home, such as an addictions counselor and a support group (Alcoholics Anonymous, for example).

What If the Older Adult Who Is Admitted to Hospital Has One or Two Very Aged Parents?

Sometimes an older adult is admitted to hospital because of particular physical or mental health problems, but the driving force behind admission is that the very aged parents can no longer care for the older adult, or, out of fear for when one or both of them dies and their need to ensure that placement of their adult child occurs. This may be because the older adult has been living with the very elderly parents all of her life due to significant mental illness, an intellectual disability, or some kind of physical disability that prohibits independence. I (AML) remember working with one older woman—Agnes—who was admitted to hospital. She was in her late 70s and had been diagnosed with schizophrenia in early adulthood. Agnes had lived with her parents all of her life and by now her parents were of very advanced years. One parent had reached the century mark, and the other was 98 years of age! Agnes was initially admitted due to a newfound "rebellion" toward her parents and the fact that her parents felt they could not handle her. The second reason for admission, however, was related to the need for placement. Agnes' parents were very afraid that they would pass away preventing them from ensuring that she had found a suitable accommodation.

Agnes absolutely loved being on the hospital unit. She developed relationships with other patients and now had a roommate that she could talk with throughout the day. Staff took an interest in her and recognized her strengths, including playing musical instruments. When time came for her to transfer to a nursing home, she screamed, begged, and pleaded. She cried out in a mournful wail that she loved the hospital unit and wanted to stay there forever. I, the psychiatrist, and a nurse tried to console Agnes and tell her that we would love to keep her, but due to the unit being in an acute care hospital, this was not possible. Our hearts and our voices were pained as we truly cared about Agnes and loved seeing her happy on the unit. Sadly, Agnes screamed all the way down the hallway, outside the hospital, and into the transfer vehicle. Initially, we were told that she was not doing well in long-term care. However, some months later we were informed that she was doing well, had adjusted to the transition, and was enjoying her new environment.

Regrettably, many aged parents fail to make caregiving plans for their aging child with a disability (Dillenburger & McKerr, 2011) or mental illness. They may be afraid that staff in an institution will not provide personalized care and also may not want to place the burden of the disabled adult child upon their other children (Gilbert, Lankshear, & Petersen, 2008). It is vital for professionals to encourage very aged parents to make future plans for their aging disabled or mentally ill children. When very aged parents have been caregiving for a child for 50 to 60 years, they may not be aware of housing options besides residential housing. Very aged parents should be aware of the waiting time on placement lists, as well as of the dangers of delaying the placement process until precipitated by a crisis, as an inappropriate option may be the only available option in an emergency (Gilbert et al., 2008).

From the perspective of developmental stages in the family life cycle, it is important to note the impact of caring for an older, intellectually disabled child, or an adult child with any significant disabilities, on a very aged couple. The couple may struggle to have the time or energy to engage in activities together that fosters a sense of "couple functioning" (Wright & Leahey, 2013, p. 109). The very elderly couple may not be able to attend to issues of preparation for their own deaths, for instance, life review, as they are too busy caring for their elderly, disabled child.

Longstanding Issues Between the Parent and Adult Child/Children

In our experience, we have found that it is not uncommon that adult children, who may be approaching their fifth or sixth decade of life, are afraid of one of their aging parents. In fact, some adult children are petrified of an older parent. The fear is not related to a current danger of being in the presence of the parent, as the parent may be frail, cognitively impaired, and quite helpless. The fear stems back to their childhood. Adult children may cry over the significant dilemma they now face; they dearly want to help the older, frail adult who needs assistance, but they have such fear and revulsion within their souls due to extensive abuse in childhood. While cognitively they recognize that the older individual is no longer the abusive individual that he or she once was, the scars are opened, the pain and horror reawakened, through contact with the parent. The predicament is this: Morally, they cannot turn their backs on the frail parent who needs help, but psychologically, spiritually, and physically, they tremble at the thought of being involved.

The work of the professional involves several aspects. First, the professional validates the fear and, sometimes, sheer terror that the adult children may be experiencing. This is important as adult children may be surprised by their overwhelming emotions; they might honestly say to the health or human service professional, "But I thought I had dealt with the abuse! Why am I feeling so terrified now?"

Second, the professional helps the adult children decide what they can and cannot do for the older parent. Perhaps the adult children can supply cigarettes and clothes for the parent but cannot come on the unit and visit the parent. This is perfectly acceptable. Or maybe they can be involved in monitoring finances through trusteeship, but cannot see the parent or can only do so sporadically. Again, this is very appropriate and the adult children should be commended for this. If the adult child does not feel that he can be involved due to painful experiences in the past, he should not be guilted or goaded into helping. If however, he wants in some way to be involved, there may be long-term benefit. For some adult children, involvement in helping an aging parent can have a healing effect. By responding in kindness toward the parent who frightened them, they finally achieve some measure of peace and closure regarding painful childhood events.

To illustrate, in one case a retired woman was afraid to visit her mother in a palliative setting due to a lifetime of emotional abuse; for this adult daughter, it was a "double bind." Ethically, she felt she could not live with herself unless she saw her mother in her dying. On the other hand, it caused profound fear. On her mother's last day, this gentle lady stood, shaking and supported by the chaplain, at the end of her mother's bed, to say "Goodbye, Mom" and "I love you." In this, she confronted her fear of seeing her mother, satisfied her deep moral and spiritual need to acknowledge her mother, and (in this situation) heard the words back from her mother, "I love you, too."

Disagreements About the Course of Action for an Aging Parent

Even when families are emotionally close and live in relative harmony, disagreements can occur regarding the course of action that should take place for an aging parent. While aging parents may be able to manage better as a pair, both in day-to-day functioning and decision-making, when one parent is placed in a facility or dies, adult children may step in to assist the one remaining parent now living alone in the community. Dissension between adult children can abound for several reasons.

First, adult siblings within the same family may hold very different views regarding how long a parent should be maintained within her home, when that parent, for a variety reasons, should be moved to an assisted living or long-term care facility. Family members, just like health care professionals, may hold varied views about the importance of maintaining autonomy by supporting the aged parent to remain in the home, or the preeminence of protecting the parent at all costs (and thus removing them from potential danger that comes with living alone). Disagreements may proliferate with end-of-life treatment decisions, as well.

Second, adult siblings who live in close proximity to the aging parent may feel that they should have more "say" in what happens with the parent than siblings who live far away. Their rationale is that because they see their parent regularly, they better understand the parent's challenges and deficits. Also, as they physically do much more for the parent, in comparison to siblings who live far away, they should have greater decision-making power.

Third, disputes regarding an appropriate course of action for the remaining parent may soon move beyond the actual disagreement and tap into power struggles of the past. Siblings who argued as children may now unwittingly enter into the dynamic in which they engaged as children. They may be certain that they are arguing for the betterment of their parent, but can actually be re-enacting power struggles of the past. Why does this happen? When individuals and families are under great stress, they often revert to previous methods of coping and interaction, even when these coping methods and patterns of interaction were unhealthy. Unknowingly, siblings can return to past methods of relating and working out arguments.

The work of health and human service professionals involves helping adult children recognize that varying opinions on what should happen with the aging parent are usually based upon care and concern; thus the adult who argues for keeping the parent at home loves his aging father no less than his sister who argues for a move into an assisted living facility. It also involves looking at how family members make decisions among themselves, who the decision-makers usually are and how they have come to resolution in the past. Further, the work of professionals involves educating family members regarding the process of placement and navigating the system. Adult children may not be aware of how long it can take to bring about placement. Once they become aware of the length of the process, as well as the steps involved, they may be able to come to a consensus. Even if family members (with input from the older adult) agree that placement in a long-term care facility is not currently necessary, this topic has been raised for discussion and the family may have a better sense of when the time will be appropriate for them.

The Influence of Grief and Guilt Upon Family Members' Decisions

Decision-making on behalf of older adults can be a perilous venture. Family members may wrestle with significant grief and guilt in the decision to place the older adult (Bern-Klug, 2008; Davis, Tremont, Bishop,

& Fortinsky, 2011; Reuss, Dupuis, & Whitfield, 2005). The emotional tur-moil family members undergo may be even greater when they feel that they had to make the decision on their own, with little support from professionals (Davies & Nolan, 2003). In our clinical experiences, family members weep over the placement process and they struggle as they make the decision to place, during the placement process, and sometimes after placement occurs.[5] Often the placement decision is delayed due to guilt and grief around placement.

Despite the magnitude of emotional turmoil that family members experience, professionals may not recognize or acknowledge the grief and guilt involved in placement (Davies, 2005). As part of a larger ethno-graphic study, Bern-Klug (2008) interviewed 44 family caregivers of older adults admitted to nursing homes in a large Midwestern American city. She found that while family members admitted to experiencing some relief with the placement of their loved one, some caregivers experienced exten-sive guilt that did not wane over time. Bern-Klug (2008) recommended that nursing home staff need to consider that each nursing home admis-sion represents a crisis to family members and that services, such as sup-port and education, need to be offered to families. If family members do not receive emotional support during the transitional period, they may feel overwhelmed and resentful (Reuss et al., 2005), thus increasing the challenges faced by nursing home staff.

For professionals working with family members, it is important to recognize that family members may have been experiencing some mea-sure of grief *for years* in relation to the older adult. This is particularly the case when the older adult is suffering from a dementia. The spouse or the parent they once knew is no longer present and they suffer as they view their spouse/parent suffering. The compounding nature of grief— watching loss after loss after loss in the older adult—with the current grief-evoking event of placement added on top, can seem overwhelming. Family members may struggle with whether they can even place the older adult, as the grief is too suffocating and they feel unable to make decisions any longer. Professionals who come alongside family members, who ver-bally recognize the grief experienced by family members, who listen to the confused thought processes of family members and help them sort out their thoughts and decision-making rationale, and who gently offer coun-sel and understanding, are invaluable.

---

5. Sometimes the weeping continues after that parent's death and can impact the decision-making for other older adult family members in the future.

Family Members May Be Exhausted

As mentioned earlier in this book, by the time adult children are examining housing and/or treatment options (e.g., palliative care) for an older parent, some or all of the children may be physically and/or emotionally exhausted. Particularly when one or both parents have/had suffered from a dementia, caregiving may have occurred for many years prior. Decades ago, Mace and Rabins wrote a book entitled *The 36 Hour Day* (1981). This was a guide for family caregivers who were providing care for an older adult with Alzheimer's disease or a related dementia. The authors outlined the various symptoms and behaviors that could be exhibited by someone with a dementia and provided practical tips for dealing with these behaviors. The notion of the "36-hour day" was an acknowledgment that caregiving occurs day and night and simply never stops, except upon the death of the older adult. As just mentioned, caregiving for a parent with dementia can be especially draining, and not only because the individual needs continuous physical assistance: The exhaustion is also emotional, as the experience is punctuated by losses, including the loss of the person the adult children once knew. Family members may be totally exhausted, yet unable to recognize the degree to which they are depleted. For their own health, they may need to access more assistance for the aging parent, yet be unable to see this, or make the decision to access more care.

Part of the role of the health or human service professional is to help the adult child (or spouse) recognize how exhausted she is, as well as understand the need for additional help to share the load of caregiving. Sometimes an adult child feels that if she places her older parent in a long-term care facility, she is reneging on her duties as a daughter and that her caregiving will end. The professional should help this woman realize that caregiving does not end just because her mother will be placed. While the relationship may change, in terms of the mother living in a facility, the caregiving continues. One of the tips we often offer to family members is that if they are going to continue to care for their aging spouse or parent, they need to care for themselves so that they will be alive and healthy to continue caring. This takes the issue of caring for the self out of the realm of selfishness (some caregivers believe that to access professional help means that they are selfish) and moves it into a caring act. By caring for themselves, adult children can continue to provide emotional and relational support to the parent.

If the older adult is relocated to an assisted living or long-term care facility, the work of health and human service professionals is to help the older adult and spouse/adult children redefine the spousal or parent/adult child relationship, in a way that still honors the older adult. One of the developmental tasks of the aging family involves "making room in the system for the wisdom and experience of the seniors" (Wright & Leahey, 2013, p. 109). This means that even if the older adult relocates to a nursing home, he still needs to feel like he is valued and that his experience is acknowledged and honored. The aging individual and his spouse or adult children can be helped to talk about how they would like their relationship to look, despite the move; this involves talking about how family members will connect, in what ways (e.g., visits, phone calls, email) and how they will continue to foster emotional bonds.

When the Older Adult Is Exhibiting Aggressive Behavior

Spouses and family members are often bewildered, devastated, and mortified when their older adult behaves aggressively toward them, health care professionals, or other patients. They express deep humiliation regarding the behaviors and are sometimes desperate to explain that the aggression is not representative of who the older adult actually is as a person. They can also experience panic when home care, hospital, or nursing home staff is unable to manage their family member's aggression. "This is not my dad!" the distressed daughter may exclaim.

   In these situations, family members require the patient understanding of health and human service professionals. Family members need to feel that the professionals involved in the care of their older adult recognize that this behavior is not indicative of the older adult, but may be caused by a dementia, delirium, or perhaps delusions (Krishnamoorthy & Anderson, 2011). Or the aggressive behavior may be in response to some unexpressed need that the older adult is not able to communicate (Keady & Jones, 2010). The work of professionals to *separate the aggressive behavior from the older adult* is key, as family members usually strongly identify with the older adult and feel that the behavior of their family member is a reflection on them. Regardless of the setting, family members need reassurance from professionals that they understand the impetus behind the aggressive behavior of the older adult and that they will assess the older adult for the triggers to this behavior. This demonstrates to family members that professionals view the older adult with respect and that they do not view the current behavior as a representation of the individual's entire life. If the older adult with aggressive behavior is still living within his home environment, it is imperative the professionals assess the safety of those living at home. If the spouse of the older aggressive adult is still living with her husband, this may necessitate a 911 call with police taking the aggressive individual to hospital for assessment. The protection of the spousal care-giver, who may be frail herself, is of paramount concern.

If the older individual is already in hospital, professionals can inform family members that they will conduct a thorough assessment of their hospitalized family member, will try a variety of non-pharmacological treatments, such as decreasing environmental stimuli (King, 2012), music (Kyomen & Whitfield, 2008), walking (King, 2012), and animal-assisted activities (Kyomen & Whitfield, 2008). If non-pharmacological approaches are not effective, medication, such as an antipsychotic, can be considered and used to decrease aggressive behaviors (Krishnamoorthy & Anderson, 2011). When professionals can verbalize a comprehensive understanding of aggressive behavior in older adults to family members, as well as knowl-edge regarding treatment options, some of the distress in family members may be assuaged.

Family members sometimes are concerned at the impact their loved one's behavior may have on the staff. It can also be helpful for profession-als to verbalize to family members that such behaviors are not taken per-sonally by them and that in situations such as these (dementia, delirium, etc.), these behaviors can occur. This can relieve family members of the sense that they need to care for staff, or "make up for" the older adult's behavior toward professional caregivers.

The following case example will demonstrate some of the concepts discussed within this chapter. We will also thread information from the case example into the subsequent section on Principles in Assessment and Intervention with Families.

Case Example

Janie is a 55-year-old woman with Down syndrome and early stage dementia.

Until just recently, she has lived with her mother and father. Her mother and father provided all of her care, with occasional help from Janie's sister and brother. Over the past number of years, Janie's parents had talked about the eventuality of one of them passing away. They worried about who would provide care for their daughter; in the earlier years of Janie's life, they could not imagine her outliving them. Ironically, the extended life span of those with Down syndrome was a mixed blessing; they loved having their daughter for a good number of years, but they worried intensely about what would happen to her when they were gone.

Within the past year, Janie's mother (Sarah) passed away. Her father, Bob, is 85 years old and has significant COPD (chronic obstructive pulmonary disease). Since Sarah's passing, Bob has worried that one morning he would not wake up, and Janie would find her father dead. Bob had spoken with both of his children regarding his worries. Janie's sister offered to provide some care for her sister, but admitted that she could not look after Janie during the day, as her work income is necessary for her and her husband to make ends meet. Janie's brother expressed reluctance to assume care for his sister, as he lives in another city and was concerned what he would do if caring for Janie proved too difficult.

Bob wondered what he should do. He was reluctant to burden his two children, figuring that their childhood was somewhat compromised by the extra care Janie needed. He was unsure whether to place Janie in a residential home or a long-term care facility: staff in residential homes might not know how to manage the challenges of dementia, but staff in long-term care might not know how to meaningfully connect with an individual with intellectual disabilities. Despite his questions regarding what placement direction he should initiate, Bob did not explore options, and his window of opportunity to make the decision himself closed.

Six months after his wife's death, Bob had a health scare and was hospitalized for almost three weeks. Janie was immediately placed in a nearby long-term care facility that had an open bed. Although Bob was discharged home with some home care support and his physical health has improved, he has been grief-stricken. He feels like he has lost his wife and his daughter, as Janie continues to reside in long-term care. At times, he cries when he visits his daughter. Although Janie is still alive, she is having trouble adjusting.

She is withdrawn and only occasionally initiates conversation; when she does communicate, she tends to abruptly and loudly call out to residents that are passing by. The residents are not comfortable with Janie; she has the characteristic facial differences that come with Down syndrome, is much younger than they are, and is ungainly in how she walks and talks.

Bob has continued to hope that circumstances will somehow work out. In the meantime, he has watched his daughter change from a previously affectionate and happy woman to a sullen and withdrawn individual.

The nursing unit manager, recreational therapist, and social worker are not sure how to help Janie. They do not know how to make sense of her behaviors. Is she grieving the death of her mother and the move to the nursing home? Is this sullen behavior just part of her Down syndrome, or is this part of her dementia?

They have decided to seek the assessment of a consulting psychiatrist. In the meantime, staff are trying very hard to reach out to Janie, and her father visits daily trying to help her adjust.

Principles in Assessment and Intervention With Families

Throughout this chapter, we have attempted to describe particular challenges that family members may encounter when faced with an older adult who is experiencing transitions related to health, and thus may be forced to examine transitions related to health, living location, or death. We offered suggestions that can guide health and human service professionals when facilitating transitions for older adults and family members. These suggestions were specific to the examples given. Now, we will suggest some general principles that can guide professionals in helping family members through transitions faced by their older adults. Throughout our discussion of principles, we will weave in our case study of Janie and her father, where applicable.

Family Systems Approach and Life Course Perspective

We agree with Wright and Leahey (2013) and Carter and McGoldrick (1989, 2005) regarding the importance of understanding individuals within the context of the family system. And as we mentioned earlier in this chapter, this tenet is particularly important with older adults because they may be quite physically and/or cognitively compromised and so most often have family involvement.

So what does a family-systems approach entail? It involves conceptualizing the older adult as part of a family system in which individuals have patterns of relating and various ways of communicating. It entails more than finding out who is in the family; it also involves examining how they support each other, instrumentally (tasks of daily living) and emotionally.

In regard to the case example, a family-systems approach includes understanding those who are in this family. Now that Janie is in long-term care, her physical needs are being largely met. However, who has she had for emotional support? Do her sister and brother provide some support? For Bob, what kinds of instrumental and emotional supports does he need? Does he need home care support? Should an occupational therapist come into his home to assess his home for safety and convenience aids? Does he have neighbors or friends who check on him on a regular basis to offer emotional support, as well as rides to appointments or to the long-term care facility?

However, a family-systems approach goes beyond merely considering the needs of single individuals within a family. It also involves looking at patterns of relationships within families (Wright & Leahey, 2013). Thus, staff within the nursing home can look at how Bob and Janie can continue their relationship as father and daughter. Staff might ask Bob and Janie about what they most enjoy in their relationship and seek to replicate, to some degree, what they enjoy together. For instance, they can consider how to support Bob and Janie in having some "private" family dinners. For instance, Bob and his other daughter (who lives in the community) may bring takeout food into the facility and have a family dinner with Janie in a room away from the busyness of the unit. Nursing staff may support these dinners by bringing coffee and tea. If Bob and Janie enjoy going out to a concert or a play, staff can make sure that Janie is ready for Bob when he comes. Besides the physical tasks of helping Janie get ready, however, they can verbally support the specialness of the event. During the day of the concert, staff can talk to Janie about her excitement about the evening's plans and her special relationship with her father. When she returns from the concert, staff can ask questions about her experience with her father at the event.

We also strongly espouse a Life Course Perspective approach. How an older adult responds to crucial transitions is not only impacted by their family context, but also by previous experiences with transitions. A history of successful or unsuccessful responses to transitions will affect how an older adult thinks about, and responds to, current transitions. As part of an individual's life history, previous experiences with health and human service professionals will also impact how this older adult seeks help in times of transition and his responses to professionals who are attempting to assist with them.

In relation to the case example of Janie, she needs to be understood within the context of her family and her life history. Due to her Down syndrome, Janie has lived with her parents almost all of her 55 years of life. As such, she has not experienced many of the transitions faced by her non-intellectually disabled counterparts. She did not leave home, go to college, get married, or have children. As she also has not previously transitioned to another location, such as a residential home, the transition to the long-term care facility is very difficult for her. She has never developed coping skills to help her manage transitions. Coupled with the lack of experience with transitions, she also has recently experienced the death of her mother and the hospitalization of her father. When her father was hospitalized and Janie was placed in long-term care, she experienced much confusion and grief. She could not understand why her father was not visiting her.

It is also important to conceptualize Bob's experiences with transitions from the Life Course Perspective. Has Bob had previous experiences with transitions that were particularly negative? For instance, if, decades earlier, his mother entered a facility and did not do well, he might be particularly frightened about this transition for Janie. Further, if he and his siblings did not help his father when his mother was placed in the facility (and subsequently passed away quickly), he may fear that his son and daughter may pay little attention to him now that his wife is gone and their sister is placed.

View families from a strengths-based perspective

As health care systems within developed countries tend to be focused upon health problems (Gottlieb, 2013) rather than strengths, it is easy for professionals working within the system to unwittingly adopt a deficit-based perspective and approach. What is a strengths-based approach? A strengths-based approach:

considers the whole person, focuses on what is working and functioning well, what the person does best, and what resources people have available to help them deal more effectively with their life, health, and health care challenges. (Gottlieb, 2013)

When working with older adults and their family members, professionals need to consciously hold onto a strengths-based approach, especially as sometimes transitions in these families are due to such extenuating and difficult situations (e.g., older husband dies; elderly wife has cognitive impairment and significant heart disease; wife is still living in the home; wife does not recognize children). This is respectful toward and empowering for the family; it enables them to recognize their resilience in what may have been years of challenging caregiving, and it also encourages them to continue to support the older adult, whether the older adult: continues to live independently within his home; moves to an assisted living facility or is placed in long-term care; or is expected to die soon and is now receiving palliative care.

It is also empowering for professionals to utilize a strengths-oriented approach. By adopting this approach, professionals are less likely to feel defeated by the degree of challenges faced by older adults and their family members, and they can remain open and curious about how best to intervene (Wright & Leahey, 2013). In embracing an open and interested stance, creativity in professionals is fostered and they are less likely to feel frustrated and angry about their work with families.

Embracing a strengths-based approach involves more than just believing families have strengths. It also involves verbally acknowledging those strengths to families so that they are aware that the professional sees them as having strengths. Health and human service professionals can ask family members how they managed to make it through previously difficult transitions. Specifically, what have been their strengths? They can then ask the family members how they can use particular strengths to make it through the current transition. By inviting them to talk about previous experiences with transitions and how those encounters can help them in the present, family members may make a mental shift. They may begin to conceptualize themselves as strong and able to face the difficulties ahead.

It may be very difficult for health and human service professionals to conceptualize those with intellectual disabilities or dementia from a strengths-oriented perspective. However, we suggest that the *greater the deficits*, the more important it is to work from the premise that individuals and families have strengths. This approach is much more than naïve idealism; it is based upon the history of the family. For example, Janie's parents have raised and supported her for 55 years. They also raised two other children. Despite the work involved to support Janie over 55 years, monitor the health conditions that are prevalent among those with Down syndrome, and help Janie with some of the challenging behaviors and mental health problems that can occur with intellectual disabilities (although these problems tend to be less with those with Down syndrome than with other intellectual disabilities) (Spendelow, 2011), Bob and Sarah prevailed. Janie, herself, was a happy individual for much of her life; her demeanor only changed when her mother passed away and she moved into the facility.

Professionals who conceptualize Bob and Janie as having strengths will seek to assess and intervene in a way that promotes these strengths. While health and human service professionals can utilize tools for assessment and intervention, unfortunately, most tools are deficit-based, rather than strengths-based. Further, most strengths-based assessment tools are designed for children (Hirst, Lane, & Stares, 2013).

However, the lack of strengths-based assessment tools does not preclude professionals from conducting a thorough assessment; based upon the assessment, they can then tailor interventions that are appropriate for the family. Professionals can ask Bob how he has managed other challenges in the past and assist him to use these positive coping methods currently. (When under stress, many individuals forego their usual methods of coping, such as reading, exercise, visiting with friends.) They may also ask Bob about how Janie copes; specifically, what can staff in the facility do to help her feel more comfortable, perhaps express her grief, and engage her in activities that are meaningful to her? They can ask Bob what activities Janie has enjoyed in the past and try to engage her in these (Brown, Dodd, & Vetere, 2010). They may also inquire if Janie has worked in the past and what this work entailed. If there are elements of a previous job that can be built into her new environment (for example, helping sweep the floor in the facility dining room), this may build self-esteem.

In an interesting Australian study, Buys, Aird, and Miller (2012) interviewed professionals who work with older adults with intellectual disabilities to ascertain their perceptions of how these intellectually disabled individuals age, and more specifically, what active aging would look like for one of their clients. They found that professionals described their clients as eager to be active and desiring to learn new things. They emphasized the importance of engaging older adults with intellectual disabilities in meaningful activities—specifically, activities that are important and valuable to individual clients. Professionals described a wide variety of possible activities, such as volunteer work, reading, arts and crafts, caring for pets, social outings, and others. The professionals stressed the importance of variety and flexibility in activities, as well as the need for productivity to continue in older age (Buys et al., 2012).

Recognize the Importance of Culture in How Families Relate

Health and human service professionals certainly cannot be knowledgeable about all or even many cultures, as not only are there many cultures within our world, there are even variations in how individuals from the same ethnic background practice culture within one country. However, within the twenty-first century, where multiculturalism is prevalent in many developed countries, it behooves professionals to recognize that culture does influence how individuals age, how the family is defined (Hines, Preto, McGoldrick, Almeida, & Weltman, 2005), how families communicate with each other and their older members, and how families view aspects of care for their elders, such as hospitalization, use of long-term care facilities, as well as accessing hospice. Further, families may vary in how much they express their cultural beliefs; for some, their cultural beliefs may not be held onto as tightly as others, as they may have adopted some beliefs within the dominant culture (Hines et al., 2005).

As part of working with families of varied cultures, health and human service professionals should assess how cultural beliefs impact family beliefs, in particular in how family members relate to each other and their aging members. Beliefs about moving older adults out of a family home into institutions of care should also be assessed. As noted in the example in Chapter 3, some cultures do not readily accept individuals placing parents into facilities (like the adult daughter in her 60s caring for her aging mother in her mid 90s). This may involve some time on the part of the professional to assess the rationale for such decision-making, for describing their professional concerns for the parent, as well as for the adult caregiver, and to look for options that might be palatable for both the adult child, as well as for them (in terms of the professional's concern about the safety and health of both the adult child and the parent). While sometimes the older adult and adult caregiver may make choices that are not in line with what the professional would choose, the health or human service professional needs to respect the self-determination of the individuals involved.

Attention to How Professionals Communicate

We do not mean to be condescending when we stress that professionals, as well as future professionals, need to attend to how they communicate. First, the importance of the *ministry of presence* (as discussed in Chapter 5) cannot be overstated. Empathy, humility, and a commitment to the family being worked with are absolutely essential.

Professionals may be excellent in *what* they communicate (content), but not necessarily attentive to *how* they communicate (nonverbal and paraverbal communication). And, the importance of attending to how one communicates cannot be exaggerated. While there is some variation regarding how much of our message is communicated verbally in comparison to nonverbally, generally, there is agreement that a significant amount of what we communicate is transmitted nonverbally or paraverbally.[6] When older adults and their family members are undergoing transition, they are often stressed and can even be feeling like they are in shock. This is particularly the case when family members are told that their parent is dying and may be moved to hospital or palliative care. They may need the information to be given a number of times, for that information to be given patiently, and to be given with sensitivity and kindness. Not only do professionals need to speak slowly and with patience, but they need to attend to the tone of their voices.

These principles about communication especially apply to older adults. Older adults are acutely sensitive to the mood and tone of voice of professionals. When professionals appear too rushed and frustrated to listen to older patients or clients, older individuals may shut down emotionally and verbally. They may stop talking out of embarrassment and a sense of not

---

6.   We use the term *paraverbal* due to our familiarity with the Crisis Prevention Institute. They define *paraverbal* as being how we say what we say. Hence, paraverbal can refer to the tone of our voice. For more information, please see the Crisis Prevention Institute (www.crisisprevention.com).

being understood (Wengryn & Hester, 2011). Professionals who work well with older adults will sit down at the same level as the older adult, maintain eye contact with the aging individual, and speak with kindness and sensitivity. They will also ask the older patient if he understands and has any questions. They will pay careful attention to factors that may hamper the understanding of an older adult, such as hearing and sight deficits, or not understanding English.

In our case example, both Janie and Bob are the "older adults." While Janie does not typically fit the older age category, she is considered to be of older age due to her Down syndrome, as individuals with Down syndrome exhibit signs of aging that non-intellectually disabled adults do not experience for another 20 or more years (Strax, Luciano, Dunn, & Quevedo, 2010). Both Bob and Janie have been experiencing shock from Bob's sudden transition to the hospital, as well as Janie's placement in the long-term care facility. They are now adjusting to living life apart after 55 years together. While literature suggests that staff in nursing homes do not always attend to the emotional challenges, including grief reactions, to the placement of family members (Givens, Prigerson, Kiely, Shaffer, & Mitchell, 2011; Perry, Dalton, & Edwards, 2010), Bob's adjustment to his daughter's move will be aided by staff who ask about how he is doing, listen to his concerns, and reassure him about the normalcy of what he is experiencing. Similarly, if staff pay extra attention to Janie and understand that she will have difficulty understanding what is happening to her (due to the Down syndrome and dementia), it may help her in beginning to adjust to the new environment.

Not only is it important what staff communicate to Janie, it is of paramount importance *how* they communicate to her. Although adults with Down syndrome generally can communicate better than what some might expect, patterns of communication will still be different from adults without an intellectual disability (Down Syndrome Education International, 2015). For instance, adults with Down syndrome often utilize shorter sentences and simple grammar (Orange & Zanon, 2005). They also have trouble comprehending the speech of others (Down Syndrome Education International, 2015). These communication challenges can be compounded by hearing deficits and early dementia. As such, professionals working with Janie need to patiently learn how she communicates and learn what kinds of communication work best for her (e.g., rephrasing questions, changing formats of questions) (Finlay & Antaki, 2012). This nuanced understanding involves time, patience, and insight.

Finlay and Antaki (2012) conducted an ethnographic study to examine how professionals communicate with adults with intellectual disabilities. They videotaped how staff interacted with adults in two residential homes and one outdoor activities setting in Britain. The researchers examined videotapes to determine how staff asked questions, how the adults with intellectual disabilities responded to the questions, and then, how staff reacted when a question failed to achieve results. (As an example, when the adult with intellectual disabilities did not respond verbally or nonverbally to the question, or when the response seemed inappropriate to the question, this was determined to be a failed question.) Professionals used various techniques to address failed questions, such as rephrasing a question, differentiating between questions that tap into intention versus desire, changing the question format (such as changing an open-ended question into a closed-ended one), and using nonverbal communication to reassert the question (Finlay & Antaki, 2012). More than just a technique, however, the sophisticated and nuanced understandings of each client's mode of communication, as well as effective professional responses, allowed for understanding and camaraderie between adults with intellectual disabilities and professionals (Finlay & Antaki, 2012). Such an approach with Janie would likely have helped her in feeling heard and cared for.

Be Prepared to Address Emotional Responses to Transitions

It is imperative for health and human service professionals to address the emotional responses of older adults and family members undergoing transitions. This seems obvious, and yet many professionals are uncomfortable with specific emotions, such as anger, or are uncomfortable with the *depth* of emotions. They may also be concerned about the amount of time it takes to listen to older adults and their family members express their grief, anger, confusion, and so on. We understand this hesitation and recognize that in many health care settings, professionals are completely strapped for time. However, we suggest that if professionals do not provide the opportunity for individuals to express their emotions, they may be forced to address these emotions in other ways. For instance, when family members are feeling much guilt around placing their older adult and they are not able to work through that guilt, they may express this through hypervigilant monitoring of the care of the older adult and outright criticism of the efforts of long-term care staff. Staff may become very frustrated and even angry with family members and consider the resident's relatives as being a "problem family." And yet staff members may not be aware of how much of the critical vigilance is actually unresolved grief.

How can grief and other emotions involved in experiencing a transition be addressed? First, we suggest that it is important for professionals to sit down with the older adult (where possible) and family members and specifically state that the transition can be filled with overwhelming emotions, such as grief, guilt, fear, and confusion. If the transition involves a move to a long-term care facility, the nursing unit manager, social worker, or Clinical Nurse Specialist can purposely meet with the family, not just to talk about specifics regarding costs, programs, and routines, but also to address family members' concerns and issues. It is important that the professional set up the meeting, as well as set the tone of the meeting, clearly stating that the transition to a facility is a life-changing event for older adults and family members that can evoke very difficult emotions; it is important that the professional verbally names the emotions that family members may experience. This process normalizes (Wright & Leahey, 2013) the overwhelming emotions that may come with this transition. When a professional informs family members that it is very common to feel guilt about placing a spouse or parent, some of the guilt may be alleviated. Family members may also give themselves the permission to feel the uncomfortable emotions, because in their minds, a knowledgeable professional has authorized the normalcy of feeling what they are feeling.

Beyond acknowledgment and normalization of these tumultuous emotions, however, there also needs to be room for *expression* of these emotions. In our experiences with older adults and their family members, there can be weeping and even wailing over transitions, whether this involves a relocation transition to hospital or a facility, or the transition of death for the older adult. When the nurse, social worker, or chaplain is able to literally just *be* with family members, talk when the family needs to talk, or sit in silence with them as they try to digest the events, this can be enormously helpful to family members. In their aloneness with grief (even in a room full of family members, each family member is alone with his or her own grief), they are not quite as alone because of the presence of the professional.

I (MBR) remember a wife who was struggling with her spouse's impending death. She had counted on her husband being healed, and it appeared that it was not happening. I spent some time with her and family members in a quiet room, where she poured out her grief to God. She wept, screamed, and shook her fists. In the presence of safe others, she came to grips with her husband's dying. (He died a few hours later.) The anger and sadness expressed was a necessary part of her process. It was not "comfortable" for this chaplain nor her family members, but it was therapeutic for her.

How do these ideas about acknowledging and encouraging the expression of grief apply to Janie and Bob? First, it is important to recognize the compounding nature of several transitions—the death of Bob's wife and Janie's mother, transitions to hospital for Bob and long-term care placement for Janie. Not only is there a compounding effect of stress caused by multiple transitions in a relatively short period of time, there is a compounding effect of grief. Both Bob and Janie are grieving the loss of Sarah and now they are grieving the loss of each other living under the same roof. Although Bob and Janie have not died, the relationship, as it once was, is now gone.

While both Bob and Janie will be grieving, the death of a parent can be catastrophic for the older adult with an intellectual disability. Not only did Janie lose the support of her mother that she had lived with since birth, the death indirectly precipitated her relocation to the facility. When Bob was hospitalized, there was no other parent who could care for her, so she had to be placed (Dodd et al., 2008; Dodd, Dowling, & Hollins, 2005). Once placed, however, Janie likely lost her main support in grieving—Bob.

Long-term care staff may not feel equipped to handle this type of loss. In working with adults such as Janie, they may feel unprepared to help with the grieving process. Or, they may believe that those with intellectual disabilities do not experience emotional responses to death. However, rather than experiencing no grief, some research suggests that older adults with intellectual disability experience *greater* emotional reactions to the death of a parent and that this grief can then progress to signs of mental illness (Dodd et al., 2008). Hence, the transition to a long-term care facility for someone like Janie is laden with grief; not only is Bob not as physically present to help her with the grief stemming from the death of her mother, but now she is in new surroundings with staff and residents who do not understand her.

Where Possible Include Older Adult in Decision-Making

Although we advocate for family involvement in assisting older adults through crucial health, moving, and life and death transitions, we feel strongly that family members' opinions should not supersede the older adult, unless the older adult is unable to make decisions due to cognitive impairment, an intellectual disability, or is unable to make decisions (e.g., is unconscious related to a medical condition). If the older adult is of sound cognition, she should be able to make her own decisions. Even in situations of early dementia, the older individual should be able to express her opinions about what she would like to see happen in her care.

If an older adult is no longer able to make decisions due to cognitive impairment, delirium, or other health problem, then the older adult's wishes can still be honored through personal directives and guardianship. These legal documents can, in essence, speak for the older adult when she is no longer able to. These forms also provide comfort and assurance for family members in that they can feel assured that their decisions are congruent with their family member's wishes.

SUMMARY

Working with older adult families can be tremendously rewarding. However, it can also be challenging, especially during times of transition. Understanding how to help older adult families during transitions can help ease the emotional turmoil for all members involved.

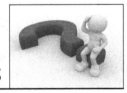

CRITICAL THINKING EXERCISES

You are the recreational therapist in the nursing home in which Janie now resides. As you walk down the nursing home hallways, you see Janie looking sad and withdrawn, and this troubles you. You decide that you will do your utmost to get Janie involved.

► How will you decide what activities are best suited for Janie?

► How will you convince her to get involved in group recreational activities? What will be your approach when you talk to her?

► When you finally convince Janie to attend and participate in an event, other residents stare and laugh at her when she attempts to participate. How will you respond to the reactions of the other residents? After the event, what will you say to Janie about the responses of others?

INTERESTING WEBSITES

▶ American Association for Marriage and Family Therapy: http://www.aamft.org

▶ Institute of Marriage and Family Canada: http://www.imfcanada.org

▶ The Vanier Institute of the Family: http://www.vanierinstitute.ca

REFERENCES

Alzheimer's Association. (2014). 2014 Alzheimer's Disease: Facts & figures. Retrieved January 8, 2015, from: http://www.alz.org/alzheimers_disease_facts_and_figures.asp

Benner Carson, V., & Koenig, H. G. (2004). *Spiritual caregiving: Healthcare as a ministry.* Philadelphia: Templeton Foundation Press.

Bern-Klug, M. (2008). The emotional context facing nursing home residents' families: A call for role reinforcement strategies for nursing homes and the community. *Journal of the American Medical Directors Association, 9*(1), 36–44. doi:10.1016/j.jamda.2007.08.010

Blanton, P. (2013). Family caregivers to frail elders: Experiences of young adult grandchildren as auxiliary caregivers. *Journal of Intergenerational Relationships, 11,* 18–31. doi:10.1080/15350770.2013.755076

Brown, J., Dodd, K., & Vetere, A. (2010). "I am a normal man": A narrative analysis of the accounts of older people with Down's syndrome who lived in institutionalised settings. *British Journal of Learning Disabilities, 38*(3), 217–224. doi:10.1111/j.1468-156.2009.00596.x

Buys, L., Aird, R., & Miller, E. (2012). Service providers' perceptions of active ageing among older adults with lifelong disabilities. *Journal of Intellectual Disability Research, 56*(12), 1133–1147. doi:10.1111/j. 1365-2788.2011.01500.x

Carter, B., & McGoldrick, M. (1989). *The changing family life cycle: A framework for family therapy.* Toronto: Allyn & Bacon.

Carter, B., & McGoldrick, M. (2005). *The expanded family life cycle: Individual, family and social perspectives* (3rd ed.). New York, NY: Pearson.

Davies, S. (2005). Meleis' theory of nursing transitions and relatives' experiences of nursing home entry. *Journal of Advanced Nursing, 52*(6), 658–671.

Davies, S., & Nolan, M. (2003). "Making the best of things": Relatives' experiences of decisions about care-home entry. *Ageing & Society, 23*(4), 429-450. doi: http://dx.doi.org/10.1017/S0144686X03001259

Davis, J., Tremont, G., Bishop, D., & Fortinsky, R. (2011). A telephone-delivered psychosocial intervention improves dementia caregiver adjustment following nursing home placement. *International Journal of Geriatric Psychiatry, 26,* 380–387.

Dillenburger, K., & McKerr, L. (2011). "How long are we able to go on?" Issues faced by older family caregivers of adults with disabilities. *British Journal of Learning Disabilities, 39*(1), 29–38. doi:10.1111/j.1468-3156.2010.00613.x

Dodd, P., Dowling, S., & Hollins, S. (2005). A review of the emotional, psychiatric and behavioral responses to bereavement in people with intellectual disabilities. *Journal of Intellectual Disability Research, 49*(7), 537–543.

Dodd, P., Guerin, S., McEvoy, J., Buckley, S., Tyrrell, J., & Hillery, J. (2008). A study of complicated grief symptoms in people with intellectual disabilities. *Journal of Intellectual Disability Research, 52*(5), 415–425. doi:10.1111/j.1365-2788.2008.01043.x

Down Syndrome Education International. (2015). Development and learning. Retrieved February 8, 2015, from: http://www.dseinternational.org/en-us/about-down-syndrome/development/

Edwards, A. P., & Graham, E. E. (2009). The relationship between individuals' definitions of family and implicit personal theories of communication. *Journal of Family Communication, 9*(4), 191–208. doi:10.1080/15267430903070147

Finlay, W. M., & Antaki, C. (2012). How staff pursue questions to adults with intellectual disabilities. *Journal of Intellectual Disability Research, 56*(4), 361–370. doi:10. 1111/j.1365-2788.2011.01478.x

Fruhauf, C. A., & Orel, N. A. (2008). Developmental issues of grandchildren who provide care to grandparents. *International Journal of Aging and Human Development, 67*(3), 209–230. doi:10.2190/AG.67.3.b

Gilbert, A., Lankshear, G., & Petersen, A. (2008). Older family-carers' views on the future accommodation needs of relatives who have an intellectual disability. *International Journal of Social Welfare, 17*(1), 54–64. doi:10.1111/j.1468-2397.2007.00485.x

Givens, J. L., Prigerson, H. G., Kiely, D. K., Shaffer, M. L., & Mitchell, S. L. (2011). Grief among family members of nursing home residents with advanced dementia. *American Journal of Geriatric Psychiatry, 19*(6), 543–550. doi:10.1097/JGP0b013e31820dcbe0

Gottlieb, L. N. (2013). *Strengths-based nursing care: Health and healing for person and family.* New York: Springer.

Hamill, S. B. (2012). Caring for grandparents with Alzheimer's disease: Help from the "forgotten" generation. *Journal of Family Issues, 33*(9), 1195–1217. doi:10.1177/0192513X12444858

Hines, P. M., Preto, N. G., McGoldrick, M., Almeida, R., & Weltman, S. (2005). Culture and the family life cycle. In B. Carter & M. McGoldrick (Eds.), *The changing family life cycle: A framework for family therapy* (3rd ed.; pp. 69–87). New York: Pearson.

Hirst, S. P., Lane, A. M., & Stares, R. (2013). Health promotion with older adults experiencing mental health challenges: Strength-based approaches. *Clinical Gerontology, 36,* 329–355.

Ihara, E. S., Horio, B. M., & Tompkins, C. J. (2012). Grandchildren caring for grandparents: Modeling the complexity of family caregiving. *Journal of Social Service Research, 38*(5), 619–636. http://dx.doi.org/10.1080/01488376.2012.711684

Keady, J., & Jones, L. (2010). Investigating the causes of behaviours that challenge in people with dementia. *Nursing Older People, 22*(9), 25–29.

King, C. (2012). Managing agitated behaviour in older people. *Nursing Older People, 24*(7), 33–36.

Krishnamoorthy, A., & Anderson, D. (2011). Managing challenging behaviour in older adults with dementia. *Progress in Neurology and Psychiatry, 15*(3), 20–27. doi:10.1002/pnp.199

Kyomen, H. H., & Whitfield, T. H. (2008). Agitation in older adults. *Psychiatric Times, 25*(8), 52–57.

Lane, A. M. (2007). *The social organization of geriatric mental health.* Unpublished doctoral dissertation, University of Calgary.

Levine, C., Hunt, G. G., Halper, D., Hart, A. Y., Lautz, J, & Gould, D. A. (2005). Young adult caregivers: A first look at an unstudied population. *American Journal of Public Health, 95*(11), 2071–2075. doi:10.2105/AJPH.2005.067702

Mace, M. L., & Rabins, P. V. (1981). *The 36 hour day: A family guide to caring for persons with Alzheimer disease, related dementing illnesses, and memory loss in later life.* Baltimore: Johns Hopkins University Press.

McGoldrick, M. (1991). Echoes from the past: Helping families mourn their losses. In F. Walsh & M. McGoldrick (Eds.), *Living beyond loss: Death in the family* (pp. 50–78). New York: W. W. Norton.

Office of the Public Guardian—Alberta Human Services. (2015). Office of the Public Guardian. Retrieved February 8, 2015, from: http://humanservices.alberta.ca/guardianship-trusteeship/office-public-guardian.html

Orange, J. B., & Zanon, M. V. (2005). Language and communication in adults with Down syndrome and dementia of the Alzheimer type: A review. *Journal of Developmental Disabilities, 12*(1), 53–62.

Perry, B., Dalton, J. E., & Edwards, E. (2010). Family caregivers' compassion fatigue in long-term facilities. *Nursing Older People, 22*(4), 26–31.

Piercy, K. W. (2007). Characteristics of strong commitments to intergenerational family care of older adults. *Journal of Gerontology: Social Sciences, 62B*(6), S381–S387.

Reuss, G. F., Dupuis, S. L., & Whitfield, K. (2005). Understanding the experience of moving a loved one to a long-term care facility: Family members' perspectives. *Journal of Gerontological Social Work, 46*(1), 17–46. doi:10.1300/J083v46n01_03

Spendelow, J. S. (2011). Assessment of mental health problems in people with Down syndrome: Key considerations. *British Journal of Learning Disabilities, 39*(4), 306–313. doi:10.1111/j.1468-3156.2010.00670.x

Statistics Canada. (2012). Portrait of families and living arrangements in Canada. Retrieved February 8, 2015, from: http://www12.statcan.gc.ca/census-recensement/2011/as-sa/98-312-x/98-312-x2011001-eng.cfm

Strax, T. E., Luciano, L., Dunn, A. M., & Quevedo, J. P. (2010). Aging and developmental disability. *Physical Medicine and Rehabilitation Clinics of North America, 21*(2), 419–427. doi:10.1016/j.pmr.2009.12.009

The Vanier Institute of the Family. (n.d.). Definition of family. Retrieved January 8, 2015, from: http://www.vanierinstitute.ca

Wengryn, M. I., & Hester, E. (2011). Pragmatic skills used by older adults in social communication and health care contexts: Precursors to health literacy. *Contemporary Issues in Communication Science & Disorders, 38*(Spring), 41–52.

Wright, L. M., & Leahey, M. (2013). *Nurses and families: A guide to family assessment and intervention* (6th ed.). Philadelphia: F. A. Davis.

CHAPTER 8

FUTURE DIRECTIONS

*Aging is not lost youth but a new stage of
opportunity and strength. (Betty Friedan, one
of the founders of the feminist movement)*

Reflective Questions

▶ In your future work with older adults, what do you think will be the most rewarding aspects of your work?

▶ What will be the most challenging facets of working with this population?

▶ In the future, what changes would you seek to enact? How would you go about this?

In the past number of decades, media advertisements for products that enhance youthful appearance, or erase—even if temporarily—the signs of aging, have burgeoned. It seems that as life spans have increased, so has the impetus to appear younger. And yet, as noted by one of the founders of the feminist movement (Betty Friedan), aging presents new opportunities and a different kind of strength. More than wishful thinking, with increasing life spans and many enjoying better health well into later life, advancing age provides individuals with many opportunities to be creative, engage in meaningful activities and causes, and move toward the end of life with strength and purpose.

In order to support older individuals to experience aging as a time of new opportunities, energy, growth, and purpose, we suggest the following strategies that are targeted at multiple levels. First, we offer ideas directed toward a grass roots level—this involves enhancing childhood experiences of and exposure to older adults. Second, we suggest changes in education for future health and human service professionals working with aging adults. We then explore future directions in services within the community and housing options for seniors, including those in various sub-populations, such as those with mental illness, who are homeless, have intellectual disabilities, those who are dying, as well as incarcerated older adults. Finally, we explore the area of advocacy; specifically, we examine older adults advocating for older adults. We recognize that these suggested directions are merely "skimming the surface" of what can and should be done in the future.

Early Age Exposure to Older Adults and Education

It is commonly acknowledged that developed countries tend to be youth-oriented and death-denying societies. Not only does this lead to some aging individuals trying valiantly to stave off signs of aging, but it can also result in a huge chasm dividing older individuals from youth. Youth may avoid older adults, particularly those who are infirmed, out of fear, and older adults may pass up opportunities to interact with youth, out of concern for being misunderstood and undervalued. By the time that youth are considering careers, they often have had little exposure to aging individuals. Thus, we wonder about when college and university programs are trying to attract professionals to work with older adults, if they are too late. At this point, young adults have formed beliefs about what aging entails; unfortunately, their beliefs may not include the humor, richness, and strength that many older adults possess. Could strategies targeted toward increasing exposure to positive aging, as well as programs aimed at integrating older adults with younger children, facilitate comfort with and interest in older adults?

Influence of the Media

As the media exerts enormous influence on children and as they watch, on average, three and a half hours of television per day (Statistic Brain, n.d.), the importance of the positive portrayal of aging cannot be overstated. There are a number of actors in their late 70s or over the age of 80 who are vibrant, excellent at their craft, and very engaging. As a few examples, Betty White is over 90 years of age and is still acting in television shows and commercials. Similarly, William Shatner is still involved in various television shows. Dame Judy Dench continues to act in movies including the *The Best Exotic Marigold Hotel*, as well as in past James Bond movies. All three actors are intelligent, very successful, and committed to their work. When these actors are interviewed on talk shows, all of them articulate that they love their work and want to work for as long as they can. Clearly, work gives them purpose and enjoyment. Their visibility helps to combat the myth that all older adults are feeble and useless. They are examples of how aging individuals can not only survive, but thrive in advancing years. Although health and human service professionals do not influence who is hired for acting roles, professional bodies can lobby against particular portrayals of older adults. A number of years ago, a provincial Alzheimer Society (in Canada) contacted a television station to complain about a documentary that portrayed an individual with Alzheimer's disease as violent. While those working within this local organization did not deny that sometimes individuals with dementia can exhibit aggressive behaviors, they opposed the notion that all individuals with dementia act aggressively. Professionals can advocate, through letters and emails, for media examples to represent aging as growth-promoting, rather than as causing dotty and infirmed, or angry and aggressive individuals.

Intergenerational Programs

Intergenerational programs are those that match older adults and children/youth together in shared activities. These programs allow children and older adults to share talents, learn from each other; they enhance the socialization of both groups, and help to combat inaccurate stereotypes about older adults (Biggs & Knox, 2014). Further, they challenge the current trend to separate programs and activities via age groups, thus separating children from older adults. They allow older adults and children/youth to see each other in a positive light. They also permit both age groupings to contribute meaningfully to society. Activities can focus on environmental concerns, such as building an electronic recycling center or helping restore a wildlife sanctuary (Steinig & Butts, 2009–10), growing gardens, and school mentoring (Cooper, 2011). Not only do children and youth report better attitudes toward older adults (Biggs & Knox, 2014), but research also suggests that older adults experience improvements in mental and physical health and overall well-being (MacCallum et al., 2010; Young & Janke, 2013).

And intergenerational education can move beyond shared activities that occur, perhaps, once a week. In 2000, an intergenerational school was started in Cleveland, Ohio (George, Whitehouse, & Whitehouse, 2011). This school has inner-city students from kindergarten to grade 8 learning alongside older adults. They even have a formal mentorship role for older adults with dementia. The older individuals with dementia are integrated into classroom curriculum, such as giving a talk on the African American experience before and during the civil rights movement. Reciprocally, adolescent students teach older adults computer skills. According to George and his colleagues (2011), the school has received an "excellent" score from the Ohio Department of Education for six out of seven years. Similar to the results of intergenerational programs just mentioned, older adults noted that they received a number of benefits from their participation, including increased cognitive stimulation and better mood, a greater sense of purpose in life and the establishment of meaningful relationships with students (George et al., 2011). This finding is not surprising, as relationships are key to meaning in life at all stages (Allemand, Steiner, & Hill, 2013).

We suggest that there needs to be more intergenerational programs available with greater advertising of and importance placed on these kinds of programs (e.g., through the media and in schools). Despite the fact that there are some intergenerational programs within developed countries, there still is a predominance of "silos" between the generations; that is, programs remain geared for single age groups, such as children, adolescents, or seniors. Further research needs to be conducted on intergenerational schools, both in the immediate, and longitudinally. For instance, graduates from these schools can be interviewed years after their attendance, in order to examine the long-term benefits of having attended this kind of school. This will provide a basis through which to evaluate aspects of the programs that have been effective or unsuccessful, thereby providing feedback for change.

Education for Current and Future Health and Human Service Professionals

Education for current and future health and human service professionals needs to accurately and meaningfully address the normal changes of aging, as well as how pathophysiological changes impact the physical, mental, and spiritual health of older individuals. In particular, it is crucial that professionals recognize how illnesses, such as depression, may present differently in older adults. Additionally, professionals should be cognizant of the impact of transitions in older adulthood, and how, despite the resilience and strength that many older adults possess, transitions may affect older adults mentally and spiritually, awakening questions about meaning and purpose in life. And it is vital that gerontological education not only address the *what* of content, but the *how* of it being delivered most effectively.

Education of Future Health and Human Service Professionals

As mentioned in Chapter 2, most future professionals, be they nurses, social workers, or physicians, do not specifically choose to work with older adults (Wray & McCall, 2007). For years, there has been ongoing discussion within the literature regarding how best to attract future professionals to gerontology. The dialogue partly focuses on whether a gerontological curriculum should be integrated into curriculum (that is, included within adult content), or if there should be stand-alone courses (Hirst, Lane, & Stares, 2012). We suggest that there is a need for older adult content to be integrated within the curriculum, as well as for stand-alone courses. This will mitigate possible pitfalls of educators teaching gerontological content when they are not knowledgeable about older adults and transitions (which may happen in integrated curriculum); it will also protect against potential problems of stand-alone courses, that being, that they are offered as options and the only students who take the courses are already committed to working with older adults or choose these courses because they fit within their timetable.

The continuous dialogue of how to attract students to careers with older adults, especially within nursing education, also concentrates on the type of clinical educational experiences students receive. The question is raised if the type of clinical placement influences students' attitudes in a negative or positive way. For instance, it was common during the 1970s and early 1980s for nursing students to experience their first clinical placement in a nursing home. Within this environment, they could learn how to give bed baths, change bed linens, and take temperatures, blood pressures, and pulses. Students tended to rate these experiences negatively and educators also wondered about the ethics of students learning basics of nursing on a vulnerable population—older individuals within long-term care facilities. Educators also began to wonder about the timing of experiences that impact how health and human service professionals feel about working with older adults. Hence, it is not just the *type* of clinical education experience, but also the *timing* of the placement that may affect attitudes (Lane & Hirst, 2012). For example, some students enjoy a placement within long-term care, not within their first year of education, but when they are in their final year. Within their final year of education, they can appreciate the complexities of providing care to older adults, can appreciate the privilege of working with families, and can understand the sophistication of skills needed to work effectively with families, as well as they have the opportunity to exercise leadership skills. Using this same reasoning, a palliative care placement is generally a student's practicum in her final year.

Although an understanding of timing of the clinical experiences with older adults begins to address the question of how to interest and excite students in gerontology, this is only a partial answer. The question is actually much more complex. Our work, as well as a search of the research, indicates that improved knowledge of and attitudes toward older adults does not necessarily translate into a desire to work with older adults (Hirst et al., 2012). Clearly, much more research needs to be conducted to further unravel the complexities of what strategies will help engage students in working with older adults.

Education for Professionals Currently Working With Older Adults

Many health and human service professionals work with older adults, but not necessarily by choice. Due to the nature of their work that cuts across age groupings, they will, regardless of preference, work with seniors. This does not mean, however, that they feel comfortable or knowledgeable enough to work with older adults. For instance, in one study, nurses and physicians admitted to not feeling confident in their assessments of pain in cognitively impaired older adults within long-term care facilities (Kaasalainen et al., 2007). In another study, delirium, a frequent and potentially life threatening condition experienced by hospitalized older adults, was recognized by less than one third of registered nurses (Dahlke & Phinney, 2008). Similarly, we have worked with social workers, ministers, and psychologists who admit to experiencing much *dis-ease* (lack of ease) in working with aging individuals or death and dying.

We believe that it is critical for these professionals to receive education about aging, illness in older adulthood (such as dementias and mental illness), and the issues faced by older individuals and their family members, including the challenges faced in transitions. While some professionals, such as social workers, registered nurses, and physicians, have mandatory continuing education requirements that are enforced by their professional bodies, other professionals do not necessarily require ongoing upgrading. For these professionals, such as the clergy, the onus to remain current in their fields is entrusted to individuals. While some may choose to educate themselves about issues outside of faith, others may not. Thus, some ministers are not knowledgeable about the signs of depression in older adults or the need for professional treatment.

Even for professionals who are mandated to update themselves yearly, the focus of the educational upgrading is not stipulated. Thus, these professionals may not choose to read about older adults or attend educational seminars on issues facing this population group. It behooves all professionals to be mindful of population trends, such as the rapid aging of developed countries, and to educate themselves so that they are prepared to respond knowledgeably to changes in demographic trends, as well as the issues and transitions faced by those who may be affected by demographic trends, such as older adults.

While clergy may not be knowledgeable about how to assess and intervene with depression in older adults (at least not to the level of other professionals, such as registered nurses, psychologists, and social workers), members of the clergy are often much more comfortable and adept in addressing existential issues than their aforementioned counterparts. As mentioned earlier in this book, many nurses and social workers do not know how to address these issues and actively steer away from them. They may not know how to talk about issues of meaning and purpose, how to bring a sense of integration to life, as well as be comfortable in discussing concerns about forgiveness of self, others, or God.

Education about how to broach these matters, even to a limited degree, should be a goal of professionals who work with older adults (Reed, 2014). Even though most professionals are not trained to advise in spiritual matters, the connection between spiritual and emotional health is strong in older adults (Ramsay, 2008), so professionals working with older adults need to know how to open up existential issues in conversation. If older adults admit to strong existential issues, professionals can then refer to clergy or other professionals who are comfortable discussing these transitional issues.

Ongoing Education for Para-Professionals

Although para-professionals[1] provide much of the direct care received by older adults within their homes (such as bathing) or within long-term care, they receive minimal education. This is a significant deficit, as individuals who provide the *most* hands-on care, have the *least* knowledge to recognize and respond to reactions to transitions in older adults, such as grief, depression, suicidal ideation, and anger. This dilemma is not fair to older adults, or to the para-professionals who work with them.

Due to the high turnover of para-professional staff in home care agencies, as well as in long-term care, education needs to be ongoing to ensure that every individual receives training. Education should focus on the challenges of transitions for older adults, such as relocation to other facilities (assisted living, long-term care, and hospice, to name a few), as well as how to address these challenges. In studies examining the impact of the transition of placement into long-term care facilities upon new residents, staff rarely talked with older adults about the challenges of relocation (Wiersma, 2010). While staff may be aware of the magnitude of the transition and the grief incurred, they reported that they just do not have the time (Wiersma, 2010). Our belief is that this is not out of callousness on the part of the staff, but rather, in addition to the overwhelming workload, they may not know how to help older adults through this life changing transition and how to address grief, depression, and confusion. Further, as will be discussed under the "Sub-Population" section of this chapter, education should be provided to para-professional staff regarding how to give effective palliative care, as some older adults choose to die within the long-term care facility (or their families make this decision), rather than be transferred to hospital or hospice.

Education for Professionals Working Within Prisons

Professionals working within the prison system should be given education about aging and its effect upon prisoners (Williams, Stern, Mellow, Safer, & Greifinger, 2012). This education can include some of the expected changes of aging, including hearing and sight impairment, as well as information on disease processes, such as arthritis, and how this affects mobility of aged prisoners (Smyer & Burbank, 2009). Health care staff in prison facilities need information and policies that guide the regular assessments

---

1. The term para-professional is used to denote health care aides or personal care attendants.

and screening (Sumner, 2012), as will be discussed in the housing section of this chapter.

Before embarking on a discussion of services within the community and housing options for aging individuals, we want to note that the changes we suggest are based upon our belief about the need to move toward more age-friendly communities, as discussed in Chapter 4. While how changes are made will depend upon the type of community and the population of that community (rural versus urban), we support the underlying premise of making living environments more meaningful and accessible for aging individuals.

Services in the Community

Services in the community should assist aging adults in preparation for retirement, help older individuals to access health services, to live independently within their homes of choice for as long as possible, and promote growth and meaning in the latter decades of life. We recognize that some communities have these types of services, but others, particularly small or rural communities, have limited services that are tailored for the needs of older adults. The kinds and amounts of rural services are often dependent upon the size of the town, as well as its proximity to a larger urban center (Niemeyer et al., 2006). The other factor is cost; depending upon the country and the health care benefits available, the cost of some of these services may be prohibitive for some individuals.

Services in Rural Areas

In some developed countries, such as Canada, the United States, and Australia, there is a larger proportion of older adults living within rural areas than in urban centers (Forbes & Edge, 2009; Niemeyer et al., 2006). It is recognized that older adults living in rural areas are at particular risk for being underserved and also, that they may underutilize what services are available. Access barriers include limited services (related in part to lack of government support for rural services), inadequate numbers of professionals who work in rural areas, difficulties securing transportation and homemaker services (Li, 2006), and limited assisted living facilities (Averill, 2012). The inability or unwillingness to access services may result in older adults delaying seeking professional help when needed. This may have deleterious effects upon health and necessitate transitions to hospitals and ultimately, to facilities which provide 24-hour care. What are some possible solutions that may assist rural older adults to maintain their health and remain in the living setting of their choice for as long as possible?

Creative and comprehensive models to organize services

There is a need for creative models that provide a balance of services in and through various modalities. These models will assist aging rural adults to access services in larger urban centers, but also provide services within their own communities. They will address the lack of gerontological professionals within rural areas, and utilize technology and other supports to counterbalance the lack of gerontological specialists. Necessary services span across the health care spectrum (health care professionals and services) and support service sectors (volunteer and paid transportation services).

There is a deficit of geriatricians, geriatric psychiatrists, and other gerontological health and human service professionals working in rural areas in developed countries. In part, this is due to limited numbers of health and human service professionals committed to working with older adults in general, but also, most geriatricians (Peterson, Bazemore, Bragg, Xierali, & Warshaw, 2011) and specifically trained gerontological health care providers work in urban centers. Besides aging individuals traveling to urban centers to receive consultation from geriatricians and geriatric psychiatrists, other options should be available. For example, teleconferencing can be utilized for physicians, nurses, and other health and human service professionals to consult with specialists about their clients. Further, teleconferencing could include older adults with geriatricians and geriatric psychiatrists. We realize that this technology is currently being used in some rural areas to benefit aging adults, but assert that these services need to be part of a larger model of care offered to rural seniors.

While the use of specialists "flying in and flying out" to remote (Margolis, 2012) or rural areas can be every effective, it is an expensive form of health care delivery. In many rural areas, the family physician provides much of the care for older adults and may feel that he or she lacks time to offer significant psychosocial or mental health care (Bocker, Glasser, Nielsen, & Weidenbacher-Hoper, 2012). Thus, the use of nurse practitioners and interprofessional teams should also be utilized (Peterson et al., 2011). And it is imperative that these professionals receive ongoing support and education in order to avoid burnout (from not being confident with decision-making in regard to their clientele) (Bulbrook, Carey,

Lenthall, Byers, & Behan, 2012). Examples of such programs include workshops to educate rural physicians on how to diagnose for Alzheimer's disease (Galvin, Meuser, & Morris, 2012), or educational sessions for nurses and other professionals on how to assess for mental illness in older adults. Additionally, health and human service professionals can offer education to rural seniors on various aspects of health care. For instance, in one study, nurses and dieticians visited with older adults through the use of telehealth to set goals with these older individuals regarding diabetes management (West, Lagua, Trief, Izquierdo, & Weinstock, 2010). This program was very successful, with 68% of the behavioral goals being met or improved upon (West et al., 2010). Similarly, nurses can utilize telecommunications or videoconferencing to educate older adults in rural areas about management of chronic heart failure (Clark et al., 2008). Additionally, telehealth can be used to provide psychosocial intervention for older adults with dementia and their caregivers (Li, Kyrouac, McManus, Cranston, & Hughes, 2012).

Telehealth services for clients, as well as teleconferencing among health and human service professionals, need to be evaluated through research. Even though they appear to be a promising and cost-effective means to offer education and consultation, there are challenges in using technology. For example, rural older adults may not have sufficient technology to access telehealth, or, they may be unfamiliar and uncomfortable in accessing this approach. Further, the usage of teleconferencing by interprofessional teams over geographical distance can result in challenges with teamwork and communication; this is especially the case when discussing complex client health or family issues (Forbes & Edge, 2009).

Pre-Retirement Education

Over the past number of decades, there have been some major changes in societal expectations surrounding retirement. For a number of years, individuals in some developed countries presumed that they would work until 65 years of age, the age at which they could access national pension plans. However, in the 1980s, some financial institutions were touting programs that could help individuals retire comfortably earlier, including some that promoted retirement at 55 years of age. Much has changed over the last several decades, though, derailing early retirement for many individuals who are approaching older age. Some of these changes make the decision to retire more complex, resulting in the importance of pre-retirement education.

One such change is that many businesses have done away with company pensions. While some employers still offer work pension plans, the numbers that do have dropped dramatically (MacEwan, 2012). If individuals approaching older age have not consciously saved for the future, they will have fewer monetary resources during their non- or reduced working years. This will not only affect their ability to enjoy recreational activities such as traveling, working out at health clubs, and eating out at restaurants on a regular basis, but may impact their access to health care services that are not covered by the government or insurance plans.

Additionally, a number of countries, such as Canada, the United States, and Australia, are pushing the current age of access to full government pensions or subsidies to a later age. As an example, Australia is implementing a change so that by 2017, Australians need to be 65.5 years of age to access the "age pension." The required age is set to increase by increments yearly, and by 2023, Australians will have to be 67 years of age to claim their age pension (Australian Government Department of Human Services, 2015). In Canada, adults who were 54 years of age and older by March 31, 2012, will still be able to claim Old Age Security Pension at the age of 65 years. However, those born in 1958 and onward, until and including January 1962, will have additional months added to the 65 years of age. Individuals born in February 1962 or later will have to wait additional time to claim the Old Age Security Pension (Service Canada, 2012). Therefore, individuals in mid-life (example 40 to 50 years of age) who do not have a company pension and are not able to save substantial monies, will need to plan on working later to receive their full pensions.

Another factor to consider is the increasing life expectancy of individuals within developed countries. With the oldest-old (those 85 years of age and older) growing at a fast rate within the older adult population in many developed countries (Statistics Canada, 2008; United States Census Bureau, 2011), adults can expect to live much longer than those decades ago. While this is considered to be positive for many individuals, a stark reality remains: How will individuals fund their longer life spans? (See Case Example further on in this chapter.)

An additional important factor to keep in mind regarding the importance of pre-retirement education is the type of opportunities that are available for older adults. Although 30% of Americans (United States Department of Labor, 2014) and 24% of Canadians age 65 years to 70 years of age continue to work (MacEwan, 2012), generally, most employment is part-time, which has lower pay scales than full-time work. There is a greater proportion of workers 65 years of age and older who work in low-paid sales and service occupations than their counterparts between the ages of 25 to 55 (25% of those over 65 years of age compared to 20% of those 25 to 54 years) (MacEwan, 2012). Although this income may be augmented by government pensions, the amounts may not be enough for some seniors to live comfortably and afford what they need to maintain enjoyable activities, such as traveling, *and* their health.

Assistance to Access Health Services

As noted earlier, older adults often have mobility challenges due to arthritis and chronic pain. Further, problems with vision, hearing, and cognition may result in the loss of a driver's license. This means that some older individuals may have difficulty accessing medical appointments, getting blood work and other tests completed, and filling prescriptions; they cannot walk lengthy distances, and neither can they drive. Transportation is a huge barrier for a number of older adults, as many Canadian neighborhoods, and some American ones, are designed for car use (Turcotte, 2012). This problem is further compounded if there are no family members available to transport the aging individual, or if the older adult lives in a rural area, on a reserve (Aboriginal), or has limited financial resources to pay for transportation services.

So what are the options for older adults? For aging individuals whose mobility is not severely compromised, they may be able to take the bus. If their city or town offers discounts for seniors' bus passes, then this can be a viable option. However, many older North American adults do not use public transit (Turcotte, 2012; United States Department of Transportation, 2010). Depending upon the size of the community in which the older adult resides, she may be able to afford a special lower cost pass for seniors, to enable her to take a taxi for appointments and errands. The challenge of this is that often older adults need to book the taxi well in advance in order to ensure availability. This may work fine for a scheduled time booked well in advance, but less well for sudden or urgent appointments. Another option is that some seniors' not-for-profit organizations will have volunteers that can drive older adults.

Transportation then, becomes much more than transportation; it is the means through which older adults can attend health care appointments and manage their physical and mental health. It also becomes the means for older adults to participate in social activities and programs, thereby decreasing their sense of isolation and loneliness within the home (Turcotte, 2012). Viable options for transportation, which are affordable and reliable for all older adults, are essential in terms of maintaining older adults within their homes, and thus decreasing premature admissions to hospitals and long-term care facilities.

Living Independently Within Their Homes

In order to live independently as long as possible within the home, some older adults need adaptations made to their living environment. These adaptations may include a shower seat, bath rails, and raised toilet seats, for example. Further, some older adults require home health aides to help them bathe or a housekeeper to clean their home. These services need to be affordable. Although the costs of these services may be based upon a sliding scale rule (cost is based upon the income of the older adult), the amount of services that are offered may not be enough for some older adults. Thus, they may need to pay more out of pocket for private services to augment the publicly offered services.

Cohabitation of Older Adults and Young Adults

Literature addressing cohabitation (sometimes termed "cohousing") of older and younger adults can include various permutations. For instance, research on intergenerational cohabiting may involve older adults and their adult children. However, research on this kind of arrangement often involves individuals living outside North America, or individuals living within North America but representing various ethnicities (Kato, 2009; Ng, Northcott, & Abu-Laban, 2007). There is also literature examining the phenomena of grandparents raising grandchildren (Copen, 2006; Poindexter, 2007; Smith & Beltran, 2003).

Intergenerational housing is also conceptualized as older adults living in vacated university dorms or living in a residence on or near an academic campus (Ward, Spitze, & Sherman, 2005). There are also reports describing specific communities/neighborhoods (such as Hope Meadows in Illinois) that were intentionally constructed for older adults and children, with the aim of older adults mentoring and helping children, and children helping older adults (Heimpel, 2011; Kennedy, 2010; Mattimore, 2006; Power, Mitchell, Eheart, & Hopping, 2011; Thomas & Blanchard, 2009).

Another variation of the cohabitation of older adults and young adults are programs that match up adults to live with older adults within their homes. These adults may be college-aged students or adults in mid-life. There are many such programs scattered throughout North America, the United Kingdom, Europe, and Australia; for example, as mentioned in Chapter 4, there are approximately 100 homesharing programs throughout the United States (Steinisch, 2007). The purpose of the match-up is for the mutual benefit of the older adult and the younger adult. The young adult lives for very little money in the home of an older adult and provides services such as grocery shopping, raking leaves, shoveling snow, driving, or other mutually agreed upon tasks. The older adult then has services done for her that she does not need to pay for, and the younger adult can live for free, or next to free, in order to facilitate studies at university or college. Proponents of these programs suggest that they delay institutionalization (e.g., Fox, 2010): the safety of having another individual in the home, as well as the services they can provide, delays the need to move to more supervised levels of care.

Anecdotally, these types of programs are believed to be very effective for older adults and young adults. However, there is a lack of research empirically proving their effectiveness. It will be important to research both the benefits and the difficulties in running such programs. For example, in one study (Rhoades & McFarland, 1999) 61 individuals (31 to 79 years of age) who shared their home with mentally ill individuals were interviewed. They were asked why they opened up their homes and lives to the mentally ill. These individuals responded with answers that were categorized by the researchers as altruism, self-actualization, and existential (life purpose). However, the homesharing individuals admitted to challenges in dealing with client disability or difficult behaviors. The second most often cited difficulty was the challenges the homesharers had in working with the program, such as bureaucracy issues causing problems in accessing resources. Because this study does not solely focus on older adults as homeowners and young adults who are engaged in post-secondary education, the application and findings need to be interpreted with caution.

However, several observations can be made. First, there needs to be more research conducted on these programs regarding the benefits for older adults and young adults. Further, besides the altruistic and existential benefits (which are important), what kind of impact does having a young adult in the home have upon delaying moves to assisted living, long-term care, or other arrangements for older adults? What are the potential risks for older adults and their younger homesharers?

Technology Within the Home

Health care has become increasingly technologically-oriented within hospitals and clinics. But what about technology in the homes to enable older adults to live independently longer? Available today are a variety of technologically advanced aids that may be used for older adults to promote independence, as well as monitor their health and safety.

Designed to allow older adults to function independently within their homes, these technological apparatuses also promote safety and monitoring. In terms of mobility devices, manual wheelchairs, powered wheelchairs, and canes are considered to be robots that aid mobility and enhance safety, both inside and outside of the home (Hirst, 2010). While powered wheelchairs may be easier for older adults to use than their non-powered counterparts, the older adult who uses a powered wheelchair still needs to perform a number of small adjustments to maneuver (Hirst, 2010). This can be tiring and difficult for some, particularly for older adults with rheumatoid arthritis or multiple sclerosis. Currently, the technology already exists for wheelchairs to automatically avoid obstructions and be partially self-navigating (Kang et al., 2010; Hirst, 2010). Similarly, there are walkers that can steer away from obstacles and be retrieved via remote control, as well as a cane that can detect when an older adult is in danger of falling (Hirst, 2010). Additionally, there are GPS (Global Positioning System) shoes that have a built-in GPS that can help track older adults who wander away from home due to Alzheimer's disease. These shoes will provide the location of the individual wearing the shoes and provide a virtual fence around the older adult, enabling him to walk in familiar places but alerting him if he is off track (Hirst, 2010).

Technology that monitors safety within the home (that is not embedded into mobility devices) includes personal emergency response systems (Mihailidis, Cockburn, Longley, & Boger, 2008), as well as sensors and motion detectors. The personal emergency response system is worn on an individual within her home, and if she is in trouble, she can push the button on the pendant or the "watch." This will alert an operator who can then talk with the individual and/or send emergency help. Similarly, sensors and motion detectors can monitor if the house door opens (safety) or if a medication cupboard door or the refrigerator is opened (offering caregivers some assurance that the older adult is taking medication and eating) (Kang et al., 2010). There are also devices that monitor health within the home; these include such implements as heart rate monitors, glucose monitors, pulse oximeters, as well as activity monitors (Kang et al., 2010).

As promising as technological advances are in helping to keep older adults within their homes longer, there are practical and ethical considerations to be taken into account (Demeris, Doorenbos, & Towle, 2009). Practically, older adults may have trouble programming some technology; for example, individuals with Alzheimer's disease may not be able to program a GPS due to cognitive deficits (Hirst, 2010). There may also be concerns regarding the reliability of the technology and that there be accessible technical support. From an ethical perspective, there are some issues. For example, older adults are concerned about privacy and confidentiality of personal information (Demeris et al., 2009). Issues regarding privacy include recordings of data, storage of data, and the possibility that in the transmission of data, personal information may be intercepted by other communication lines, such as telephone lines. Ethically, who should make the decision about using technology, such as a GPS system, for aging individuals with dementia (Landau, Auslander, Werner, Shoval, & Heinik, 2011)? Informed consent can be ethically sticky when there is a concern about capacity in the older adult (Demeris et al., 2009). Thus, we suggest that policies and procedures need to guide how technology is used and monitored. As well, research needs to examine the ethical issues involved in the use of technology to enhance the safety of older adults within their homes, including possible solutions to address the dilemmas.

Case Example

Bertha is an 86-year-old woman currently residing outside a small town in Kansas. She has experienced extreme anxiety for years, as well as ongoing depression, for which she has been hospitalized periodically over the decades. Throughout their lives, Bertha and her husband Jake have coped with her mental illness very well and continued to function in their family business, as parents, and as members of the community.

Currently, however, Bertha is experiencing greater problems managing her anxiety, in part because of her concerns about Jake. Jake is 88 years old and has Parkinson's disease. He has fallen twice recently, including once when he hit his head and sustained a concussion. Bertha and Jake's daughter, Emma, is concerned about how long her parents can remain in their home. Although an occupational therapist assessed the home several years ago and implemented changes such as raised toilet seats, bath seats, and so on, Emma believes that her parents are no longer safe.

Emma contacted a home care nurse who conducted an assessment with Bertha and Jake. Within the assessment, Emma and her parents talked about their concerns for their health and well-being residing in their home. Emma spoke about the problems in getting health care aide support for bathing Jake, as well as to perform some household duties, such as cleaning. Although their municipality had resources in the past to provide these services at a subsidized cost, they currently have no staff to provide these services. Further, finances are now a problem. As Emma stated in exasperation, "When Mom and Dad sold their business, they got a lot of money! We thought they would be set for life! Now, they don't have enough money to keep on living in their home!" In response to her daughter's statements, Bertha responded quietly, "What can we do? We never thought we would live this long."

Personal Growth and Meaning

Programs that promote personal growth and meaning are imperative for older adults. As previously stated in this chapter, intergenerational programs where seniors are mentors for children or youth add to their sense of meaning and purpose. The sense of meaning helps with transitions such as retirement or changes in health. In fact, older adults report better mental and physical health when their lives are imbued with meaning.

Post-secondary education

Some states/provinces offer university or college courses to older adults for free or reduced rates. This allows older adults to study topics of interest, to learn, and, perhaps, to fulfill an unrealized dream—to achieve a university or college degree. In one study examining life regrets and pride among older adults with lower income, almost half of the older respondents stated they wished they could have, or would have, finished high school or college education (Choi & Jun, 2009). Post-secondary learning can be deeply fulfilling for some older adults; not only do they enjoy learning for the sake of learning (rather than learning for the sake of obtaining future employment), they garner a sense of purpose in and structure to their lives. By learning in a post-secondary setting, they also have the satisfaction of repairing regrets from the past; this chance is meaningful to older adults, as they may feel that due to their age, their opportunities to rectify past decisions are limited, as compared to younger adults (Choi & Jun, 2009).

Volunteer work or paid work

As one strategy for addressing personal growth in aging, some older adults volunteer (as discussed in Chapter 5). Not only does the volunteer work provide a sense of structure and offer personal meaning, it can also become part of the self-identity of individuals. This may be especially significant for older adults who feel that they lost some of their identity upon retirement. As mentioned earlier, the gains of volunteer work include improved physical and mental health. However, the benefits can also include improved cognition. In one study, the impact of late life volunteering or work activities upon the mental health of older adults from Singapore was examined (Schwingel, Niti, Tang, & Ng, 2009). Volunteering and work had a very positive effect upon the mental health of aging individuals from Singapore, but also, both had significant impact on cognitive functioning (Schwingel et al., 2009). As such, there should be advertisements about volunteering, information about volunteer agencies that connect older adults with opportunities, as well as literature that promotes the rewards. As noted in the research, sometimes older adults are not aware of the volunteer possibilities in their vicinity.

There is a problem, however. Most of the time, volunteering by older adults is predicated upon good physical and mental health. What about older adults whose health or mobility is significantly compromised? Can they volunteer and what are the benefits? In one study, the impact of volunteering upon older adults with fair health was examined (Barron et al., 2009). Within this study, the researchers investigated how intensive volunteering (greater than 15 hours per week) in a Baltimore, Maryland, elementary school affected 174 older adults who reported their health as "good," "fair," or "poor." Although most of the volunteers in each category showed improvement in strength and energy, those in the "fair" category demonstrated the greatest level of improvement. Most individuals in this category exhibited greater speed in climbing stairs than those in the excellent or good category and a number became faster in walking speed (Barron et al., 2009). Although this is just one study, the findings suggest that older adults can benefit greatly from volunteer experiences, even when their health may not be strong and when the volunteer experience requires extensive involvement. Obviously, more research should be conducted on the impact of volunteering upon older adults who have a number of health conditions.

What about older adults who want to volunteer, but are limited in mobility or are housebound? Older adults can still volunteer through offering phone support to socially isolated older adults (Cattan, Kime, & Bagnall, 2011), or can become involved in "virtual" volunteerism (Mukherjee, 2010). Studies reveal that older adults who volunteer through virtual or phone work have a sense of purpose and a feeling like they are giving something back to society. They also report feeling less isolated (Cattan et al., 2011). As we noted in an earlier chapter, reducing social isolation is important as this can lessen depression in housebound older adults.

So what are some future considerations with regard to volunteer opportunities for older adults? First, attention needs to be given as to how to best interest older adults in volunteering and make them aware of opportunities, including those that are episodic, those that require minimal levels of commitment, and those that are time intensive. Generally speaking, adolescents and younger adults are more aware of opportunities through their schools or work situations and thus have more chances to volunteer than their older counterparts (Morrow-Howell, 2010). Older adults who are poorly informed of the varieties of experiences and the variations in time commitment may be less inclined to volunteer, not because of a lack of interest, but because of a lack of knowledge. By becoming more knowledgeable about the types of experiences (both the focus and the work), as well as the time commitments involved, older adults can select opportunities that resonate with their life philosophies, belief systems, and passions.

Second, we propose that research and attention needs to be directed not only toward recruitment of older adults to volunteer work, but also toward retention factors. Specifically, what factors in their volunteer experiences assist older adults to remain committed and interested? At the present time, research has largely focused on specific characteristics of older individuals that motivate them to volunteer. There is a need for research to address the organizational aspects that impact the volunteer experience for older adults, as well as how life transitions—such as cessation of work, caregiving, and health changes—impact volunteering for older adults (Morrow-Howell, 2010).

Third, we suggest that organizations examine how volunteer programs can be geared toward older individuals who have significant health and mobility issues. This means that organizations that rely upon volunteers can begin programs that involve outreach through the Internet or phones. These organizations need to build in mechanisms not only to assess the satisfaction of older volunteers who provide phone or Internet support to others, but also, the benefits received by clients. Further, there should be research into the best means to reward and thank these volunteers that are largely unseen by the organization's staff members.

Housing Options

Over the last several decades, more housing options have become available for older adults within the United States, Canada, and other developed countries. However, housing options are much more readily available in large urban centers than in rural areas. Also, the stipulations for admission, as well as the costs incurred, may prohibit some older adults from accessing various kinds of housing. Further, with the significant increase in the older adult population within developed countries, finding appropriate housing for older adults may become more difficult in the decades to come. Some of the options include seniors' complexes (these can be low-cost housing or condominiums that are designed for higher-income seniors), lodges, assisted living, and long-term care facilities. Seniors' low-income housing is available in many large urban areas, but often the waiting lists for these facilities are long; some older adults have to wait years for this option. Also, group homes for older adults exist in some cities, but often availability is limited and accessibility is limited to those with specific illnesses or conditions. We suggest the following changes in housing options for older adults.

Independent or Semi-Independent Living Arrangements

Seniors' low-cost housing provides a nice option for aging adults who are on fixed incomes. Individuals rent low-cost condominiums or apartments that are often in a complex. This provides both privacy and community, if older adults desire the companionship of others. While these arrangements are a good alternative to older adults renting a single home dwelling (house with yard to tend to and walks to shovel), the waiting lists are often very long. More low-cost seniors' complexes should be created to address the current need for seniors' housing, as well as help to meet the future need with the projected explosive growth in the older adult population.

Assisted living facilities provide very nice accommodations, and like seniors' complexes, allow for privacy and togetherness. However, as some assisted living facilities are privately owned, the cost may be prohibitive for older adults on fixed incomes (Lane, 2007). We propose that there need to be more assisted living facilities that are government subsidized, so that this option is accessible to aging individuals with lower incomes. Further, all assisted living facilities should have 24-hour health care support on-site. We recognize that some assisted living facilities have a health care professional on-site throughout the day and night, but others do not. Continual health care presence in facilities would provide assurance and safety for older adults who experience tenuous health, and who otherwise might need to enter a long-term care facility.

Aside from cost and the presence/absence of a health care professional, there are differences in the particulars of the services. For instance, home care services may include helping an elderly resident dress in the morning. However, the services do not include "cueing" the older individual to dress. There is a significant difference, as cueing involves letting the older adult dress himself, with prompts from the professional, rather than dressing the individual (Lane, 2007). Not only does cueing promote self-mastery and autonomy on the part of the aging individual, but it also maintains functional abilities longer.

Dependent Living Arrangements

Older adults often do not enter long-term care until very frail, significantly cognitively impaired, or very elderly. These facilities provide daily support and care for older adults when they are unable to care for themselves due to physical illness or cognitive impairment.

Person-centered care

Originally, long-term care facilities were organized according to a hospital model. This meant that, like in hospitals, there were specific times to rise in the morning and to retire in the evening. Bath and shower times were regulated and care was often governed by routines. However, in the last number of years, there has been a move toward a culture of person-centered care. While there are still routines that guide some of the work of staff in facilities (to enhance the smooth running of a unit), there is much more attention paid to acknowledging the uniqueness of individuals and enabling residents to make choices in their daily living. We applaud this move toward a person-centered culture within long-term care, especially as these facilities often become the permanent *home* of older adults.

Obviously, *how* the person-centered culture is operationalized will differ from facility to facility. We advocate, therefore, for the widespread adoption of the person-centered culture that maximizes, as much as possible, autonomy of and choices for older residents.

While routines are a fact of institutional life, owing to the large numbers of older adults that need care, we propose that routines continue to be relaxed to promote individuality within these facilities. When older adults have more control over how they regulate their daily activities, autonomy is promoted, which may then enhance mental health. In order to enhance the person-centered culture in long-term care (nursing *homes*), where the home is somewhat closer to the notion of "home" that older adults espouse, there would need to be *fewer policies* dictating routines and *more staff* to facilitate individual choice. Understandably, this will cost governments more money (or companies, for privatized nursing homes). However, residents and family members may be much happier and less likely to pursue legal avenues due to events where staff and residents are caught in conflict, trying to carry out institutional routines.

Single occupancy rooms

Also, we believe that there should be a move toward more single occupancy rooms within long-term care facilities (Lane, 2007). Not only can this decrease acts of aggression between roommates, particularly when individuals have dementia and misread the behavioral cues and intents of others, but single occupancy spaces allow for residents to personalize their space. Personal space promotes privacy in an environment where there is limited privacy. Residents can also exercise autonomy about when they want to watch TV or when they want the room lights out, for example, without concern about disturbing a roommate.

Presence of pets

As part of making long-term care less medicalized, more person-centered, and more like a home, we fully support the movement toward animals within facilities. In Chapter 4, we discussed the importance of pets for some aging adults living within their homes. In order to create a friendly, home-like environment within long-term care facilities, we advocate for resident cats, visits by dogs, or other options. While some facilities have animals that can be petted and lie on residents' laps, not all do. Additionally, some facilities have pets, generally cats or birds, which reside full-time in

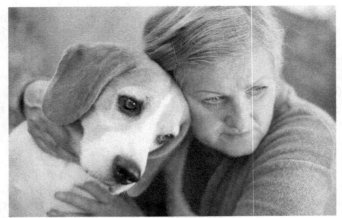

Halfpoint/Shutterstock, Inc.

the facility,[2] while others have animals, such as dogs, that come for time-limited visits. What is the impact of such programs upon aging residents?

In an interesting study, researchers compared the effects of dog visits (with a volunteer) as compared to human visits (Lutwack-Bloom, Wijewickrama, & Smith, 2005). By using the Geriatric Depression Scale and the Profile of Mood Disorders, the researchers compared residents in two facilities over a six-month period; one group received visits without a dog and the other group received visits from a volunteer who brought a dog. The results revealed that the residents who received regular visits from the dog showed a significant positive effect upon their mood. Further, the residents receiving dog visits also experienced improvement in depression, although the results were not significant (Lutwack-Bloom et al., 2005).

How do pets affect aging adults with Alzheimer's disease or related dementias? While there is limited research examining the impact of pets upon older adults with dementia, a couple of older studies address their effectiveness. Baun and McCabe (2003) suggested that dogs can be helpful for individuals with Alzheimer's disease who pace. They can go on walks with the dog, although someone else will actually have to handle the pet. They can also toss a ball or object to the dog to discharge the energy that is normally managed through pacing. Dogs are also known to calm the agi-

---

2. As a humorous note, in one long-term care facility, the live-in cat, named Bartholomew, is enjoyed so much by residents that he has become very obese ("Too many nibbles!" exclaimed one elderly woman). Signs were put up throughout the facility asking residents to avoid feeding him, as he had been put on a diet!

tated behaviors of those with Alzheimer's disease (McCabe, Baun, Speich, & Agrawal, 2002). Further, as language abilities become compromised in individuals with dementia, dogs will still maintain eye contact with the affected persons and provide companionship. When the aging adult with dementia becomes bedridden, a dog (or cat) can lie next to the person and provide warmth, security, and comfort (Baun & McCabe, 2003).

Beyond research results, anecdotal reports of the impact of animals upon older adults, particularly very vulnerable older adults, abound within the literature. Stories also emerge from clinical practice. I (AML) have one such anecdote. A number of years ago, I supervised a geriatric mental health unit. My husband (Dave) and I had a new dog—Suzie, a basset hound. Staff on my unit wanted to see her. One day near the end of the shift Dave brought Suzie up to the unit. Suzie was just a young puppy and Dave was carrying her in his arms. Suzie had the typical sad expression of the basset hound, facilitated in part by sad eyes set within square eye sockets (which gave the appearance of drunkenness), long floppy, soft ears, and gigantic paws (in relation to her size). A fair distance across the unit a patient spied Suzie. This woman had frontal lobe dementia and could be very verbally, and even physically, aggressive. Even though she was physically frail and used a cane, she shuffled amazingly quickly across the unit to us. Her normally hard and angry face appeared soft, even tender, and awestruck. She quietly, even reverently asked, "Where did you get that dog?" "How much did you pay for her?" As she gently petted Suzie and the three of us talked about her, the woman was kind, respectful, and truly serene. As Dave and I reflected upon the experience and shared what had happened with my sister (MBR) afterward, Marlette responded, "Suzie did the work of God that humans could not do." We agreed. The ability of Suzie to produce gentleness and serenity within this woman was in stark contrast to our best efforts as professionals. Suzie, as an innocent and gentle puppy, touched an area in this woman's heart and soul that was unreachable by professionals.

Costs

Another issue about long-term care facilities is cost. The cost of long-term care can vary between the United States and Canada, even between regions in the same country. Often, the difference in cost is related to whether the facility is private or public, with private facilities being more expensive than public ones. And differences in cost are also related to funding differences between the United States and Canada. However, even in Canada where health care is publicly funded, there can be differences in cost according to region. For instance, while the Canada Health Act covers medically required costs and some costs related to residency in long-term care, some aspects of life in facilities are left up to provinces and territories to determine what is funded (Fernandes & Spencer, 2010). And while provinces and territories foot a significant part of the cost of residency within long-term care facilities, there are some private costs that are assumed by residents and families. In their study examining long-term care cost disparities across Canada, Fernandes and Spencer (2010) found that private costs incurred were dependent upon where residents lived, their marital status, and income level. Thus, a single older adult living in Atlantic Canada with an average income will pay double the cost than his or her counterpart in Quebec. Further, a couple living in Newfoundland with one member in care will pay almost four times more than a similar couple in Alberta (Fernandes & Spencer, 2010). This means that even though a number of the costs of residency in long-term care facilities are covered for aging adults in Canada, the remaining costs may still be considerable for some living in the Atlantic region. Regardless of country or region, cost disparities for long-term care should be reduced and quality care should be available for all adults, irrespective of income.

Education for para-professionals

As mentioned earlier within this chapter, para-professionals within nursing homes should have regular education. This education should cover the issue of how to work with older adults with dementia, but also, how to work with sub-populations of older adults that may increasingly come into long-term care, such as the mentally ill, those with HIV/AIDS (Lane, Hirst, & Reed, 2013), older adults who have intellectual disabilities (Hirst, Lane, & Seneviratne, 2013) and aging individuals who are dying.

Housing Options for Sub-Populations of Older Adults

The above section addressed general issues related to housing for older adults. However, there is increased recognition about sub-populations that fall between the housing cracks. In light of this, we will discuss several sub-populations of older adults that require housing, but face access challenges. While some may question why housing should be provided for those who cannot afford it, housing and health are undeniably linked. If older adults do not have secure housing, their health suffers.

Shelters for older adults experiencing abuse

Abuse of older adults within developed countries is becoming more widely recognized (Solomon & Reingold, 2012). Sometimes aging individuals continue to live with an abusive relative, because the older person does not have anywhere else to go. In order to provide a safe place to flee, shelters for abused aging adults have opened. The first shelter to be opened in North America for abused older adults was the Kerby Rotary House in Calgary, Alberta, Canada (Special Senate Committee on Aging, 2009). However, since the opening of the Kerby Rotary House in Calgary, more shelters have sprung up across North America. These shelters may be housed within long-term care facilities (not-for-profit nursing homes in the United States) (Reingold, 2006; Solomon, 2006; Solomon & Reingold, 2012). Older adults receive crisis intervention, assistance from an interprofessional team, including legal advice, as well as housing (Reingold, 2006; Solomon, 2006). These services provide the space and opportunity for aging individuals to make decisions about future living options. More of these kinds of shelters need to be available for older adults, as many aging individuals do not feel comfortable in shelters that service younger, homeless adults.

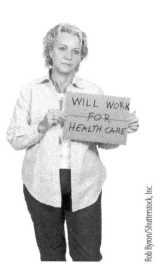

Rob Byron/Shutterstock, Inc.

Mentally ill older adults

Depending upon the geographical location, housing options for mentally ill older adults may be limited. If older, mentally ill individuals behave in a socially unacceptable manner, they may not be considered appropriate for assisted living facilities (Lane, 2011). Additionally, if mental illness has been persistent and severe over a number of years, they most likely do not have the money to afford an assisted living facility. Some older, mentally ill individuals have lived in precarious living situations for much of their lives; they may have spent time on the streets and in homeless shelters, as well as lived in unsuitable apartments for short periods of time.

At some point in time, mentally ill older adults may be brought to hospital for a mental health assessment. If deemed to be mentally or physically unable to care for themselves, these individuals may be admitted to hospital for further assessment and planning for alternate housing arrangements. As discussed in Chapter 3, however, finding appropriate living arrangements for these older adults can be difficult. Assisted living facilities may be reluctant to accept those with mental illness out of concern that these individuals may be too disruptive (Lane, 2011). Although living in a group home could be an option, depending upon the geographical location, availability may be an issue.

Further, long-term care facilities may be reluctant to accept older adults with mental illness. In my doctoral research, I (AML) examined the process of placing older adults from hospital mental health units in a western Canadian city into long-term care facilities (Lane, 2007). Staff working on mental health units (physicians, nurses, social workers) spoke about the difficulty of placing older adults, due in part to the reluctance of staff in these facilities to accept them. The professionals on hospital units discussed how some staff within long-term care facilities expressed fear that those with mental illness are violent.

Professionals who were interviewed also described how the requirements of placement, in terms of the degree of physical and cognitive incapacitation necessary for long-term care, precluded this option. Ironically, some older adults with mental illness are too well to be admitted to facilities, and too ill (mentally) to live independently. By virtue of being able to dress themselves, eat independently, and take care of bodily functions, they do not fit the requisites (as stipulated by assessment forms) to be placed (Lane, McCoy, & Ewashen, 2010). We propose that exceptions to the usual requirements of long-term care placement (extreme physical and functional difficulties) need to be made for those with mental illness in order to ensure that they have safe housing (Lane, 2011).

We also suggest that within larger urban settings, some long-term care units be designated for older adults with mental illness. This would promote ongoing staff education for those working with individuals with such issues. Education would not only include the pathophysiology of mental illness, but also how to respond to the behavioral manifestations of mental illness, such as the delusional utterances of residents. Education may decrease apprehension to work with this sub-population of older adults and may therefore enhance the retention of staff.

Older adults with intellectual disabilities

As discussed in Chapter 7, some individuals with intellectual disabilities are now living into their 50s and 60s, which for this population is considered old (Hirst et al., 2013). According to the American Association on Intellectual and Developmental Disabilities (2013), the term *intellectual disability* refers to "significant limitations in intellectual functioning" and in "adaptive behaviors." This term is commonly used for disorders such as Down syndrome. The loss of a parent is often the impetus for placement of older adults with intellectual disabilities. As noted in Chapter 7, however, family members often fear placement, wondering about how the aging adult with an intellectual disability will adjust. The concerns are well-founded, because group homes for individuals with intellectual disabilities are often geared for younger adults and workers may lack knowledge of how aging and dementia impacts their clients. Similarly, staff in long-term care facilities may be uncertain of how to effectively work with someone with an intellectual disability. With the growth in this sub-population of older adults, staff working in group homes need education on how aging and dementia impact their clients, and staff in long-term care should receive education on how to provide effective care to aging individuals with intellectual disabilities. Further, as individuals with intellectual disabilities often have trouble communicating and describing sensations or symptoms experienced, it is imperative that staff are educated on how to patiently and astutely assess these clients (Hirst et al., 2013).

Further, future directions should also include research on what kinds of living environments are best suited for aging individuals with intellectual disabilities. If one kind of setting is deemed to be more effective than another (for example, group homes considered better than long-term care facilities), then this type of living option could be designated for aging individuals with intellectual disabilities. This would not only promote staff education, but might also enhance the comfort level of individuals with intellectual disabilities, as others around them would be similar in age and also understand their functional deficits.

Homeless older adults

Older age in homeless adults is often considered to be about 50 years of age (Donley, 2010); this benchmark can vary, however, depending upon the researcher or clinician; for some, the suggested older age may range from 50 to 65 years of age (Brown & Steinman, 2013). The criteria for old age is set earlier, as the stress of living on the streets results in premature aging and problems such as cardiac disease, diabetes, respiratory problems, and communicable diseases, as well as substance abuse and mental illness (Brown & Steinman, 2013). Older adults who are homeless may have been homeless for many years (perhaps due to issues such as severe mental illness) or may have become homeless in later life.

When individuals become homeless in later life, this is generally related to marital breakdown, alcoholism, widowhood, death of a family member (Gonyea, Mills-Dick, & Bachman, 2010), and sometimes, retirement (in particular, when housing is attached to employment). Homeless older adults who are in their 50s are in a particularly vulnerable situation, because they are not eligible for full government pensions (Donley, 2010). They also tend to have many more health problems than their younger homeless counterparts (Kushel, 2012). This sub-population of older adults has been relatively invisible for policymakers, professionals who work in programs for the homeless, and health care providers (Gonyea et al., 2010). However, with the burgeoning of the older adult population in developed countries, the homeless older adult population is expected to grow.

In order to address the complex challenges of homeless older adults, there needs to be better communication between governmental departments, both *within* state (or provincial) governments and also *between* state/provincial and federal governments. Departments responsible for services that assist individuals to remain in their homes should collaborate with the departments responsible for housing in order to develop policies that enhance the chances of these individuals to be housed. For instance, in one Canadian study, the researchers examined the impact of a housing program to assist older adults who were homeless or at risk of becoming homeless (e.g., being evicted due to living in squalor) (Ploeg, Hayward, Woodward, & Johnston, 2008). The housing support workers in the program found that older adults who were at risk of being evicted from current living environments could not access appropriate homemakers to clean their apartments. They were therefore at risk for eviction. If they had been able to access appropriate homemaking services (prior to the cuts to services), their home environments might have been clean enough to avert eviction. Thus, a lack of coordination between government departments/programs works against vulnerable, homeless, or nearly homeless, older adults (Ploeg et al., 2008).

Additionally, there needs to be more low-income housing available within the United States, Canada, and other developed countries (Gonyea et al., 2010; Kushel, 2012; Ploeg et al., 2008). Typically, there are long wait lists to access low-income housing (Donley, 2010; Ploeg et al., 2008). This is problematic, as older homeless adults cannot, or may not necessarily want to, access the shelters that their younger counterparts use. They may not be eligible for shelters accommodating women with young children, and they may fear exposure to illness and violence at shelters for the general adult population. Further, McDonald, Dergal, and Cleghorn (2007) suggested that the housing needs of the recently homeless elderly should be addressed quickly in order to prevent these individuals from becoming rooted in the homeless life.

In general, housing options for vulnerable older adults (not including the situation of incarcerated seniors that will be discussed momentarily) need to be affordable and available in both urban and rural locations (in order that vulnerable seniors can remain close to their support systems, such as family and friends) (Weeks & LeBlanc, 2010). Housing should be suitable for the health and social situations of the elderly adults, so that those with disabilities can live as independently as possible, for as long as possible. Further, services should be available and affordable that aging adults can maintain their homes (Weeks & LeBlanc, 2010).

Dying older adults

Currently only a small percentage of dying older adults receive specialized palliative care (Lee, Coakley, Dahlin, & Carleton, 2009). For instance in Canada, depending upon the region, only 16–30% of dying individuals have access to palliative care (Canadian Hospice Palliative Care Association, 2012). As we have emphasized in this text, the population of developed countries is living longer, so providing appropriate holistic care to dying people is vital. Not only is it vital, we suggest that such provision of care during dying is a basic human right. That being said, owing to the pressures on the health care systems in developed countries, some are skeptical that such care will be delivered to more aging individuals. Scottish geriatrician Colin Douglas (1992) caused a great stir in the United Kingdom when he said, "The hospice movement is too good to be true and too small to be useful" (p. 579).

A number of studies have called for better palliative methods in a number of different settings (Arnup, 2013; Field & Addington-Hall, 2000; Sidell, Samson Katz, & Komaromy, 2000). The variety of settings for palliative care is growing. For instance, in North America, there are a number of options for palliative care in different settings: free standing residential hospices, hospices attached to nursing homes, palliative wards within hospitals, hospices within the hospital setting, and palliative home care. Often, however, these services are generally available in large urban centers, with few options in smaller towns. Like others, we believe that palliative care must be accessible for those in rural settings, not just for dying older adults in larger cities (Ley & van Bommel, 1994). Further, comprehensive palliative care should reach into the worlds of those who are sequestered from the mainstream, such as the incarcerated (addressed later in this chapter) as well as those who are marginalized (Ley & van Bommel, 1994), such as the mentally ill (Kissane & Kelly, 2000) and those with intellectual disabilities.

As a number of North American older adults will die in long-term care facilities on the units where they have resided for years, there is a recognition that effective palliative care needs to be provided.[3] However, for this to occur, much education needs to take place on multiple levels. First, there needs to be greater awareness of what palliative care entails and who is entitled to this type of care. Predominantly, palliative care is still conceptualized as measures taken at the end of a *cancer* patient's life (Sidell et al., 2000), though many Canadian and American hospices have patients with a variety of terminal conditions residing therein. Also, in the United States the definition of palliative care includes comfort measures for those with serious illness who are not dying (Jackson, 2015). The health care community and the public needs to become aware about the importance of multifaceted care for older adults and ask for it. Second, staff need to be prepared to deal effectively with their palliative patients. In all health settings where the dying are present—home, hospitals, long-term care facilities—staff need to be able to recognize the signs of pain and delirium and deal with them (Nunn, 2014). They need to have the skills and presence to speak to and be with dying people and their families (Benner Carson & Koenig, 2004; Reed, 2014; Ryan, 2005). And they need to have resources to turn to, when they encounter situations they cannot handle on their own, such as in the case of specialized medical needs, or complex spiritual distress (Benner Carson & Koenig, 2004; Reed, 2014).

In this day and age of monetary pressures on health care systems, can this be done? Sidell and colleagues (2000) believed this aspiration to be attainable. Others put it more strongly: "[P]alliative care is the only moral, intellectual and practical way forward" (George & Sykes, 1997, p. 252). Despite the hopefulness and moral imperatives implied by these comments offered decades ago, there is still much to be done to operationalize palliative care for older adults.

Incarcerated older adults

As mentioned in Chapter 2, there is a sub-population of older adults within the prison systems of the United States, Canada, and other developed

---

3. An American study cited that 30% of older adults dying in long-term care facilities within the US have accessed some hospice services (Unroe et al., 2013)

countries that have been incarcerated for years. These adults are usually in their 50s, but are considered to be old due to the health problems that they have related to lifestyle choices (e.g., smoking) and incarceration (Higgins & Severson, 2009).

Prisons were not designed for older inmates, so the current living environments are unsuitable for some older prisoners (Duffin, 2010). They may need walkers or wheelchairs, oxygen, raised toilet seats, commodes, and hospital beds (Duffin, 2010). The doorways may be too small for older prisoners to navigate through with a wheelchair. The noise of the prison may be confusing and upsetting for those with Alzheimer's disease or other types of dementia.

Public policies should address issues of safety for aging prisoners. For instance, prisons need to make accommodations to help older adults navigate through the hallways safely. There also need to be changes in routine to accommodate older inmates, such as affording them a longer time span to get to the dining room or allowing them to bring food back to their cell if they are unable to finish their meals. Hearing-impaired inmates may have trouble with noise at visiting times, so they can be accommodated by situating them away from other prisoners and their visitors (Sumner, 2012). Other important adaptations include large-print informational brochures that enable sight-impaired older inmates to receive the information they need, as well as large-print books (Sumner, 2012). Additionally, there should be educational and recreational programs designed specifically for older adults, rather than expecting older adults to fit into programs designed for healthier and stronger inmates (Snyder, van Wormer, Chadha, & Jaggers, 2009).

As part of policy and procedure, older inmates need regular preventive health care and screening. Some authors suggest screening upon entry to the prison (if 55 years of age or older) and yearly screening thereafter for sensory impairment (sight, hearing) and dementia (Williams et al., 2012). Women need regular mammography and cervical screening (Duffin, 2010). Stress management programs are also recommended (Smyer & Burbank, 2009).

Prison units that are designated for physically frail individuals or for older adults may be helpful and desirable for some (Smyer & Burbank, 2009). The units can include adaptations such as handrails, wheelchair accessible ramps, and showers. As noted by Williams and colleagues (2012), however, older prisoners should have a choice as to whether they want to be placed within these units or stay within the general population. Although they could have easier access to assistance in the geriatric unit, they may prefer to stay with their friends (Williams et al., 2012).

Some older adults will be released from prison into general society. If they have spent years in prison, they are generally unprepared to reintegrate into everyday life; they often have little education, few job skills, and may have no family (Smyer & Burbank, 2009). Months prior to release, there should be regular consultation between the prison officer who is responsible for resettlement, the prison health care department, and the parole officer (Sumner, 2012). Transitional work should involve helping older inmates connect with health care, social services, and case management in the community prior to their release. Then, when in the community, follow-up should occur to make certain that older adults have accessed services and support (Roberts, Kennedy, & Hammett, 2004).

A number of older inmates die within the prison, and as the older population within correctional facilities grows, more are expected to die within custody. In response to this reality, there is beginning recognition within the literature that better palliative care services are needed within the correctional system (Reviere & Young, 2004). Even when prisons have some kind of end-of-life care, most likely the number of services offered will be fewer than those offered through hospice care in the community (Turner, Payne, & Barbarachild, 2011). Staff in both areas—palliative care and corrections—may feel intimated about the challenges in providing care to the dying incarcerated. Health care staff in prisons often have little experience in palliative care, and sometimes even less experience in grief and spiritual support, thus requiring education and guidance in providing end-of-life care (Turner et al., 2011). Prison staff may also be concerned about dying prisoners distributing pain medication to other prisoners, either because they are pressured or for the money. As such, there should be an interface between hospice care and prison health care to facilitate the care of aging, dying prisoners within custody (Turner et al., 2011). In the United States, the National Prison Hospice Association was established in the 1990s to address the issues of prisoners dying with AIDS and standards of practice were formulated; however, this is not the case for all developed countries (Bolger, 2005).

Aging prisoners who are very frail may be given compassionate release and discharged early to a long-term care facility if very frail or to a hospice, if terminally ill (Duffin, 2010). Compassionate release may be given when the prison environment is believed to cause serious deleterious effects to the physical or mental health of the aging prisoner. However, as noted by Beckett and colleagues (2003), the early release of prisoners for compassionate reasons is controversial; the general population may question why grace is extended to individuals who have committed violent crimes, even if committed decades earlier. Also, receiving institutions, such as long-term care facilities, may be reluctant to accept released prisoners (Beckett, Peternelj-Taylor, & Johnson, 2003).

Support for Families (Caregivers)

As illustrated throughout this text, family members provide much care, and expend much physical and emotional energy in caring for their aging members. They truly provide the bulk of care for aging individuals (Arnup, 2013; Special Senate Committee Report on Aging, 2009). Although provision of care by family members helps maintain bonds between older members and their spouses/adult children/relatives, and friends, it is not without cost to the caregivers. As recognized in the 1990s by the proliferation of research conducted on caregiver burden, caregiving for older adults—whether they are experiencing cognitive, physical, or mental challenges—exacts a toll. With the burgeoning of the older adult population, in concert with fewer adult children available to care for aging parents (from factors such as decreased birth rates, increased geographical mobility, and increased numbers of women in the workforce), the stress upon family caregivers may become greater. This is particularly the case when family caregivers themselves are elderly, whether they are spouses or adult children. Not only do family caregivers need supportive services such as respite care for older adults (Special Senate Committee Report on Aging, 2009), they also need direct support themselves, through support groups (e.g., Alzheimer Society chapters), telephone-based support (Glueckauf et al., 2007), and financial support for caregiving (as provided by other countries, such as the Netherlands, Germany, the United Kingdom, and Australia) (Special Senate Committee Report on Aging, 2009).

Further, it is imperative that nurses and other professionals provide supportive understanding for caregivers, especially aging caregivers as they make decisions for their younger, yet aging children. Aging caregivers of adult children with severe mental illness and intellectual disabilities (Gilbert, Lankshear, & Petersen, 2008) often struggle greatly regarding the decision to place their children, when relocation becomes a reality. Professionals need to respond to these diligent parents with gracious awareness of their commitment to their children, balancing the impact that caregiving may be having on their health and their abilities to provide care to their children.

Advocacy: By Older Adults for Older Adults and the Vulnerable

The importance of advocating for vulnerable populations cannot be overstated. Some older adults feel marginalized and believe that government and society are not recognizing their issues and strengths. For instance, 60% of older adults in the UK believe that there is age discrimination (Age Concern and Help the Aged, 2009). Sixty-eight percent of older adults in the UK believe that politicians do not give priority to the issues of older adults. Further, 76% of UK adults believe that their talents and skills are not being recognized or used by their country (Age Concern and Help the Aged, 2009).

Generally speaking, we tend to assume that the role of advocacy is assumed by health or human service professionals or by younger adults, and certainly, this is important. However, we propose that *advocacy for older adults be conducted by older adults*. Older adults can advocate for changes to housing options for older adults, as well as for other conditions that impact their age cohort. The beauty of older adults advocating for other older adults is multifold. First, in this way older adults are involved in meaningful activities that add purpose to their lives (and hence address some existential issues). Second, older adults can experientially understand some of the issues faced by older adults. While they may not be homeless or have a particular illness or condition, they can understand the changes that occur with aging and how illness or other challenging circumstances could impact the changes they have encountered with aging. Third, by virtue of being retired or working part-time, older adults may have more time for advocacy than middle-aged adults.

An interesting example of older adults advocating for older adults includes grandmothers in Canada advocating for grandmothers in Africa. In the *Grandmothers to Grandmothers* campaign, Canadian grandmothers advocate for African women who are raising their grandchildren, due to their adult children dying from AIDS. These older women have gone to Parliament to advocate for the responsibility of Canada to send medications to Africa to assist in the AIDS crisis (see http://grandmothers campaign.org). Another example involves older adults advocating for homeless older adults. In the early 1990s, seven older woman who had had extensive experience in housing, health, and human services pooled their knowledge and formed the Committee to End Elder Homelessness in the United States (Gonyea et al., 2010). In 2005 the name of this organization was changed to Hearth, Inc. This organization offers over 100 long-term supportive housing units for formerly homeless older adults in the Boston area (Gonyea et al., 2010).

Older adults may also advocate for those who are aging by participating in a movement toward making cities age-friendly (as discussed in Chapter 4). An interesting example of this was offered by McGarry and Morris (2011). They described how Manchester, England, was chosen by the World Health Organization (WHO) in 2010 to sign a commitment to move toward being an age-friendly city (after they had established a *Valuing Older People* program). Since the establishment of the *Valuing Older People* program, as well as making the agreement with WHO, aging individuals have taken an active, consultant role in project design and delivery to make Manchester a more age-friendly city for older adults. They have and are currently partnering with community agencies, being active leaders in the process (McGarry & Morris, 2011).

Advocacy roles for older adults can be for other vulnerable populations besides those who are aging, and these "populations" do not necessarily have to be human. Recreational staff within assisted living facilities (whose residents tend to be stronger physically) can arrange a dog assistance program. Within such a program, aging adults may volunteer weekly to walk dogs that are currently staying in an animal shelter. Not only do these older adults get exercise, they share in the camaraderie of working together for the good of vulnerable animals. Hence, this activity addresses physical, social, and existential needs.

SUMMARY

Older adults experiencing transitions can be very vulnerable. How health and human service professionals respond to their health needs, their psychological needs as they progress through the transitions, the issues regarding relocation for older adults and their family members, as well as their concerns about life's meaning, can impact how older adults experience their transitions. Becoming aware of the significance of transitions for older adults as well as the challenges involved in these transitions can better equip health and human service professionals to respond in meaningful and effective ways. However, changes need to be made in service delivery, the education of health care professionals, as well as in the development of policies and procedures at a governmental, as well as service level, if the needs of older adults experiencing transitions are to be adequately addressed in the coming years with the significant growth of the aged population. All of this ideally occurring within a society that becomes more attuned to and valuing of older adults, will allow old age to be a "new stage of opportunity and strength" (Betty Friedan).

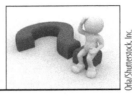

CRITICAL THINKING EXERCISES

▶ Review the case example of Bertha and Jake again. If you were the nurse assessing this couple, what conclusions would you come to in terms of placement options?

▶ Consider where you live. What does your state/province and municipality have for services for individuals such as Bertha and Jake?

INTERESTING WEBSITES

▶ Grandmothers to Grandmothers Campaign: http://grandmotherscampaign.org

▶ i2i Intergenerational Society: http://www.intergenerational.ca/

▶ Road Scholar—Intergenerational Programs: http://www.roadscholar.org/programs/intergenerational_default.asp

▶ WHO Age Friendly Cities: http://www.who.int/ageing/projects/age_friendly_cities/en/

REFERENCES

Age Concern and Help the Aged. (2009). *One voice: Shaping our aging society*. Retrieved January 12, 2015, from: www.ageuk.org.uk

Allemand, M., Steiner, M., & Hill, P. (2013). Effects of a forgiveness intervention for older adults. *Journal of Counseling Psychology, 60*(2), 279–286.

American Association on Intellectual and Developmental Disabilities (2013). Retrieved February 8, 2015, from: http://aaidd.org/intellectual-disability/definition#.VNfb- 005CUk

Arnup, K. (2013). *Death, dying and Canadian families*. Ottawa, ON: Vanier Institute.

Australian Government Department of Human Services. (2015). Retrieved March 30, 2015, from: http://www.humanservices.gov.au/customer/services/centrelink/age-pension

Averill, J. B. (2012). Priorities for action in a rural older adults study. *Family & Community Health, 35*(4), 358–372. doi:10.1097/FCH.0b013e318266686.e

Barron, J. S., Tan, E. J., Yu, Q., Song, M., McGill, S., & Fried, L. P. (2009). Potential for intensive volunteering to promote the health of older adults in fair health. *Journal of Urban Health: Bulletin of the New York Academy of Medicine, 86*(4), 641–653. doi:10.1007/s11524-009-9353-8

Baun, M. M., & McCabe, B. W. (2003). Companion animals and persons with dementia of the Alzheimer's type: Therapeutic possibilities. *American Behavioral Scientist, 47*(1), 42–51. doi:10.1177/0002764203255211

Beckett, J., Peternelj-Taylor, C., & Johnson, R. L. (2003). Growing old in the correctional system. *Journal of Psychosocial Nursing & Mental Health Services, 41*(9), 12–18.

Benner Carson, V., & Koenig, H. G. (2004). *Spiritual caregiving: Healthcare as a ministry.* Philadelphia: Templeton Foundation Press.

Biggs, M. J., & Knox, K. S. (2014). Lessons learned from an intergenerational volunteer program: A case study of a shared life model. *Journal of Interpersonal Relationships, 12*(1), 54–68. doi:10.1080/15350770.2014.869981

Bocker, E., Glasser, M., Nielsen, K., & Weidenbacher-Hoper, V. (2012). Rural older adults' mental health: status and challenges in care delivery. *Rural and Remote Health, 12*(4), 1–13. www.rrh.org.au

Bolger, M. (2005). Dying in prison: Providing palliative care in challenging environments. *International Journal of Palliative Nursing, 11*(12), 619–621.

Brown, R. T., & Steinman, M. A. (2013). Characteristics of emergency department visits by older adults versus younger homeless adults in the United States. *American Journal of Public Health, 103*(6), 1046–1051. doi:10.2105/AJPH2012.301006

Bulbrook, K. M., Carey, T. A., Lenthall, S., Byers, L., & Behan, K. P. (2012). Treating mental health in remote communities: What do remote health practitioners need? *Rural and Remote Health, 12*(4), 1–3. www.rrh.org.au

Canadian Hospice Palliative Care Association (2012). Fact sheet: Hospice palliative care in Canada. Canadian Hospice Palliative Care Association. Retrieved February 2, 2015, from: http://www.chpca.net/media/7622/fact_sheet_hpc_in_canada_may_2012_final.pdf

Cattan, M., Kime, N., & Bagnall, A. M. (2011). The use of telephone befriending in low level support for socially isolated older people—an evaluation. *Health and Social Care in the Community, 19*(2), 198–206. doi:10.1111/j.1365-2524.2010.00967.x

Choi, N. G., & Jun, J. (2009). Life regrets and pride among low-income older adults: Relationships with depressive symptoms, current life stressors and coping resources. *Aging & Mental Health, 13*(2), 213–225. doi:10.1080/13607860802342235

Clark, A. M., Freydberg, N., Heath, S. L., Savard, L., McDonald, M., & Strain, L. (2008). The potential of nursing to reduce the burden of heart failure in rural Canada: What strategies should nurses prioritize? *Canadian Journal of Cardiovascular Nursing, 18*(4), 40–46.

Cooper, C. (2011). Jefferson Area Board for Aging intergenerational programs in development. *Journal of Intergenerational Relationships, 9*(4), 481–484. doi: 10.1080/15350770.2011.619914

Copen, C. (2006). Welfare reform: Challenges of grandparents raising grandchildren. *Journal of Aging & Social Policy, 18* (3/4), 193–209. doi:10.1300/J031v18n03_13

Dahlke, S., & Phinney, A. (2008). Caring for hospitalized older adults at risk for delirium: The silent, unspoken piece of nursing practice. *Journal of Gerontological Nursing, 34*(6), 41–47.

Demeris, G., Doorenbos, A. Z., & Towle, C. (2009). Ethical considerations regarding the use of technology for older adults: The case of telehealth. *Research in Gerontological Nursing, 2*(2), 128–136.

Donley, A. M. (2010). Sunset years in sunny Florida: Experiences of homelessness among the elderly. *Case Management Journals, 11*(4), 239–244. doi:10.1891/1521-0987.11.4.239

Douglas, C. (1992). For all the saints. *British Medical Journal,* (February 29), *304,* 579.

Duffin, C. (2010). Doing time: Health care in the criminal justice system. *Nursing Older People, 22*(10), 14–18.

Fernandes, N., & Spencer, B. G. (2010). The private cost of long-term care in Canada: Where you live matters. *Canadian Journal on Aging, 29*(3), 307–316. doi:10.1017/S0714980810000346

Field, D., & Addington-Hall, J. (2000). Extending specialized palliative care to all? In D. Dickinson, M. Johnson, and J. Samson Katz (Eds.), *Death, dying and bereavement* (pp. 91–106). London: Sage.

Forbes, D. A., & Edge, D. S. (2009). Canadian home care policy and practice in rural and remote settings: Challenges and solutions. *Journal of Agromedicine, 14*(2), 119–124. doi:10.1080/10599240902724135

Fox, A. (2010). HomeShare—An intergenerational solution to housing and support needs. *Housing, Care and Support, 13*(3), 21–26. doi:10.5042/hcs.2010.0707

Galvin, J. E., Meuser, T. M., & Morris, J. C. (2012). Improving physician awareness of Alzheimer disease and enhancing recruitment: The Clinician Partners Program. *Alzheimer Disease and Associated Disorders, 26*(1), 61–67. doi:10.1097/WAD.0b013e3182c0df

George, D., Whitehouse, C., & Whitehouse, P. (2011). A model of intergenerativity: How the model of intergenerational school is bringing the generations together to foster collective wisdom and community health. *Journal of Intergenerational Relationships, 9*(4), 389–404. doi:10.1080/15350770.2011.619922

George, R., & Sykes, J. (1997). Beyond cancer. In S. Ahmehdzai, D. Clark, and J. Hockley (Eds.), *New themes in palliative care* (pp. 239–254). Buckingham: Open University Press.

Gilbert, A., Lankshear, G., & Petersen, A. (2008). Older family-carers' views on future accommodation needs of relatives who have an intellectual disability. *International Journal of Social Welfare, 17*(1), 54–64. doi:10.1111/j.1468-2397.2007.00485.x

Glueckauf, R. L., Sharma, D., Davis, W. S., Byrd, V., Stine, C., Jeffers, S. B., Massey, A., et al. (2007). Telephone-based cognitive-behavioral intervention for distressed rural dementia caregivers: Initial findings. *Clinical Gerontologist, 31*(1), 21–41. doi:10.1300/J018v31n01_03

Gonyea, J. G., Mills-Dick, K., & Bachman, S. S. (2010). The complexities of elder homelessness, a shifting political landscape and emerging community responses. *Journal of Gerontological Social Work, 53*(7), 575–590. doi:10.1080/01634372.2010.510169

Heimpel, D. (2011). A hub of innovation in Easthampton. *CWLA, 20*, 4.

Higgins, D., & Severson, M. (2009). Community reentry and older adult offenders: Redefining social work roles. *Journal of Gerontological Social Work, 52*(8), 784–802. doi:10.1080/01634370902888618

Hirst, S. P. (2010). *Health promotive technologies: Life in my own home.* NGNA National Conference, Palm Springs, CA.

Hirst, S. P., Lane, A. M., & Seneviratne, C. C. (2013). Growing old with a developmental disability. *Indian Journal of Gerontology, 27*(1), 38–54.

Hirst, S. P., Lane, A. M., & Stares, B. (2012). Gerontological content in Canadian nursing and social work programs. *Canadian Geriatrics Journal, 15*(1), 8–15. doi:http://dx.doi.org/10.5770/cgj.15.21

Jackson, V. (2015). Navigating discussions of prognosis: Balancing honesty with hope. Schwartz Center Webinar Series (January 13, 2015). Information available at www.theschwartzcenter.org/media/Navigating-Discussions-of-Prognosis-HANDOUT.pdf

Kaasalainen, S., Coker, E., Dolovich, L., Papaioannou, A., Hadjistavropoulos, T., Emili, A., & Ploeg, J. (2007). Pain management decision making among long-term care physicians and nurses. *Western Journal of Nursing Research, 29*(5), 561–580. doi:10.1177/0193945906295522

Kang, H. G., Mahoney, D. F., Hoenig, H., Hirth, V. A., Bonato, P., Hajjar, I., & Lipsitz, L. A. (2010). In situ monitoring of health in older adults: Technologies and issues. *Journal of the American Geriatrics Society, 58*(8), 1579–1586. doi:10.1111/j.1532-5415.2010.02959.x

Kato, A. (2009). The relationship between aged parents and cohabiting unmarried children: Results from the Tokorozawa Living Arrangement study. *Journal of Intergenerational Relationships, 7*(1), 78–83. doi:10.1080/15350770802629032

Kennedy, C. (2010). The city of 2050—An age-friendly, vibrant, intergenerational community. *Generations, 34*(3), 70–75.

Kissane, D. W., & Kelly, B. J. (2000). Demoralisation, depression and desire for death: Problems with the Dutch guidelines for euthanasia of the mentally ill. *Australian and New Zealand Journal of Psychiatry, 34*(2), 325–333. doi:10.1046/j.1440-1614.2000.00692.x

Kushel, M. (2012). Older homeless adults: Can we do more? *Journal of General Internal Medicine, 27*(1), 5–6.

Landau, R., Auslander, G. K., Werner, S., Shoval, N., & Heinik, J. (2011). Who should make the decision on the use of GPS for people with dementia? *Aging & Mental Health, 15*(1), 78–84. doi:10.1080/13607861003713166

Lane, A. M. (2007). *The social organization of placement in geriatric mental health.* Unpublished doctoral dissertation, University of Calgary.

Lane, A. M. (2011). Placement of older adults from hospital mental health units into nursing homes: Exploration of the process, system issues, and implications. *Journal of Gerontological Nursing, 37*(2), 49–55.

Lane, A. M., & Hirst, S. P. (2012). Placement of undergraduate students in nursing homes: Careful consideration versus convenience. *Journal of Nursing Education, 51*(3), 145–149. doi:10.3928/01484834-20120127-04

Lane, A. M., Hirst, S. P., & Reed, M. B. (2013). Housing options for North American older adults with HIV/AIDS. *Indian Journal of Gerontology, 27*(1), 55–68.

Lane, A. M., McCoy, L., & Ewashen, C. (2010). The textual organization of placement into long term care: Issues for older adults with mental illness. *Nursing Inquiry, 17*(1), 3–14. doi:10.1111/j.1440-1800.2009.00470.x

Lee, S. M., Coakley, E. E., Dahlin, C., & Carleton, P. F. (2009). An evidence-based nursing program in geropalliative care. *Journal of Continuing Education in Nursing, 40*(12), 536–542.

Ley, D., & van Bommel, H. (1994). *The heart of hospice.* Toronto: NC Press Limited.

Li, H. (2006). Rural older adults' access barriers to in-home and community-based services. *Social Work Research, 30*(2), 109–118.

Li, H., Kyrouac, G. A., McManus, D. Q., Cranston, R. E., & Hughes, S. (2012). Unmet home care service needs of rural older adults with Alzheimer's disease: A perspective of informal caregivers. *Journal of Gerontological Social Work, 55*(5), 409–425. doi:10.1080/01634372.2011.650318

Lutwack-Bloom, P., Wijewickrama, R., & Smith, B. (2005). Effects of pets versus people visits with nursing home residents. *Journal of Gerontological Social Work, 44*(3–4), 137–159. doi:10.1300/J083v44n03_09

MacCallum, J., Palmer, D., Wright, P., Cumming-Potvin, W., Brooker, M., et al. (2010). Australian perspectives: Community building through intergenerational exchange programs. *Journal of Interpersonal Relationships, 8*(2), 113–127. doi:10.1080/15350771003741899

MacEwan, A. (2012). *Working after age 65: What is at stake?* Alternative federal budget 2012 technical paper. Canadian Centre for Policy Alternatives. Retrieved March 30, 2015, from: https://www.policyalternatives.ca/publications/reports/working-after-age-65

Margolis, S. A. (2012). Is fly in/fly out (FIFO) a viable interim solution to address remote medical workforce shortages? *Rural and Remote Health, 12*(3), 1–6. www.rrh.org.au

Mattimore, H. (2006). Agency briefs: It takes an intergenerational village to raise kids in care. *Children's Voice, 15*(4), 6.

McCabe, B. W., Baun, M. M., Speich, D., & Agrawal, S. (2002). A resident dog in the special care unit: Its effect on problem behaviors of persons with AD. *Western Journal of Nursing Research, 24*(6), 684–696. doi:10.1177/019394502320555421

McDonald, L., Dergal, J., & Cleghorn, L. (2007). Living on the margins: Older homeless adults in Toronto. *Journal of Gerontological Social Work, 49*(1/2), 19–46. doi:10.1300/J083v49n01_02

McGarry, P., & Morris, J. (2011). A great place to grow older: A case study of how Manchester is developing an age-friendly city. *Working with Older People, 15*(1), 38–46. doi:10.5042/wwop.2011.0119

Mihailidis, A., Cockburn, A., Longley, C., & Boger, J. (2008). The acceptability of home monitoring technology among community-dwelling older adults and baby boomers. *Assistive Technology, 20*(1), 1–12.

Morrow-Howell, N. (2010). Volunteering in later life: Research frontiers. *Journal of Gerontology: Social Sciences, 65B*(4), 461–469. doi:10.1093/geronb/gbq024

Mukherjee, D. (2010). An exploratory study of older adults' engagement with virtual volunteerism. *Journal of Technology in Human Services, 28*(3), 188–196. doi:10.1080/15228835.2010.508368

Ng, C. F., Northcott, H. C., & Abu-Laban, S. M. (2007). Housing and living arrangements of south Asian immigrant seniors in Edmonton, AB. *Canadian Journal on Aging, 26*(3), 185–194. doi:10.3138/cja.26.3.185

Niemeyer, S. M., Cook, C. C., Memken, J., Crull, S., Bruin, M., Laux, S., White, B. J., & Yust, B. (2006). Local housing and service decisions: Planning for aging adults. *Journal of Housing for the Elderly, 20*(4), 5–22. doi:10.1300/J081v20n04_02

Nunn, C. (2014). It's not just about pain: Symptom management in palliative care. *Nurse Prescribing, 12*(7), 338–344.

Peterson, L. E., Bazemore, A., Bragg, E. J., Xierali, I., & Warshaw, G. A. (2011). Rural-urban distribution of U.S. geriatrics physician workforce. *Journal of the American Geriatrics Society, 59*(4), 699–703. doi:10.1111/j.1532-5415.2011.03335.x

Ploeg, J., Hayward, L., Woodward, C., & Johnston, R. (2008). A case study of a Canadian homelessness intervention programme for elderly people. *Health and Social Care in the Community, 16*(6), 593–605. doi:10.1111/j.1365-2524.2008.00783.x

Poindexter, C. C. (2007). Older persons parenting children who have lost a parent due to HIV. *Journal of Intergenerational Relationships, 5*(4), 77–95. doi:10.1300/J194v05n04_06

Power, M. B., Mitchell, E., Eheart, B. K., & Hopping, D. (2011). The power of language: Practice in a shared site. *Journal of Intergenerational Relationships, 9*(3), 281–292. doi:10.1080/15350770.2011.593438

Ramsay, J. L. (2008). Forgiveness and healing in later life. *Generations, 32*(2), 51–54.

Reed, M. B. (2014). Me and my shadow: Interprofessional training in and modeling of spiritual care in the palliative setting, *Indian Journal of Gerontology,* (November), *28*(4), 501–518.

Reingold, D. A. (2006). An elder abuse shelter program. *Journal of Gerontological Social Work, 46*(3–4), 123–135. doi:10.1300/J083v46n03_07

Reviere, R., & Young, V. D. (2004). Aging behind bars: Health care for older female inmates. *Journal of Women & Aging, 16*(1/2), 55–69. doi:10.1300/J074v16n01_05

Rhoades, D. R., & McFarland, K. F. (1999). Caregiver meaning: A study of caregivers of individuals with mental illness. *Health & Social Work, 24*(4), 291–298.

Roberts, C., Kennedy, S., & Hammett, T. M. (2004). Linkages between in-prison and community-based health services. *Journal of Correctional Health Care, 10*(3), 333–368. doi:10.1177/107834580301000306

Ryan, P. Y. (2005). Approaching death: A phenomenologic study of five older adults with advanced cancer. *Oncology Nursing Forum, 32*(6), 1101–1108. doi:10.1188/05.ONF.1101-1108

Schwingel, A., Niti, M. M., Tang, C., & Ng, T. P. (2009). Continued work employment and volunteerism and mental well-being of older adults: Singapore longitudinal ageing studies. *Age and Ageing, 38*(5), 531–537. doi:10.1093/aging/afp089

Service Canada. (2012). Sustainable social programs and a secure retirement. Retrieved February 6, 2015, from: http://www.budget.gc.ca/2012/plan/chap4-eng.html

Sidell, M., Samson Katz, J., & Komaromy, C. (2000). The case for palliative care in residential and nursing homes. In D. Dickinson, M. Johnson, & J. Samson Katz (Eds.), *Death, dying and bereavement* (pp. 107–121). London: Sage.

Smith, C. J., & Beltran, A. (2003). The role of federal policies in supporting grandparents raising grandchildren families: The case of the U.S. *Journal of Intergenerational Relationships, 1*(2), 5–20. doi:10.1300/J194v01n02_02

Smyer, T., & Burbank, P. M. (2009). The U.S. correctional system and the older prisoner. *Journal of Gerontological Nursing, 35*(12), 32–37.

Snyder, C., van Wormer, K., Chadha, J., & Jaggers, J. W. (2009). Older adult inmates: The challenge for social work. *Social Work, 54*(2), 117–124.

Solomon, J. (2006). Sounding the shofar: A wake-up call to the epidemic of elder abuse. *Journal of Jewish Communal Service, 81*(3/4), 211–218.

Solomon, J., & Reingold, D. A. (2012). Creating an elder abuse shelter: A best-practice model for nonprofit nursing homes. *Generations, 36*(3), 64–65.

Special Senate Committee Report on Aging. (2009). *Canada's aging population: Seizing the opportunity.* Retrieved February 2, 2015, from: www.parl.gc.ca/Content/SEN/Committee/402/agei/rep/AgingFinalReport-e.pdf

Statistic Brain. (n.d.). Television watching statistics. Retrieved February 8, 2015, from: http://www.statisticbrain.com/television-watching-statistics/

Statistics Canada. (2008). Census snapshot of Canada—Population (age and sex). Ottawa: Statistics Canada—Catalogue No. 11-008.

Steinig, S. Y., & Butts, D. M. (2009–10). Generations going green: Intergenerational programs connecting young and old to improve our environment. *Generations, 33*(4), 64–69.

Steinisch, M. (2007). Senior homesharing a win-win. Retrieved March 30, 2015, from: http://hffo.cuna.org/32383/article/1802/html

Sumner, A. (2012). Assessment and management of older prisoners. *Nursing Older People, 24*(3), 16–21.

Thomas, W. H., & Blanchard, J. M. (2009). Moving beyond place: Aging in community. *Generations, 33*(2), 12–17.

Turcotte, M. (2012). Profile of seniors' transportation habits. *Statistics Canada, Catalogue no. 11-008.* Ottawa: Statistics Canada.

Turner, M., Payne, S., & Barbarachild, Z. (2011). Care or custody? An evaluation of palliative care in prisons in North West England. *Palliative Medicine, 25*(4), 370–377. doi:10.1177/0269216310393058

United States Census Bureau. (2011). Census Bureau releases comprehensive analysis of fast-growing 90-and-older population. Retrieved January 11, 2015, from: http://www.census.gov/newsroom/releases/archives/aging_population/cb11-194.html

United States Department of Labor. (2014). Labor for statistics from the current population survey. Retrieved January 11, 2015, from: http://www.bls.gov/cps/cpsaat03.htm

United States Department of Transportation. (2010). Attracting senior drivers to public transportation: Issues and concerns. Retrieved January 11, 2015, from: http:www.fta.dot.gov/research

Unroe, K. T., Sachs, G. A., Hickman, S. E., et al. (2013). Hospice use among nursing home patients. *Journal of the American Medical Directors Association, 14,* 254–259.

Ward, R. A., Spitze, G. D., & Sherman, S. R. (2005). Attraction to intergenerational housing on a university campus. *Journal of Housing for the Elderly, 19*(1), 93–111. doi:10.1300/J081v19n01_07

Weeks, L. E., & LeBlanc, K. (2010). Housing concerns of vulnerable older Canadians. *Canadian Journal on Aging, 29*(3), 333–347. doi:10.1017/S0714980810000310

West, S. P., Lagua, C., Trief, P. M., Izquierdo, R., & Weinstock, R. S. (2010). Goal setting using telemedicine in rural underserved older adults with diabetes: Experiences from the Informatics for Diabetes Education and Telemedicine Project. *Telemedicine and e-Health, 16*(4), 405–416. doi:10.1089/tmj.2009.0136

Wiersma, E. C. (2010). Life around . . . : Staff's perceptions of residents' adjustment into long-term care. *Canadian Journal on Aging, 29*(3), 425–434. doi:10.1017/S0714980810000401

Williams, B. A., Stern, M. F., Mellow, J., Safer, M., & Greifinger, R. B. (2012). Aging in correctional custody: Setting a policy agenda for older prisoner health care. *American Journal of Public Health, 102*(8), 1475–1481. doi:10.2105/AJPH.2012.300704

Wray, N., & McCall, L. (2007). Plotting careers in aged care: Perspectives of medical, nursing, allied health students and new graduates. *Educational Gerontology, 33*(11), 939–954. doi:10.1080/03601270701364636

Young, T. L., & Janke, M. (2013). Perceived benefits and concerns of older adults in a community intergenerational program: Does race matter? *Activities, Adaptation & Aging, 37*(2), 121–140.

AFTERWORD

We began this text with an explanation of transitions. We stated that to transition is to *cross over, to undergo or cause to undergo a process*; it involves *adaptation* and *metamorphosis*. We posited that if one encounters a circumstance of change, but does not adapt herself, she herself is changed by the position she takes in not transitioning. In Chapter 5 we had the chutzpah to endeavor to "rattle the bars on the cage" of your existence (using Robert Fulghum's expression).

In all of this, our motivation was four-fold:

- ► To increase your knowledge of the kinds and numbers of transitions experienced by older adults;
- ► To sensitize you to the complexities of the transitions faced by aging individuals;
- ► To raise concerns and issues that you yourself will encounter as you age;
- ► To motivate you, as one training to be a health or human service professional, to choose to work with this marvelous age group; as they have greatly enriched our lives, so they will enrich yours!

We hope that we have succeeded, at least in some measure; and we leave you, the reader, with the following words:

Old age is not a disease—it is strength and survivorship, triumph over all kinds of vicissitudes and disappointments, trials and illnesses.
(Maggie Kuhn)

and

Those who love deeply never grow old; they may die of old age, but they die young.
(Dorothy Canfield Fisher)

May the transitions of your life result in strength and survivorship and triumph—loving life and others deeply, so that in your final transition, you may cross over as one who is young at heart!

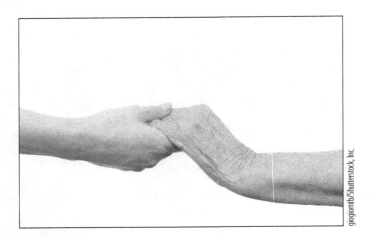

giogiombr/Shutterstock, Inc.

INDEX

CPSIA information can be obtained
at www.ICGtesting.com
Printed in the USA
LVHW03s0225140718
583593LV00007B/71/P